A Clinical Guide to Pediatric HIV

Tiffany Chenneville
Editor

A Clinical Guide to Pediatric HIV

Bridging the Gaps Between Research and Practice

Springer

Editor
Tiffany Chenneville
University of South Florida St. Petersburg
St. Petersburg, FL
USA

ISBN 978-3-319-49702-0 ISBN 978-3-319-49704-4 (eBook)
DOI 10.1007/978-3-319-49704-4

Library of Congress Control Number: 2016957699

Printed on acid-free paper

This Springer imprint is published by Springer Nature
The registered company is Springer International Publishing AG
The registered company address is: Gewerbestrasse 11, 6330 Cham, Switzerland

This book is dedicated to young people across the world living with or affected by HIV.

Preface

A Clinical Guide to Pediatric HIV: Bridging the Gaps Between Research and Practice examines the impact of HIV on children, adolescents, and their families. Written by experts in the field, this book covers issues of concern to clinicians and researchers working in the area of pediatric HIV. Beginning with an overview of pediatric HIV epidemiology and the medical, developmental, and psychosocial concerns facing children and adolescents with HIV, this book offers a description of the unique challenges associated with HIV within families and schools. In addition, this book provides the latest research on topics of relevance to clinicians and researchers working in this area to include but not limited to disclosure, antiretroviral adherence, and ethical issues surrounding pediatric HIV. It concludes with a discussion of cross-cultural issues, HIV prevention, and HIV-related stigma. This book is an invaluable resource for researchers, academics, and clinicians working with children with HIV and their families as well as graduate students in the fields of psychology, social work, sociology, mental health, and public health. Although there are many resources focusing on HIV, this book's exclusive focus on pediatric HIV makes it an essential compendium for pediatric clinicians and researchers.

St. Petersburg, FL, USA Tiffany Chenneville

Acknowledgement

I would like to acknowledge Hunter Drake for his contributions to this book.

Contents

Editor and Contributors

About the Editor

Tiffany Chenneville, Ph.D. is an Associate Professor and Graduate Program Director in the Psychology Department at the University of South Florida St. Petersburg. She has a joint appointment in the USF Department of Pediatrics where she has been involved for many years as a clinician and as a researcher in the pediatric/adolescent HIV program. Historically, Dr. Chenneville's research focused on issues of law, policy, and ethics with a particular emphasis on the decisional capacity of children with HIV to participate in treatment and research. She continues with this line of inquiry but, more recently, also has begun community-based participatory research in the area of HIV-related stigma among youth. Because HIV is a global disease, Dr. Chenneville is interested in cross-cultural research. She has worked in India and currently is working in Kenya. In addition to her research, Dr. Chenneville is collaborating with a filmmaker on a documentary about pediatric HIV.

Contributors

Jamie N. Albright University of Virginia, Charlottesville, VA, USA

Miriam R. Arbeit University of Virginia, Charlottesville, VA, USA

Tiffany Chenneville University of South Florida St. Petersburg, St. Petersburg, FL, USA

Kristina Decker University of Memphis, Memphis, TN, USA

Ralph J. DiClemente Emory University, Druid Hills, GA, USA

Patricia Emmanuel University of South Florida, Tampa, FL, USA

Cynthia D. Fair Elon University, Elon, NC, USA

Celia B. Fisher Fordham University, Bronx, NY, USA

Susan L. Gillespie Baylor College of Medicine, Baylor International Pediatric AIDS Initiative at Texas Children's Hospital, Houston, TX, USA

Robin Hardin University of Memphis, Memphis, TN, USA

Danielle Harris University of California, Los Angeles, CA, USA

Audra St. John Walsh University of South Florida, Tampa, FL, USA

Manisha Joshi University of South Florida, Tampa, FL, USA

Celia M. Lescano University of South Florida, Tampa, FL, USA

Courtney Lynn University of South Florida, Tampa, FL, USA

Stephanie L. Marhefka University of South Florida, Tampa, FL, USA

Christy Newman National Centre in HIV Social Research, University of New South Wales, Sydney, Australia

Sharon Nichols University of California, San Diego, CA, USA

Kimberly O'Leary University of South Florida, Tampa, FL, USA

Nihari Patel Emory University, Druid Hills, GA, USA

Guitele J. Rahill University of South Florida, Tampa, FL, USA

Carina Rodriguez University of South Florida, Tampa, FL, USA

Mary Jane Rotheram-Borus University of California, Los Angeles, CA, USA

Kirsty Sievwright International Center for Research on Women, Washington, DC, USA

Anne Stangl International Center for Research on Women, Washington, DC, USA

Idia B. Thurston University of Memphis, Memphis, TN, USA

DeAnne E. Turner University of South Florida, Tampa, FL, USA

Katherine L. Wesley University of South Florida, Tampa, FL, USA

Maryann Koussa Youssef University of California, Los Angeles, CA, USA

Chapter 1
Epidemiology of Pediatric HIV Infection

Susan L. Gillespie

Epidemiology of Pediatric HIV Infection

The HIV epidemic among children and adults alike has seen a stabilization and a reversal of the overall growth of the global AIDS epidemic resulting in fewer new infections, better health outcomes and fewer AIDS-related deaths. These improvements are due to the scale-up of HIV testing, availability of more efficacious combination antiretroviral therapy (cART) and more effective preventive measures. In the pediatric population, however, there have been gaps in prevention of mother-to-child transmission (PMTCT) efforts, and access to lifesaving cART treatment for children lags behind that of adults. In addition, there are increasing numbers of youth infected with HIV who face many challenges that interfere with their ability to optimally manage their infections and thereby put the hard-won gains in the fight against AIDS at risk.

Perinatal HIV Infection

Acquisition of HIV in children and youth can occur through mother-to-child transmission (MTCT), through sexual contact and through other mechanisms that have been described as "non-vertical, non-sexual" and include unsafe injection practices (Cotton et al. 2012). In the US and other developed countries, the number of children newly infected with HIV has decreased dramatically as a consequence of successful interventions to prevent mother-to-child HIV transmission (Centers for Disease Control and Prevention 2012). The CDC estimates the number of

S.L. Gillespie (✉)
Baylor College of Medicine, Baylor International Pediatric AIDS Initiative at Texas Children's Hospital, Houston, TX, USA
e-mail: slg@bcm.edu

T. Chenneville (ed.), *A Clinical Guide to Pediatric HIV*,
DOI 10.1007/978-3-319-49704-4_1

infants born with HIV annually in the US dropped from 1650 in 1991 to fewer than 200 starting in 2004. Globally, in 2014, the number of newly infected children was 170,000, a 40% reduction from 2009, but still unacceptably high (Joint United Nations Programme on HIV/AIDS (UNAIDS) 2015a).

Mother-to-child transmission accounts for the majority (~90%) of pediatric HIV cases and for 5–10% of HIV infections in patients of all ages. MTCT can occur in utero during pregnancy, during labor and delivery and postnatally through breast-feeding. Maternal risk factors for MTCT include acute HIV infection during pregnancy, detectable plasma viral load, low CD4 count and advanced stage of HIV infection. Mode of delivery, premature delivery, duration of membrane rupture >4 h and inflammation in the birth canal increase the risk of transmission during delivery. Postnatal risks include mixed infant feeding, maternal mastitis and practices such as premastication or prechewing of food fed to infants (Gaur et al. 2009). Without preventive therapy, the risk of an infant contracting HIV from the mother ranges from 15 to 25% in formula-fed infants and from 25 to 40% among infants who are breast-fed (De Cock et al. 2000). In the absence of breast-feeding, about 30% of infant HIV infections occur in utero and 70% occur during the passage of the fetus through the birth canal when the infant is exposed to the virus in maternal blood, amniotic fluid and/or cervical and vaginal secretions. Exposure to HIV through breast-feeding confers an additional 15–30% risk of HIV transmission from mother to child (De Cock et al. 2000).

Efforts to prevent mother-to-child transmission include a sequence of interventions focused on the reproductive health of girls and women that begin with primary prevention of HIV infection, early detection of HIV infection, provision of adequate preconception care and family planning services, early identification HIV infection in pregnant women through universal prenatal screening and provision of adequate prenatal care for women including treatment of HIV-infected pregnant women with cART to assure maximal suppression of viral load throughout pregnancy (Nesheim et al. 2012).

Antiretroviral-based interventions have transformed the management of pregnant women with HIV infection and the prevention of HIV transmission to their infants. Treatment of all pregnant women regardless of CD4 count is the most effective intervention for PMTCT particularly when cART is started before conception and plasma viral load is maximally suppressed throughout pregnancy. In a study in France, there were no infections among 2651 infants born to women with HIV who received ART that was initiated before conception and who had a plasma viral load of less than 50 copies/ml at delivery (Mandelbrot et al. 2015).

Current recommended interventions for PMTCT in well-resourced settings include the routine use of cART during pregnancy to maximally suppress viral load, cesarean delivery when maternal viral load is not maximally suppressed, provision of neonatal antiretroviral prophylaxis and avoidance of breast-feeding. In the US and other well-resourced settings when all applicable PMTCT interventions are used, MTCT risk can be reduced to <1% (Whitmore et al. 2012).

It is important for preventive interventions to be considered within the social and economic contexts of the mother–infant dyad. The issue of breast-feeding is illustrative. In well-resourced settings, where infant formula and clean water are available, women with HIV infection are advised not to breast-feed to minimize ongoing exposure of the infant to the HIV virus. The majority of children born to mothers with HIV, however, live in resource-limited settings where infant replacement feeding and clean water are inconsistently available and breast-feeding is a critical component of infant survival. In these settings, the risk of HIV infection is outweighed by the risk of dying from malnutrition and diarrheal diseases (McIntyre 2010).

In resource-limited settings, PMTCT programs also emphasize treating pregnant women with combination antiretroviral medications and neonatal prophylaxis, but it is the antiretroviral management of the mother–infant dyad, providing antiretroviral therapy to lactating mothers or extending prophylactic antiretroviral medications to breast-feeding infants, that has enabled infants to receive lifesaving nutritional and immunologic benefits of breast-milk while reducing the risk of HIV infection. With the use of these interventions the rate of postnatal transmission can be reduced to less than 2% (White et al. 2014). A major gap in the goal to eliminate new infections among children is reflected in the fact that only 77% of pregnant women with HIV received ART during pregnancy worldwide in 2014 (Joint United Nations Programme on HIV/AIDS (UNAIDS) 2015a).

Perinatally Infected Children

With greater access to HIV testing and effective treatment, children with HIV are surviving longer and with fewer opportunistic infections, transforming HIV infection from a clinical emergency to a manageable chronic disease. Of the 36.9 million people worldwide living with HIV or AIDS at the end of 2014, 3.2 million were children under the age of 15 years (Joint United Nations Programme on HIV/AIDS (UNAIDS) 2015b). In 2014, 176 children younger than age 13 years were newly diagnosed with HIV in the US; 128 (73%) of whom were perinatally infected. At the same time, new pediatric AIDS cases and AIDS deaths also have plummeted, in large part due access to powerful combinations of antiretroviral drugs (Centers for Disease Control and Prevention 2014).

Natural History of HIV

The clinical course of HIV infection depends upon whether effective cART is provided. Although access to care and treatment services for children with HIV in resource-limited settings is expanding, it is estimated that worldwide, only 31% of children in need received lifesaving antiretroviral therapy in 2014 (Joint United Nations Programme on HIV/AIDS (UNAIDS) 2015a).

Without antiretroviral therapy, HIV infection is characterized by progressive immunosuppression, caused by HIV virus-mediated depletion of CD4 + lymphocytes, leaving patients at risk of developing opportunistic infection (OI) and other HIV-related disorders. The rate of disease progression among children who acquired the infection perinatally is variable. North American and European cohorts demonstrate a bimodal pattern of disease progression. A minority (15–20%) of children have rapidly progressive disease with severe immunosuppression, OI and encephalopathy within the first year of life, while most children (about 75%) develop severe immunosuppression by 10 years of age (Blanche et al. 1997; Gray et al. 2001). A similar pattern of disease progression is also seen in resource-limited settings, but with a faster rate of disease progression with mortality of 26–45% by age one year, 45–53% by age two years and 50–62% by age five years (Newell et al. 2004; Spira et al. 1999). Many children with perinatally acquired HIV with slowly progressing untreated disease present for the first time in adolescence (Ferrand et al. 2010).

In most children with perinatally acquired HIV, the first year of life is characterized by the development of mild and nonspecific signs and symptoms (e.g., lymphadenopathy, hepatosplenomegaly, parotitis) followed by clinical and immunologic deterioration. Disease progression and immunosuppression are associated with increased susceptibility to OI, the most common being serious bacterial infections, such as pneumonia and bacteremia, followed by herpes zoster, disseminated Mycobacterium avium complex infections and invasive candidal infections of the esophagus or tracheobronchial tree (Krasinski et al. 1989).

Timing of HIV transmission from mother to child is an important determinant of disease progression. Children infected in utero or within the first one to two months of life have a higher mortality rate at 12 months than those infected later as through breast-feeding (Mbori-Ngacha et al. 2001; Newell et al. 2004). Among a small South African cohort of infants with HIV born to mothers who received antiretroviral medications to prevent mother-to-child transmission of HIV, 35, 70 and 80% of infants progressed to severe immunosuppression within 3, 6 and 12 months of life, respectively. Rapid progression was inversely related to maternal CD4 count and more common in infants with intrauterine infection (Mphatswe et al. 2007). Other factors, including early onset of HIV-related conditions, failure to thrive and generalized lymphadenopathy, were all poor prognostic features, whereas lymphoid interstitial pneumonia was associated with milder illness (Spira et al. 1999).

HIV Infection Treated with ART

Two developments in ART have had the greatest impact on the natural history of pediatric HIV infection: (1) the availability and use of combination antiretroviral therapy (cART, previously referred to as highly active ART or HAART), particularly regimens including protease inhibitors, and (2) the early initiation of ART in infants infected with HIV.

Treatment of HIV with combination ART has changed the natural history of the infection by halting and reversing the progressive immunodeficiency that characterizes the infection. Combination ART is associated with improvement in virologic, immunologic and clinical health for adults and children with HIV (Chiappini et al. 2009; de Martino et al. 2000; Guillen et al. 2010; Le Doare et al. 2012; Palella et al. 1998).

Population studies in the US have demonstrated marked reductions in morbidity and mortality in children and adults infected with HIV-1 since the mid-1990s, temporally associated with increased use of HAART. Early studies in adult patients in the US demonstrated a steep decline in the mortality of patients treated with ART from 29.4 deaths per 100 person-years in 1995 to 8.8 deaths per 100 person-years in 1997. Moreover, there was a stepwise reduction in mortality over time as the intensity of ART increased from none to monotherapy and then to combination antiretroviral therapy (Palella et al. 1998). A similar effect was seen among children and adolescents as use of combination ART regimens, and particularly combination ART regimens containing protease inhibitors, increased (de Martino et al. 2000; Gortmaker et al. 2001). Benefits of combination ART in children and adolescents with HIV include improved growth, improvement in immune function and a marked decrease in the incidence of opportunistic infections, hospitalization and risk of death (Gona et al. 2006; Gortmaker et al. 2001; Peacock-Villada et al. 2011; Sauvageot et al. 2010).

Cohort studies from the US, UK and Europe have all demonstrated improved survival of children with HIV over time and were associated with HAART treatment (Agwu et al. 2013; Berti et al. 2015; Brady et al. 2010; Judd et al. 2007; Van Dyke et al. 2011). Combination ART was associated with prolongation of life; among children who died, the age at death increased from 8.9 years in 1994 to 18.2 years in 2006 (Brady et al. 2010). Risk factors for death have included absolute CD4 cell count <200, CD4 percentage <15, having an AIDS-defining condition at study entry, younger age at entry and belonging to an early birth cohort. Ninety-seven percentage of deaths were directly attributable to HIV infection. Over time, the proportion of deaths caused by opportunistic infection and central nervous system disease have declined, and the proportion of deaths due to end-stage AIDS, sepsis and renal failure have increased (Hazra et al. 2010).

Resource-Limited Settings

Several reports have used data pooled from a number of different cohorts to describe similar improvements in the outcomes of children with HIV treated with combination ART in resource-limited settings (Ciaranello et al. 2009; Davies et al. 2009; Fenner et al. 2010; Kids-Art-Linc Collaboration 2008). Mortality rates in these studies were 4.5% at one year (Fenner et al. 2010), 6.9% at two years (Kids-Art-Linc Collaboration 2008) and 7.7% at three years (Davies et al. 2009). The effectiveness of ART in resource-limited settings was further illustrated in an analysis of data pooled from cohorts from 15 countries in Asia, Africa and the Caribbean. In this analysis, after 12 months of ART therapy, 70% of children attained virologic suppression (HIV RNA < 400 copies/mL) and had an increase of 13.7% in CD4 percentage (Ciaranello et al. 2009; De Beaudrap et al. 2013).

Despite increasing access to ART and these encouraging outcomes, mortality remains high for children with HIV in low- and middle-income countries even among children treated with ART. Overall post-HAART mortality was 7.6% in resource-limited countries compared to 1.6% in developed countries (Peacock-Villada et al. 2011). Mortality is particularly high in the first year after ART initiation. Risk factors for mortality in the first year of ART treatment include young age, low CD4% or advanced clinical disease (Bolton-Moore et al. 2007; Davies et al. 2014; Fenner et al. 2010; Kids-Art-Linc Collaboration 2008; Walker et al. 2012). Anemia and low weight for age Z score (WAZ) have also been found to predict mortality in the first year of life (Davies et al. 2014).

Advanced disease at the start of ART is associated with poorer outcomes. In resource-limited settings, there is a high prevalence of advanced clinical disease and/or severe immunosuppression at the start of ART. According to a large collaborative study including 34,706 children younger than age 16 years from cohorts across the globe, in 2010, approximately two-thirds of children in low- and middle-income countries already had severe immunodeficiency at the initiation of ART (Koller et al. 2015). Prognostic modeling suggests that mortality in the first year of ART in children was 40% higher in children with advanced disease [World Health Organization (WHO) clinical stage 3 or 4] than in children with milder disease (WHO clinical stages 1 or 2). Similarly, mortality in children starting ART with CD4% >10% was about half that of children with CD4% < 5% (Davies et al. 2014). The risk of disease progression associated with a specific CD4 cell count or percentage varies with the age of the child. Infants in the first year of life experience higher risks of progression or death than older children. Early diagnosis and treatment of infants with HIV dramatically decrease morbidity and prolong survival. The Children with HIV Early Antiretroviral Therapy (CHER) study (Violari et al. 2008) is a landmark study that validates early initiation of HAART to reduce morbidity and mortality in infants with perinatally acquired HIV. This study demonstrated a 75% reduction in early mortality in children with normal immune function (CD4% $\geq$ 25) initiating HAART before 12 weeks of age when compared with delaying HAART initiation until the child met clinical or immune criteria. Based in part on results from the CHER study, the WHO revised its treatment recommendations to include virologic testing of all infants exposed to HIV at four to six weeks of age and treatment of all children with HIV less than 12 months of age, regardless of immunologic or clinical stage (World Health Organization 2015).

Early infant diagnosis and prompt initiation of ART remain a challenge in resource-limited settings. In pooled analyses, the median age of children treated with ART ranged from 42.3 months to 4.9 years with less than 30% of patients <18 months of age (Kids-Art-Linc Collaboration 2008) and only 12–24% of patients age <12 months (Davies et al. 2009; Fenner et al. 2010). The small proportion of young children who are treated with ART in resource-limited settings highlights the continued need to scale-up programs for the early identification of infants exposed to and infected with HIV to assure appropriate follow-up and timely initiation of treatment.

Adolescents and Young Adults with HIV

Youth with HIV are a diverse population comprised of two distinct populations: young people who were infected perinatally and those who acquired HIV horizontally, either by risk behaviors including sexual activity and intravenous drug use or, less commonly, through transfusion of blood products.

In the US, by the end of 2013, an estimated 11,130 individuals of all ages living with HIV were classified as having become infected perinatally. Over 80% of children with perinatal HIV infection had aged into adolescence and adulthood and were older than 13 years of age (Centers for Disease Control and Prevention 2014). Youth aged 13–24 years are also vulnerable to acquiring HIV infection and accounted for an estimated 26% (12,200) of all new HIV infections (47,500) in the US in 2010.

In the US, most new infections among youth occur in young men who have sex with men (YMSM) who accounted for 72% of new HIV infections in this age group in 2010. Black youth accounted for an estimated 57% (7000) of all new infections among youth in the US, followed by Hispanic/Latino (20%, 2390) and white (20%, 2380) youth. It is estimated that over 50% of youth with HIV in the US do not yet know that they are infected (Centers for Disease Control and Prevention 2015).

Globally, 35.3 million people were living with HIV at the end of 2012, including 2.1 million adolescents aged 10–19 years. The vast majority (>80%) of youth with HIV live in sub-Saharan Africa, and in contrast to the pattern observed in the US, the majority (56%) of youth with HIV in sub-Saharan Africa are girls. This difference can be attributed to the fact that adolescent girls and young women are disproportionately acquiring new infections. Young women acquire HIV infection in their early teens, five to seven years before men, who generally acquire HIV in their mid-20s. In 2012, more than 80% of adolescents newly infected with HIV were girls in South Africa, Sierra Leone and Gabon (Idele et al. 2014). Factors that may be related to girls acquiring HIV at such a high rate include early sexual debut, which may be related to gender-based violence or involvement in transgenerational relationships, economic vulnerability, lack of access to education, lack of access to medical services and legal and social policies that interfere with girls and women exercising their human rights (Joint United Nations Programme on HIV/AIDS (UNAIDS) 2014).

The global data collected for youth with HIV combine perinatal infections with infections acquired through unprotected sex or intravenous drug use. HIV acquisition in youth through men who have sex with men (MSM) behavior is under-reported in part due to the criminalization of same sexual practices in many countries. Young MSM (YMSM) may experience stigma, discrimination and social exclusion that prevent them from seeking prevention, care and treatment services (Joint United Nations Programme on HIV/AIDS (UNAIDS) 2014).

Whether in well-resourced or resource-limited settings, adolescence is a developmental stage characterized by rapid physical, psychological and physiological changes that present complications for adolescents who are also facing challenges related to HIV infection. These challenges may include adherence to daily ART;

acceptance of HIV diagnosis; disclosure of HIV status to family, friends and romantic/sexual partners; stigma and discrimination associated with HIV status; cognitive dysfunction and education attainment, psychiatric illness and substance abuse; sexual, reproductive and gender health; orphan status or foster care; and socioeconomic status with food and housing instability.

Youth with HIV are challenged by every stage of the HIV care and treatment cascade, which follows a population of individuals with HIV through testing and diagnosis, engagement in medical care, retention in care to viral suppression. Viral suppression is the ultimate goal of comprehensive HIV care because it promotes immune reconstitution, prevents development of drug resistance and disease progression and decreases the risk of onward transmission (Frieden et al. 2015). In the US, it is estimated that as few as 6% of youth with HIV remain virally suppressed as they follow a cascade that begins with only 41% of youth who are infected aware of their infection (Zanoni and Mayer 2014). This estimate is much less than a similar analysis of adults with HIV in the US, which suggests as many as 30% remain virally suppressed, but in that analysis, it was estimated that 80% knew their infection status (Bradley et al. 2011).

Achieving an AIDS-free generation of youth requires interventions at every step of the HIV care and treatment cascade. First, by increasing routine screening and targeted testing, more youth will be aware of their HIV status. Identifying acute HIV infections is particularly important because acute infection is associated with higher viral loads and higher infectivity than chronic infection (Cohen et al. 2011). Initiating ART in acute infection will decrease onward infection. Subsequent partner notification is important in identifying individuals who are at risk for acquiring HIV and providing ART pre-exposure prophylaxis to those who are not yet infected. Once HIV infection is diagnosed, linking youth to medical care is critical for the initiation of treatment. Current US guidelines recommend treatment for all people with HIV regardless of clinical stage. Treatment, ideally leading to viral suppression, benefits the individual with HIV by improving or sustaining their health and is also a public health intervention for interrupting transmission. A major barrier for youth with HIV is accessing youth-friendly medical care and the likelihood that they will fail to engage or become lost to follow-up.

There are increasing numbers of potent antiretroviral medications with fewer associated side effects and simpler dosing regimens, including daily single pill fixed-dose combinations available for adolescents and adults. Poor adherence to these medications, however, raises the risk for the development of drug resistance with resultant disease progression and ongoing HIV transmission. Youth with perinatally acquired HIV are often highly treatment-experienced and in need of complex salvage combination ART regimens that involve higher pill burdens, with multiple doses per day. Maintaining ART adherence in this subpopulation is particularly challenging.

As youth with perinatally acquired HIV age, they are more likely to develop detectable HIV viremia and advanced immunosuppression (CD4 count <200 cells/mm^3), both factors that are associated with disease progression, poorer clinical outcomes and ongoing transmission. Youth with HIV are also more likely to become lost to follow-up as they get older, sometimes related to transitioning from receiving care in a pediatric clinic to adult model care but also continuing as youth age through 25 years (Agwu et al. 2013). Among youth non-perinatally infected, less than 45% of youth remained in care for one year and less than 25% remained in care for three years (Farmer et al. 2016).

Potential barriers to retention in care for youth with both perinatally and behaviorally acquired HIV may include lack of transportation to appointments, poor health literacy and a perceived lack of a youth-friendly atmosphere (Farmer et al. 2016). Youth also struggle with the intertwined issues of adherence, stigma, disclosure, negotiation of sexual relationships and transitioning to adult care. Psychosocial support is a key component to multidisciplinary comprehensive care and is a critical resource to assist youth with HIV successfully navigate potential barriers so that they will remain engaged in medical care and adherent to lifesaving antiretroviral therapy (Martinez et al. 2014). The American Academy of Pediatrics recommends addressing the needs of youth with HIV by providing confidential comprehensive care with sensitivity in a youth-friendly medical home. In this setting, the structural barriers to health care should be addressed so that youth can access mental health services, drug and alcohol treatment, transportation and housing (Martinez et al. 2014).

Future Directions

Worldwide, infants, children and youth with HIV infection remain underserved, lagging behind adults in terms of diagnosis, engagement in child- and youth-friendly care, access to antiretroviral (ARV) treatment and prevention. Increasing HIV testing and diagnosis is the gateway to treatment. Ongoing surveillance is essential to better monitor and evaluate current care and treatment programs. Expanding access to ART for all in need is a challenge but especially affects infants and children who must be maintained on appropriate weight-based doses and for whom medication preparation and palatability may be barriers to adherence. Medication adherence is critical in preventing the development of viral drug resistance and particularly affects children and youth. Access to simpler regimens and development long-acting preparations of ART may also improve adherence to ART for treatment and prevention for youth. Retention of infants, children and youth in care remains challenging. Poor adherence to medication and attrition of children from care may potentially reverse gains in health and survival made through other interventions. Supporting youth as they transition from pediatric to adult care is key to maintaining their health and preventing ongoing transmission. Improved testing and engagement in care of young women of childbearing age not only affects the health and well-being of the woman but also of her children. Improving access of women to medications for PMTCT and improving the timely testing of infants to ensure prompt initiation of ART in infants infected with HIV may bring us closer to ending the pediatric HIV epidemic. Age disaggregation of existing cohort and surveillance data is needed to improve understanding of adolescent-specific issues and needs. It is also important to collect surveillance data from vulnerable pediatric populations such as MSM and intravenous drug user (IVDU), populations that are growing and may threaten the progress made in the general population.

Conclusion

There have been many achievements in pediatric HIV prevention and treatment resulting in the transformation of HIV from a life-threatening emergency to a chronic illness. There exist many gaps and missed opportunities to prevent HIV transmission and provide effective ART to children and youth that thwart the goal to achieve an -free generation. Continued efforts are required to improve PMTCT coverage for pregnant women with HIV and their infants; to improve access to lifesaving ART for children with HIV; to prevent new infections among adolescent girls and boys; and to retain youth in care.

Annotated Bibliography

AIDS*info* | Information on HIV/AIDS Treatment, Prevention and Research. (n.d.). Retrieved from https://www.aidsinfo.nih.gov/. AIDS*info* is a federally funded website that offers access to the latest, federally approved HIV/AIDS medical practice guidelines, HIV treatment and prevention clinical trials, and other research information for US health care providers, researchers, people affected by HIV/AIDS, and the general public.

CDC | HIV/AIDS. (2016). Retrieved from http://www.cdc.gov/hiv/. The US Centers for Disease Control and Prevention (CDC) website provides up to date information on basic HIV information for health professionals and for the general public. It is also a resource for US statistics and fact sheets.

HIV/AIDS. (n.d.). Retrieved from http://www.who.int/topics/hiv_aids/en. The World Health Organization website provides up to date information on HIV/AIDS clinical guidelines, statistics, and operational guidance for HIV care and treatment programs.

UNAIDS. (n.d.). Retrieved from http://www.unaids.org/. UNAIDS is the Joint United Nations Programme on HIV/AIDS, an organization that advocates for the accelerated, comprehensive and coordinated global action on the HIV/AIDS epidemic. The website features up-to-date reports on the global HIV/AIDS epidemic as well country-specific information.

References

Agwu, A. L., Fleishman, J. A., Rutstein, R., Korthuis, P. T., & Gebo, K. (2013). Changes in Advanced Immunosuppression and Detectable HIV Viremia Among Perinatally HIV-Infected Youth in the Multisite United States HIV Research Network. *Journal of the Pediatric Infectious Diseases Society, 2*(3), 215–223. doi:10.1093/jpids/pit008

Berti, E., Thorne, C., Noguera-Julian, A., Rojo, P., Galli, L., de Martino, M., et al. (2015). The new face of the pediatric HIV epidemic in Western countries: Demographic characteristics, morbidity and mortality of the pediatric HIV-infected population. *The Pediatric Infectious Disease Journal, 34*(5 Suppl 1), S7–S13. doi:10.1097/INF.0000000000000660

Blanche, S., Newell, M. L., Mayaux, M. J., Dunn, D. T., Teglas, J. P., Rouzioux, C., et al. (1997). Morbidity and mortality in European children vertically infected by HIV-1. The French Pediatric HIV Infection Study Group and European Collaborative Study. *Journal of Acquired Immune Deficiency Syndromes & Human Retrovirology, 14*(5), 442–450. doi:10.1097/00042560-199704150-00008

Bolton-Moore, C., Mubiana-Mbewe, M., Cantrell, R. A., Chintu, N., Stringer, E. M., Chi, B. H., … & Stringer, J. S. (2007). Clinical outcomes and CD4 cell response in children receiving antiretroviral therapy at primary health care facilities in Zambia. *JAMA, 298*(16), 1888–1899. doi:10.1001/jama.298.16.1888

Bradley, H., Hall, H. I., Wolitski, R. J., Van Handel, M. M., Stone, A. E., LaFlam, M., … & Valleroy, L. A. (2011). Vital Signs: HIV diagnosis, care, and treatment among persons living with HIV–United States, 2011. *MMWR. Morbidity and Mortality Weekly Report, 63*(47), 1113–1117.

Brady, M. T., Oleske, J. M., Williams, P. L., Elgie, C., Mofenson, L. M., Dankner, W. M., … & Pediatric, A. C. T. G. C. T. (2010). Declines in mortality rates and changes in causes of death in HIV-1-infected children during the HAART era. *Journal of Acquired Immune Deficiency Syndromes, 53*(1), 86–94. doi:10.1097/QAI.0b013e3181b9869f

Centers for Disease Control and Prevention. (2012). HIV Among Pregnant Women, Infants, and Children, from http://www.cdc.gov/hiv/group/gender/pregnantwomen/index.html

Centers for Disease Control and Prevention. (2014). HIV Surveillance Report. *26*.

Centers for Disease Control and Prevention. (2015). HIV Among Youth. Retrieved 3 Jan 2016, from http://www.cdc.gov/hiv/group/age/youth/

Chiappini, E., Galli, L., Tovo, P. A., Gabiano, C., Lisi, C., Bernardi, S., … & de Martino, M. (2009). Five-year follow-up of children with perinatal HIV-1 infection receiving early highly active antiretroviral therapy. *BMC Infectious Diseases, 9*, 140. doi:10.1186/1471-2334-9-140

Ciaranello, A. L., Chang, Y., Margulis, A. V., Bernstein, A., Bassett, I. V., Losina, E., et al. (2009). Effectiveness of pediatric antiretroviral therapy in resource-limited settings: A systematic review and meta-analysis. *Clinical Infectious Diseases, 49*(12), 1915–1927. doi:10.1086/648079

Cohen, M. S., Shaw, G. M., McMichael, A. J., & Haynes, B. F. (2011). Acute HIV-1 Infection. *New England Journal of Medicine, 364*(20), 1943–1954. doi:10.1056/NEJMra1011874

Cotton, M. F., Marais, B. J., Andersson, M. I., Eley, B., Rabie, H., Slogrove, A. L., … & Mehtar, S. (2012). Minimizing the risk of non-vertical, non-sexual HIV infection in children–beyond mother to child transmission. *Journal of the International AIDS Society, 15*(2), 17377. doi:10.7448/IAS.15.2.17377

Davies, M. A., Keiser, O., Technau, K., Eley, B., Rabie, H., van Cutsem, G., … & International Epidemiologic Databases to Evaluate, A. S. A. C. (2009). Outcomes of the South African National Antiretroviral Treatment Programme for children: The IeDEA Southern Africa collaboration. *South African Medical Journal, 99*(10), 730–737.

Davies, M. A., May, M., Bolton-Moore, C., Chimbetete, C., Eley, B., Garone, D., … & Ie, D. E. A. S. A. C. (2014). Prognosis of children with HIV-1 infection starting antiretroviral therapy in Southern Africa: A collaborative analysis of treatment programs. *The Pediatric Infectious Disease Journal, 33*(6), 608–616. doi:10.1097/INF.0000000000000214

De Beaudrap, P., Boulle, C., Lewden, C., Gabillard, D., Nacro, B., Diagbouga, S., … & Group, A. M. M. S. (2013). Morbidity after antiretroviral therapy initiation in HIV-1-infected children in West Africa: Temporal trends and relation to CD4 count. *The Pediatric Infectious Disease Journal, 32*(4), 354–360. doi:10.1097/INF.0b013e318278b222

De Cock, K. M., Fowler, M. G., Mercier, E., de Vincenzi, I., Saba, J., Hoff, E., ... & Shaffer, N. (2000). Prevention of mother-to-child HIV transmission in resource-poor countries: Translating research into policy and practice. *JAMA, 283*(9), 1175–1182. doi:10.1001/jama.283.9.1175

de Martino, M., Tovo, P. A., Balducci, M., Galli, L., Gabiano, C., Rezza, G., et al. (2000). Reduction in mortality with availability of antiretroviral therapy for children with perinatal HIV-1 infection. Italian Register for HIV Infection in Children and the Italian National AIDS Registry. *JAMA, 284*(2), 190–197. doi:10.1001/jama.284.2.190

Farmer, C., Yehia, B. R., Fleishman, J. A., Rutstein, R., Mathews, W. C., Nijhawan, A., ... & Network, H. I. V. R. (2016). Factors Associated With Retention Among Non-Perinatally HIV-Infected Youth in the HIV Research Network. *Journal of the Pediatric Infectious Diseases Society, 5*(1), 39–46. doi:10.1093/jpids/piu102

Fenner, L., Brinkhof, M. W., Keiser, O., Weigel, R., Cornell, M., Moultrie, H., ... & International epidemiologic Databases to Evaluate, A. i. S. A. (2010). Early mortality and loss to follow-up in HIV-infected children starting antiretroviral therapy in Southern Africa. *Journal of Acquired Immune Deficiency Syndromes, 54*(5), 524–532. doi:10.1097/QAI.0b013e3181e0c4cf

Ferrand, R. A., Munaiwa, L., Matsekete, J., Bandason, T., Nathoo, K., Ndhlovu, C. E., ... & Corbett, E. L. (2010). Undiagnosed HIV infection among adolescents seeking primary health care in Zimbabwe. *Clinical Infectious Diseases, 51*(7), 844–851. doi:10.1086/656361

Frieden, T. R., Foti, K. E., & Mermin, J. (2015). Applying public health principles to the HIV epidemic-how are we doing? *New England Journal of Medicine, 373*(23), 2281–2287. doi:10.1056/NEJMms1513641

Gaur, A. H., Dominguez, K. L., Kalish, M. L., Rivera-Hernandez, D., Donohoe, M., Brooks, J. T., et al. (2009). Practice of feeding premasticated food to infants: A potential risk factor for HIV transmission. *Pediatrics, 124*(2), 658–666. doi:10.1542/peds.2008-3614

Gona, P., Van Dyke, R. B., Williams, P. L., Dankner, W. M., Chernoff, M. C., Nachman, S. A., ... & Seage, G. R., 3rd. (2006). Incidence of opportunistic and other infections in HIV-infected children in the HAART era. *JAMA, 296*(3), 292–300. doi:10.1001/jama.296.3.292

Gortmaker, S. L., Hughes, M., Cervia, J., Brady, M., Johnson, G. M., Seage, G. R., III, ... & Oleske, J. M. (2001). Effect of combination therapy including protease inhibitors on mortality among children and adolescents infected with HIV-1. *New England Journal of Medicine, 345*(21), 1522–1528. doi:10.1056/NEJMoa011157

Gray, L., Newell, M. L., Thorne, C., Peckham, C., Levy, J., & European Collaborative, S. (2001). Fluctuations in symptoms in human immunodeficiency virus-infected children: The first 10 years of life. *Pediatrics, 108*(1), 116–122. doi:10.1542/peds.108.1.116

Guillen, S., Garcia San Miguel, L., Resino, S., Bellon, J. M., Gonzalez, I., Jimenez de Ory, S., ... & Madrid Group for Research on Pediatric, H. I. V. I. (2010). Opportunistic infections and organ-specific diseases in HIV-1-infected children: A cohort study (1990–2006). *HIV Medicine, 11*(4), 245–252. doi:10.1111/j.1468-1293.2009.00768.x

Hazra, R., Siberry, G. K., & Mofenson, L. M. (2010). Growing up with HIV: Children, adolescents, and young adults with perinatally acquired HIV infection. *Annual Review of Medicine, 61*, 169–185. doi:10.1146/annurev.med.050108.151127

Idele, P., Gillespie, A., Porth, T., Suzuki, C., Mahy, M., Kasedde, S., et al. (2014). Epidemiology of HIV and AIDS among adolescents: Current status, inequities, and data gaps. *Journal of Acquired Immune Deficiency Syndromes, 66*(Suppl 2), S144–S153. doi:10.1097/QAI.0000000000000176

Joint United Nations Programme on HIV/AIDS. (2014). *The Gap Report 2014*. Retrieved from http://www.unaids.org/en/resources/documents/2014/20140716_UNAIDS_gap_report

Joint United Nations Programme on HIV/AIDS. (2015a). *2015 Progress Report on the Global Plan*. Retrieved from http://www.unaids.org/sites/default/files/media_asset/JC2774_2015ProgressReport_GlobalPlan_en.pdf

Joint United Nations Programme on HIV/AIDS. (2015b). *AIDS by the numbers 2015.* Retrieved from http://www.unaids.org/sites/default/files/media_asset/AIDS_by_the_numbers_2015_en.pdf

Judd, A., Doerholt, K., Tookey, P. A., Sharland, M., Riordan, A., Menson, E., … & Duong, T. (2007). Morbidity, mortality, and response to treatment by children in the United Kingdom and Ireland with perinatally acquired HIV infection during 1996–2006: Planning for teenage and adult care. *Clinical Infectious Diseases, 45*(7), 918–924. doi:10.1086/521167

Kids-Art-Linc Collaboration. (2008). Low risk of death, but substantial program attrition, in pediatric HIV treatment cohorts in Sub-Saharan Africa. *Journal of Acquired Immune Deficiency Syndromes, 49*(5), 523–531. doi:10.1097/QAI.0b013e31818aadce

Koller, M., Patel, K., Chi, B. H., Wools-Kaloustian, K., Dicko, F., Chokephaibulkit, K., … & studies, I. C. (2015). Immunodeficiency in children starting antiretroviral therapy in low-, middle-, and high-income countries. *Journal of Acquired Immune Deficiency Syndromes, 68* (1), 62–72. doi:10.1097/QAI.0000000000000380

Krasinski, K., Borkowsky, W., & Holzman, R. S. (1989). Prognosis of human immunodeficiency virus infection in children and adolescents. *The Pediatric Infectious Disease Journal, 8*(4), 216–220.

Le Doare, K., Bland, R., & Newell, M. L. (2012). Neurodevelopment in children born to HIV-infected mothers by infection and treatment status. *Pediatrics, 130*(5), e1326–e1344. doi:10.1542/peds.2012-0405

Mandelbrot, L., Tubiana, R., Le Chenadec, J., Dollfus, C., Faye, A., Pannier, E., … & Group, A.-E. S. (2015). No perinatal HIV-1 transmission from women with effective antiretroviral therapy starting before conception. *Clinical Infectious Diseases, 61*(11), 1715–1725. doi:10.1093/cid/civ578

Martinez, J., Chakraborty, R. and American Academy of Pediatrics Committee on Pediatric AIDS (2014). "Psychosocial support for youth living with HIV." Pediatrics 133(3): 558–562. doi:10.1542/peds.2013-4061

Mbori-Ngacha, D., Nduati, R., John, G., Reilly, M., Richardson, B., Mwatha, A., … & Kreiss, J. (2001). Morbidity and mortality in breastfed and formula-fed infants of HIV-1-infected women: A randomized clinical trial. *JAMA, 286*(19), 2413–2420. doi:10.1001/jama.286.19.2413

McIntyre, J. (2010). Use of antiretrovirals during pregnancy and breastfeeding in low-income and middle-income countries. *Current Opinion in HIV and AIDS, 5*(1), 48–53. doi:10.1097/COH.0b013e328333b8ab

Mphatswe, W., Blanckenberg, N., Tudor-Williams, G., Prendergast, A., Thobakgale, C., Mkhwanazi, N., … & Goulder, P. (2007). High frequency of rapid immunological progression in African infants infected in the era of perinatal HIV prophylaxis. *AIDS, 21*(10), 1253–1261. doi:10.1097/QAD.0b013e3281a3bec2

Nesheim, S., Taylor, A., Lampe, M. A., Kilmarx, P. H., Fitz Harris, L., Whitmore, S., … & Mermin, J. (2012). A framework for elimination of perinatal transmission of HIV in the United States. *Pediatrics, 130*(4), 738–744. doi:10.1542/peds.2012-0194

Newell, M. L., Coovadia, H., Cortina-Borja, M., Rollins, N., Gaillard, P., & Dabis, F. (2004). Mortality of infected and uninfected infants born to HIV-infected mothers in Africa: A pooled analysis. *The Lancet, 364*(9441), 1236–1243. doi:10.1016/S0140-6736(04)17140-7

Palella, F. J., Jr., Delaney, K. M., Moorman, A. C., Loveless, M. O., Fuhrer, J., Satten, G. A., … & Holmberg, S. D. (1998). Declining morbidity and mortality among patients with advanced human immunodeficiency virus infection. HIV Outpatient Study Investigators. *New England Journal of Medicine, 338*(13), 853–860. doi:10.1056/NEJM199803263381301

Peacock-Villada, E., Richardson, B. A., & John-Stewart, G. C. (2011). Post-HAART outcomes in pediatric populations: Comparison of resource-limited and developed countries. *Pediatrics, 127*(2), e423–e441. doi:10.1542/peds.2009-2701

Sauvageot, D., Schaefer, M., Olson, D., Pujades-Rodriguez, M., & O'Brien, D. P. (2010). Antiretroviral therapy outcomes in resource-limited settings for HIV-infected children <5 years of age. *Pediatrics, 125*(5), e1039–e1047. doi:10.1542/peds.2009-1062

Spira, R., Lepage, P., Msellati, P., Van De Perre, P., Leroy, V., Simonon, A., ... & Dabis, F. (1999). Natural history of human immunodeficiency virus type 1 infection in children: A five-year prospective study in Rwanda. Mother-to-Child HIV-1 Transmission Study Group. *Pediatrics, 104*(5), e56. doi:10.1542/peds.104.5.e56

Van Dyke, R. B., Patel, K., Siberry, G. K., Burchett, S. K., Spector, S. A., Chernoff, M. C., ... & Pediatric, H. I. V. A. C. S. (2011). Antiretroviral treatment of US children with perinatally acquired HIV infection: Temporal changes in therapy between 1991 and 2009 and predictors of immunologic and virologic outcomes. *Journal of Acquired Immune Deficiency Syndromes, 57* (2), 165–173. doi:10.1097/QAI.0b013e318215c7b1

Violari, A., Cotton, M. F., Gibb, D. M., Babiker, A. G., Steyn, J., Madhi, S. A., ... & Team, C. S. (2008). Early antiretroviral therapy and mortality among HIV-infected infants. *New England Journal of Medicine, 359*(21), 2233–2244. doi:10.1056/NEJMoa0800971

Walker, A. S., Prendergast, A. J., Mugyenyi, P., Munderi, P., Hakim, J., Kekitiinwa, A., ... & teams, A. t. (2012). Mortality in the year following antiretroviral therapy initiation in HIV-infected adults and children in Uganda and Zimbabwe. *Clinical Infectious Diseases, 55* (12), 1707–1718. doi:10.1093/cid/cis797

White, A. B., Mirjahangir, J. F., Horvath, H., Anglemyer, A., & Read, J. S. (2014). Antiretroviral interventions for preventing breast milk transmission of HIV. *Cochrane Database of Systematic Reviews, 10*, CD011323. doi:10.1002/14651858.CD011323

Whitmore, S. K., Taylor, A. W., Espinoza, L., Shouse, R. L., Lampe, M. A., & Nesheim, S. (2012). Correlates of mother-to-child transmission of HIV in the United States and Puerto Rico. *Pediatrics, 129*(1), e74–e81. doi:10.1542/peds.2010-3691

World Health Organization. (2015). *Guideline on When to Start Antiretroviral Therapy and on Pre-Exposure Prophylaxis for HIV.* Retrieved from http://apps.who.int/iris/bitstream/10665/186275/1/9789241509565_eng.pdf?ua=1

Zanoni, B. C., & Mayer, K. H. (2014). The adolescent and young adult HIV cascade of care in the United States: Exaggerated health disparities. *AIDS Patient Care STDS, 28*(3), 128–135. doi:10.1089/apc.2013.0345

Chapter 2
Medical Implications of HIV Among Children and Adolescents

Carina Rodriguez and Patricia Emmanuel

Introduction

The Biology and Evolution of HIV Infection

In 1983, a new human retrovirus was isolated from a culture derived from a lymph node biopsy sample of a patient with generalized lymphadenopathy (Barre-Sinoussi et al. 2004). Within that year, similar viruses had been isolated from patients with AIDS (Popovic et al. 1984) and a serological test had been developed, which confirmed that HIV causes AIDS (Gottlieb 1984).

The HIV epidemic arose after zoonotic infections with simian immunodeficiency viruses from African primates. Bush meat hunters were probably the first group to be infected with HIV (Sharp and Hahn 2011). The four groups of HIV-1 represent three separate transmission events from chimpanzees (M, N, and O), and one from gorillas (P). Groups N, O, and P are restricted to West Africa. Group M, originated over 100 years ago, is the cause of the global HIV pandemic (Hemelaar et al. 2011) and consists of nine subtypes: A–D, F–H, J, and K. Subtype C predominates in Africa and India. Subtype B predominates in Western Europe, the Americas, and Australia. HIV-2 is largely confined to West Africa and causes a similar illness to HIV-1, but immunodeficiency progresses more slowly. HIV-2 is less transmissible

C. Rodriguez (✉) · P. Emmanuel
University of South Florida, Tampa, FL, USA
e-mail: crodrig1@health.usf.edu

P. Emmanuel
e-mail: pemmanue@health.usf.edu

T. Chenneville (ed.), *A Clinical Guide to Pediatric HIV*,
DOI 10.1007/978-3-319-49704-4_2

and has distinct resistance to antiretrovirals. This chapter will focus primarily on HIV-1 infection unless otherwise specified.

HIV-1 and HIV-2 are cytopathic lentiviruses that belong to the family Retroviridae, and they are closely related to the simian immunodeficiency viruses. The HIV genome has both conserved and highly variable domains. Three principal genes (gag, pol, and env) encode the major structural and enzymatic proteins, and six accessory genes regulate gene expression and aid in assembly and release of infectious virions. The envelope glycoprotein interacts with CD4 receptors and one of two major co-receptors (CCR5 and CXCR4). The main steps in the HIV-1 replication cycle are: (1) binding to the CD4 receptor and co-receptors; (2) fusion with the host cell membrane; (3) uncoating of the viral capsid; (4) release of the HIV RNA and proteins into the cytoplasm; (5) reverse transcription of HIV RNA to DNA; (6) formation of the pre-integration complex; (7) integration of viral DNA into the host DNA; (8) transcription and translation of new viral RNA and viral proteins; (9) translocation to the cell surface, and assembly into new immature virus forms; (10) budding and release of new viruses; and (11) finally, during maturation, the protease enzyme cleaves the structural polyprotein to form mature gag proteins, resulting in the production of new infectious virions. The marked genetic diversity of HIV-1 is a consequence of the error-prone function of the reverse transcriptase, which results in a high mutation rate. The major families of antiretroviral drugs target different steps of the life cycle, and its combination decreases the likelihood of developing resistance to therapy.

Humans are the only known reservoir for HIV-1 and HIV-2. Latent viruses persist in peripheral blood mononuclear cells, and in cells of the brain, bone marrow, and genital tract even when plasma viral load is undetectable. Only blood, semen, cervicovaginal secretions, and human milk have been implicated in transmission of infection. Modes of transmission include: (1) sexual contact (vaginal, anal, or orogenital); (2) percutaneous blood exposure; (3) mucous membrane exposure to contaminated blood or body fluids; (4) mother-to-child transmission during pregnancy, labor, and delivery and postnatally through breastfeeding; and (5) transfusion with contaminated blood. As a result of highly effective screening methods, the later mode of transmission has been virtually eliminated since 1985. In addition, cases of transmission from caregivers with HIV to their infants through feeding blood-tinged pre-masticated food have been reported in the US (Gaur et al. 2009).

HIV Pathogenesis

The main target of HIV is activated CD4 T lymphocytes which results in progressive depletion of CD4 T cells because of reduced production and increased destruction. Other cells bearing CD4 and chemokine receptors are also infected, including resting CD4 T cells, monocytes and macrophages, and dendritic cells. Later after the discovery of HIV infection, research groups identified the main co-receptors of HIV: CXC-chemokine receptor 4 (CXCR4) and CC-chemokine receptor 5 (CCR5) (Feng et al. 2011). Binding to these chemokine receptors was found to lead to the conformational changes that are necessary for entry of X4-tropic HIV-1 (which uses CXCR4) and R5-tropic HIV-1 (which uses CCR5). Interesting, a rare group of individuals with a homozygous CCR5 deletion was later identified and found to be resistant to HIV-1 infection. In these individuals, as the transmitted virus is typically R5-tropic, the *CCR5Δ32* mutation blocks viral entry conferring resistance to HIV infection (Liu et al. 1996; Samson et al. 1996). This concept is being further explored using T cells from these individuals as a potential cure strategy (Tebas et al. 2014; Hütter et al. 2009). Other cells, not CD4 dependent, are also infected such as astrocytes and renal epithelial cells. This has an important role in the pathogenesis of HIV-associated neurocognitive disorder and nephropathy. Transmission of HIV across mucosal membranes is usually established by one founder virus, followed by a rapid increase in HIV replication and induction of inflammatory cytokines and chemokines. CD4 T cells are eliminated by direct infection, and effects of immune activation, proliferation, and senescence. In early infection, a transient reduction in circulating CD4 T cells is followed by some degree of recovery. The most important effect on T cell homoeostasis happens very early, in the gastrointestinal tract, which has a massive depletion of activated CD4 T cells and is linked to microbial translocation, and alteration of the microbiome. The impact of microbial translocation in HIV disease progression and immune activation is an area of extensive research (Wallet et al. 2010).

After the initial peak in viremia, the viral load decreases to a viral set point, the level of which is established by innate and adaptive immune responses and is predictive of disease progression. Typically, HIV-infected infants and children had a higher viral set point as a result of their immature immune responses. HIV-specific CD8 T cells develop soon after infection, and the potent adaptive immune response to HIV selects for the emergence of mutations in key epitopes, leading to immune escape. Response is also affected by HLA types; for example, individuals with *HLA-B27* allele display a more effective immune response and may present as long-term non-progressors. In addition, neutralizing antibodies arise approximately three months following transmission. Broadly neutralizing antibodies, which can neutralize many HIV-1 subtypes, are produced by about 20% of patients. These antibodies are being explored both as therapeutic and preventive tools against HIV-1 infection, including for the prevention of mother-to-child transmission (Fouda et al. 2015). Other characteristics of HIV infection include hyper-gammaglobulinemia due to polyclonal activation of B cells, CD4+ T cells lymphopenia, decreased delayed hypersensitivity skin test response to recall antigens, neutropenia, decreased phagocytosis, and poor serological responses following vaccination. This is the result of failure to prime for immunological memory, and/or loss of immunological memory. For example, hepatitis B vaccination in patients infected with HIV has been associated with low seroconversion rate (35–45% in children) and a more rapid serum antibody decline. Reports of immunogenicity after administration of pneumococcal and Haemophilus influenzae type b conjugate vaccines have demonstrated lower antibody concentrations in children with HIV compared with children without HIV. Patients on highly active antiretroviral therapy (HAART) with immune reconstitution may exhibit a more favorable and persistent antibody response. HAART initiation within the first year of life is correlated with a normal development of memory B cells and to longevity of antibody response (Sutcliffe and Moss 2010). A recent study showed poor response to measles, rubella, and mumps vaccine in children with HIV-1 if the vaccine was administered prior to virologic control with subsequent need for revaccination (Siberry et al. 2015). Other infections may also impact the clinical presentation and disease progression. The serologic status for infections such as cytomegalovirus, toxoplasmosis, hepatitis B, hepatitis C, varicella-zoster, and syphilis are important for further management in individuals with HIV. For example, the absence of varicella-zoster antibodies despite a history of disease was found to be a predictive factor in individuals with HIV who developed zoster during immune reconstitution on HAART.

The pathogenesis of HIV infection in children with HIV has unique considerations including: (1) effects of acquisition of infection through perinatal exposure for most children who are infected; (2) in utero, intrapartum, and/or postpartum neonatal exposure to ARV drugs in most children who are perinatally infected; (3) need for use of HIV virologic tests to diagnose perinatal HIV infection in infants younger than 18 months; (4) age-specific interpretation of CD4 T lymphocyte (CD4) cell counts; (5) higher viral loads in infants who are perinatally infected than in adolescents and adults who are HIV infected; (6) changes in pharmacokinetic (PK) parameters with age caused by the continuing development and maturation of organ systems involved in drug absorption, distribution, metabolism, and clearance; (7) differences in the clinical manifestations and treatment of HIV infection; and (8) special considerations associated with adherence to ARV treatment.

Chronic Inflammation and HIV Infection

An important area of research is currently focused on the role of a generalized immune activation state that occurs in HIV infection and how it affects the microbiome and its detrimental impact on long-term survival. Several pro-inflammatory cytokines and chemokines are elevated in HIV infection triggered in part by the microbial translocation of bacterial products in the gut following HIV infection (Brenchley et al. 2006). This chronic systemic inflammation has a detrimental impact on the cardiovascular and neurocognitive health of patients. As a result of high levels of pro-inflammatory cytokines, patients with HIV are more prone to development of arterial plaques leading to heart disease and stroke at an earlier age. Unfortunately, use of antiretroviral therapy does not adequately control this chronic state of inflammation. Several drugs that are available for other indications (e.g., statins, aspirin) have the potential to reduce HIV-associated inflammation; however, no significant clinical effect has been observed so far in clinical trials.

Clinical Course and Manifestations of HIV Infection

The natural history and clinical manifestations of HIV infection differs between children and adults, with more rapid disease progression in infancy and a predilection for recurrent, common viral and bacterial infections over opportunistic infections. The more rapid progression is due to the impact of the virus on an immature immune system, and the effect of viral replication and inflammation on somatic and neurodevelopmental growth. The opportunistic infections that result from immune deficiency in children with HIV are often primary, not reactivation disease, thereby resulting in greater morbidity. Despite these challenges, the great strides made in the treatment of children with HIV have positively impacted disease progression and immune capacity, which continue to improve survival rates and quality of life.

HIV Progression in the First Year of Life

Maternal-to-child transmission accounts for the majority of pediatric HIV, and as discussed in the perinatal prevention section, all high-risk pregnant women should be counseled and tested for HIV so that maternal HIV prophylaxis can be initiated as early as possible. In the US, there is negligible transmission via breastfeeding or transfusions; however, these modes still occur in resource-poor countries. While neonates with HIV infection are usually asymptomatic, maternal comorbidities may contribute to perinatal conditions such as prematurity, low birth weight, fetal alcohol syndrome, opioid withdrawal, anemia, and concomitant perinatal infections, including congenital syphilis, cytomegalovirus, hepatitis B, and hepatitis C co-infections. Infants who are vertically infected usually do not present with the acute HIV syndrome that is seen in adults or adolescents with behaviorally acquired HIV; therefore, all exposed infants should be tested with nucleic acid testing before symptoms occur (Havens and Mofenson 2009). Common presentations for infants infected with HIV include chronic diarrhea, oral candidiasis, failure to thrive, and respiratory symptoms, with early central nervous system findings such as loss or delay in motor skills, irritability, and poor head growth.

Prior to the widespread use of antiretrovirals, 10–20% of US and European infants presented with early symptoms of AIDS and died within the first two years of life (Prendergast et al. 2007). They often presented with failure to thrive, oral candidiasis, pneumonia, and encephalopathy. *Pneumocystis jiroveci* pneumonia (PJP) was the most common presenting opportunistic infection prior to the establishment of routine HIV prenatal testing programs and trimethoprim-sulfamethoxazole prophylaxis; mortality rates were high for infants who developed PJP (Simpson et al. 2000). HIV should always be in the differential of infants presenting with interstitial pneumonia and hypoxia. Symptomatic early disease is associated with in utero transmission of HIV, advanced maternal disease, high maternal viral burden, malnutrition and co-infection (Prendergast et al. 2007; Abrams et al. 2003; Lambert et al. 1997). There is no standardized method to identify infants who will progress rapidly. CD4 T cell counts are naturally high in infants; therefore, normal values must be reviewed when interpreting laboratory results. Although CD4 percentages tend to be more stable in young children, there is no difference in prognostic value and absolute counts can be used to follow progression (Boyd et al. 2010). Progression risk is greatest during infancy, regardless of CD4 count, and CD4 counts and viral loads can be poor predictors of progression in this population. Children less than five have higher mortality rates at all levels of immune status (Yin et al. 2014). In settings with limited resources, as many as 50% of infants will present with early symptoms and die by age two (Spira et al. 1999). Infants with early onset symptoms such as failure to thrive and diarrhea are more likely to die or have continued progression, with diarrheal illness or pneumonia being the most common causes of death. A study from Zaire reported that infants infected with HIV with persistent diarrhea had an 11-fold higher risk of death than uninfected infants (Thea et al. 1993). Co-trimoxazole prophylaxis is efficacious in preventing some infectious illnesses in untreated infants infected with HIV (Church et al. 2015). Co-infection with tuberculosis (TB) occurs in 30–50% of cases of HIV infection in TB-endemic areas, further contributing to morbidity and mortality (Ciaranello et al. 2014). Figure 2.1 depicts the cycle of viremia, inflammation, and immune dysregulation that drives disease progression in infants.

Strong and consistent data indicate that infants infected with HIV benefit from early antiretroviral therapy. HIV viral loads increase quickly in the first few months of life and can remain high during infancy—in progressors and non-progressors—

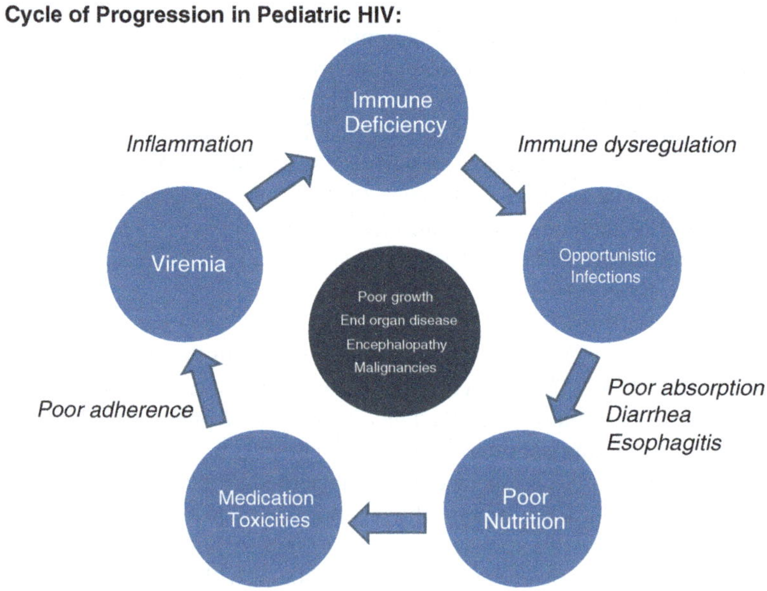

Fig. 2.1 Pathogenesis of HIV progression

therefore, they are not strongly predictive unless associated with low CD4 counts. In the South Africa's CHER study, asymptomatic infants were randomized to receive antiretroviral therapy beginning at 12 weeks of age or when CD4 counts declined or clinical symptoms appeared. Infants in the early treatment group had a 76% decrease in death rates and a 75% decrease in progression to AIDS; infants often died from their first clinical event, with gastroenteritis or pneumonia being the most common causes (Violari et al. 2008). The results from this study confirm the need for close follow-up of exposed infants, early HIV testing, and prompt access to antiretroviral therapy. A recent systematic review confirmed that infants benefit greatly from early HAART; however, there is less evidence to start medications on asymptomatic infants between age one and three years (Penazzato et al. 2014). Current US guidelines recommend that all infants and children be treated regardless of CD4 count or viral load. Many studies have shown that children who start antiretroviral therapy while asymptomatic are much more likely to survive for five years than children who do not start treatment until they reach the Centers for Disease Control (CDC) Category C disease category of illness (Gray et al. 2001). In a review of mortality from HIV, infants who started HAART within six months had a 6-year survival rate of 94% (Kapogiannis et al. 2011).

HIV Progression After the First Year of Life

The rate of HIV disease progression decreases after the first two years of life, with further, but slower, decreases after five years of age. After age five, HIV progression is similar to adults and associated with lower mortality (Yin et al. 2014). CD4 count and viral load have better predictive value in older children, and they are independent predictors of disease progression. Children infected with HIV who are not diagnosed in the perinatal period and who do not die in the first two years often present between 36 and 60 months of age. Recurrent and acute respiratory infections are a common presentation; these children have increased susceptibility to bacterial pathogens such as *Streptococcus pneumoniae* and *Haemophilus*, in addition to more prolonged viral respiratory diseases. Serious recurrent bacterial infections were the most common pediatric AIDS-defining illness and occurred at relatively high CD4 counts (Boyd et al. 2010). Case series conducted in endemic areas revealed that TB, both pulmonary and extra-pulmonary, was present in 30–50% of cases at diagnosis and was the most common opportunistic infection. Patients with lymphoid interstitial pneumonitis (LIP), which can mimic TB in its symptoms and X-ray findings, can present with chronic cough, tachypnea, clubbing, and interstitial reticulo-nodular infiltrates on chest X-ray. LIP can result in pulmonary hypertension, but has been associated with a milder course of HIV (Spira et al. 1999).

Other clinical presentations that are associated with poorer prognosis include malnutrition, encephalopathy, anemia, and chronic diarrhea, in addition to stage 4 World Health Organization (WHO) criteria and other CDC stage 3 opportunistic infections. In a cohort of children perinatally infected in Italy, 44% who were diagnosed with a stage 3 disease died within one year (Galli et al. 2000). As expected, children with mild symptoms, previously called CDC Category A diagnoses, had the best survival: 62% at eight years in this group with mixed exposure to antiretroviral therapy. See Table 2.1 for the revised CDC staging of HIV based on CD4 count and clinical stage 3 diseases.

Table 2.1 Stage -3 -Defining Opportunistic Infections in HIV

Bacterial infections, multiple or recurrent[a]
Candidiasis of bronchi, trachea, or lungs
Candidiasis of esophagus
Cervical cancer, invasive[b]
Coccidioidomycosis, disseminated or extrapulmonary
Cryptococcosis, extrapulmonary
Cryptosporidiosis, chronic intestinal (>1 month of duration)
Cytomegalovirus disease (other than liver, spleen, or nodes), onset at age >1 month
Cytomegalovirus retinitis (with loss of vision)
Encephalopathy attributed to HIV[c]
Herpes simplex: chronic ulcers (>1 month of duration) or bronchitis, pneumonitis, or esophagitis (onset at age >1 month)
Histoplasmosis, disseminated or extrapulmonary
Isosporiasis, chronic intestinal (>1 month of duration)
Kaposi sarcoma
Lymphoma, Burkitt (or equivalent term)
Lymphoma, immunoblastic (or equivalent term)
Lymphoma, primary, of brain
Mycobacterium avium complex or *Mycobacterium kansasii*, disseminated or extrapulmonary
Mycobacterium tuberculosis of any site, pulmonary[b], disseminated, or extrapulmonary
Mycobacterium, other species or unidentified species, disseminated or extrapulmonary
Pneumocystis jirovecii (previously known as "*Pneumocystis carinii*") pneumonia
Pneumonia, recurrent[b]
Progressive multi-focal leukoencephalopathy
Salmonella septicemia, recurrent
Toxoplasmosis of brain, onset at age >1 month
Wasting syndrome attributed to HIV[c]

Adapted from CDC (2014)

[a]Only among children aged <6 years

[b]Only among adults, adolescents, and children aged ≥ 6 years

[c]Suggested diagnostic criteria for these illnesses, which might be particularly important for HIV encephalopathy and HIV wasting syndrome, are described in the following references: CDC. 1994 Revised classification system for human immunodeficiency virus infection in children less than 13 years of age. MMWR 1994;43(No. RR-12). CDC. 1993 Revised classification system for HIV infection and expanded surveillance case definition for AIDS among adolescents and adults. MMWR 1992;41(No. RR-17)

In addition to clinical staging, the CD4 count and HIV viral load are important for assessing a child's individual risk and need for treatment. While both are independent predictors of progression and risk of death, a CD4 count of less than 15% has stronger prognostic value than high viral load (Mofenson et al. 1997). The Pediatric Prognostic Markers Collaborative Study, which pooled longitudinal data from multiple cohorts in the US and Europe, showed that after five years of age, rates of progression to AIDS were similar between children and adults with the same CD4 count (HIV, P. P. M. C. S. 2006). As with adults, when the CD4 count falls to 200 cells/μl, the risk of progression to AIDS increases to 4% per year. A risk calculator that is based on data from the HIV Pediatric Prognostic Markers Collaborative Study can be used to derive estimates of individual patient's risk of progression to AIDS or death based on age plus CD4 count, lymphocyte count, or viral load (Dunn 2003).

Slow Progressors—Late Presentation of HIV

Children with HIV may not present until the first or even second decade, and they may not have had a long history of previous illnesses. These late-presenting patients can be diagnostic challenges, presenting with immune thrombocytopenic purpura, anemia, recurrent parotitis, chronic diarrhea, cardiomyopathy, encephalopathy, or stroke. Family history may help to identify HIV risk factors, such as a mother's death.

Late-presenting patients are slow progressors, also referred to as long-term non-progressors (LTNP). They are a heterogeneous group, and the etiology of the delayed progression can be viral polymorphisms that impact replication and virulence, host genetic factors, and immune factors. Definitions of LTNP vary, including no progression of disease in the first ten years of life, CD4 percentages at or above 25% at ten years (Ofori-Mante et al. 2007), and median survival of 12–13 years compared to the usual six years (Ferrand et al. 2009). Depending on the definition used, 3–25% of all children can be considered slow progressors (Warszawski et al. 2007). Although these children may have had few significant illnesses prior to presentation, they often present with AIDS-defining events and subsequently have rapid disease progression if untreated. There is insufficient data to determine whether LTNPs respond differently to antiretroviral therapy. HIV infection should be part of the differential diagnosis during the adolescent years since late perinatal disease, sexual abuse and early behavioral-acquired transmissions can occur.

Survival to Adulthood

The broad uptake of early HAART therapy has changed the epidemiology of disease in the US and Europe. Hospitalization and mortality rates have declined dramatically, as have rates of opportunistic infections (OIs) (Brady et al. 2010). Despite significant progress, the mortality rate in the US cohort is 0.6–0.8 per 100,000, which is 30–50 times higher than in uninfected children (Kapogiannis et al. 2011). Deaths due to OI have decreased, and multi-organ failure due to end-stage AIDS is the most common cause of death. Many of these children were from earlier birth cohorts who entered care late. The mean age of most US and European pediatric cohorts is now over 18 years, and many are transitioning into adult care. Mental health is frequently affected in children and adolescents infected with HIV, as a result of a chronic illness, social disparities, history of substance abuse, and loss of caregiver due to HIV/AIDS. A more detailed description of the impact of HIV infection in behavioral health is included in other sections of this book.

Along with the long-term survival of children perinatally infected are reports of pregnancy in young women (Byrne et al. 2014). A US study reported a high rate of premature rupture of membranes and delivery; however, outcomes were still good, and only one out of ten infants acquired HIV infection (Williams et al. 2009). Most studies have not shown a substantially different risk of mother-to-child transmission in women perinatally infected; however, the numbers are very limited. The long-term consequences for mothers and infants require further study.

Youth with Behaviorally Acquired HIV

Although there is a growing population of adolescent and young adults perinatally infected, the majority of youth infected acquired HIV through high-risk behaviors. Young people age 13–24 accounted for 22% of all new infections in 2012, with the vast majority occurring in minority men who are bisexual or men who have sex with men (MSM) (Centers for Disease Control and Prevention n.d. a). It is estimated that almost 40% of these youth are not aware of their diagnosis. Adolescents are also less likely to link into care once diagnosed. The clinical presentations of HIV mirror the adult population. Acute HIV syndrome can present with flu-like symptoms, fevers, lymphadenopathy, oral ulcers, and leukopenia; it is often missed in the acute care setting (Weintrob et al. 2003). More often youth are diagnosed during testing and evaluation of other sexually transmitted infections (STIs) such as chlamydia, gonorrhea, and syphilis. A smaller percentage of youth can present with classic opportunistic infections such as pneumocystis pneumonia and recurrent candidiasis. Caring for the adolescent infected with HIV requires a multi-disciplinary approach due to complex psychosocial issues and mental health comorbidities that interfere with linkage and retention in care (Philbin et al. 2016). Although the response to antiretroviral therapy is good, adherence and viral suppression are lower than in other age groups. Transition to adult care should be a stepwise formal process that facilitates retention in care (Judd et al. 2016).

Antiretroviral Therapy

Mortality in children with perinatal HIV infection has decreased by more than 80–90% since the introduction of protease inhibitor-containing combinations, and opportunistic and other related infections in children have significantly declined in the era of HAART (Gona et al. 2006; Brady et al. 2010). ARV drug resistance testing has enhanced the ability to choose effective initial and subsequent regimens. Treatment strategies continue to focus on timely initiation of HAART regimens capable of maximally suppressing viral replication in order to prevent disease progression, preserve or restore immunologic function, and reduce the development of drug resistance. Availability of new drugs has led to more potent regimens with lower toxicity, lower pill burdens, and less frequent medication administration. The use of ARV drugs in pregnant women with HIV has resulted in a dramatic decrease (to less than 2%) in the rate of HIV transmission to infants in the US. In addition, as children and youth living with HIV infection are growing older, new challenges related to adherence, drug resistance, reproductive health planning, transition to adult medical care, and the potential for long-term complications from HIV and its treatments require special attention (Hazra et al. 2010). Several trials in both symptomatic as well as asymptomatic adults have provided evidence of benefit with initiation of ART regardless of CD4 cells expanding the recommendation of HAART to all HIV-positive patients. Similarly, improved outcomes have been shown with initiation of ART in asymptomatic infants between 6 and 12 weeks of age. Although there are fewer available data on the risks and benefits of immediate therapy in asymptomatic children with HIV than in adults, data from the multinational START and PENPACT1 trials served as the background on current ART recommendation for all children with HIV regardless of clinical symptoms, viral load, or CD4 T lymphocyte (CD4) count.

Table 2.2 depicts the current recommendations for therapy in children and adolescents including preferred and alternative regimens. Baseline genotype testing is recommended for all patients at HIV diagnosis, at initiation of antiretroviral therapy and when virologic failure is suspected. In addition, newest resistance testing using next-generation sequencing (GenoSure Archive) amplifies cell-associated HIV-1 DNA from infected cells and provides valuable information when considering regimen changes in virologically suppressed patients due to side effects, regimen simplification, or regimen intolerance. In patients with known or suspected complex drug resistance mutation patterns, the addition of phenotypic to genotypic testing is preferred. Drug resistance testing in the setting of virologic failure should be performed while the patient is taking ARVs or, if not possible, within four weeks after discontinuing therapy to enhance the chance of detection of resistant viruses.

Options for treatment-experienced patients may be more limited, and consultation with a pediatric HIV expert should be sought. In addition, potential side effects, drug interactions, palatability, and type of formulation available based on age influence the clinician decision when constructing the drug regimen. Table 2.3

Table 2.2 Selection of antiretroviral therapy by class and age

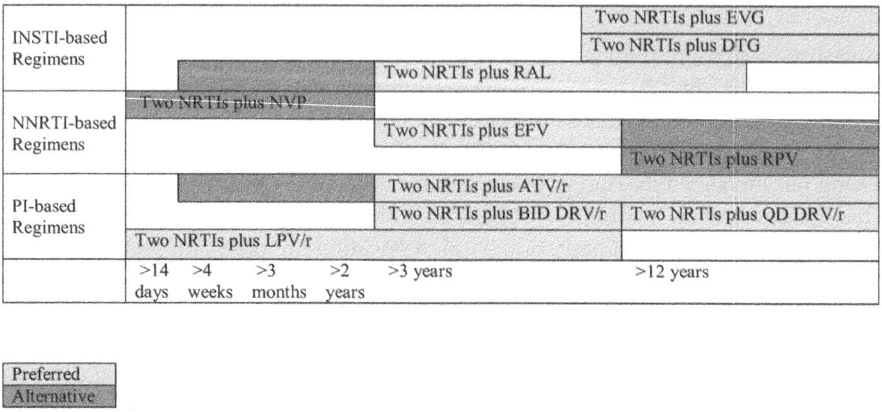

NRTI:	Nucleoside reverse transcriptase inhibitor	RPV:	Rilpivirine
NNRTI:	Non-nucleoside reverse transcriptase inhibitor	QD:	Once daily
PI:	Protease inhibitor	NPV:	Nevirapine
INSTI:	Integrase inhibitor	EFV:	Efavirenz
EVG:	Elvitegravir	ATV/r:	Boosted atazanavir
DTG:	Dolutegravir	DRV/r:	Boosted darunavir
RAL:	Raltegravir	BID:	Twice a day

Adapted from panel on antiretroviral therapy and medical management of HIV-infected children. Guidelines for the use of antiretroviral agents in pediatric HIV infection. Available at http://aidsinfo.nih.gov/contentfiles/lvguidelines/pediatricguidelines.pdf. Accessed July 1, 2016

shows most common side effects related to HIV drug classes. As this field rapidly changes, it is recommended to refer to the most updated guidelines (www.aidsinfo.nih.gov).

The timing for initiation of HAART should be discussed at length with the patient and family in order to provide the best acceptable and long-term option. Immune reconstitution inflammatory syndrome (IRIS) may complicate the initiation of antiretroviral therapy, as do interactions between therapy for other co-infections such as TB and antiretroviral therapy. IRIS presents as a result of the restoration of immune competence by administration of ART, resulting in an exuberant host response to other infections (TB, Cryptococcus, Mycobacterium avium) and/or antigens. IRIS occurs in two forms: unmasking (clinical manifestation of an active infection; for example, TB occurs soon after ART is started) and paradoxical (worsening of clinical symptoms after ARV is started in patients who are already receiving therapy for the co-infection; for example, TB). Predictors of IRIS include C4 count < 50 cells/mm; higher on ART CD4 counts; high pre-ART and lower on ART HIV viral loads; severity of co-infection; and less than 30-day interval between initiation of co-infection therapy and HIV treatment. Most IRIS occur within three months of the start of co-infection therapy. Depending on CD4 count and presentation, delaying initiation of ART for two to eight weeks may reduce the

Table 2.3 Summary of advantages and disadvantages of antiretroviral agents used for HIV therapy in children and adolescents

ARV class	Class side effects	Advantages	Disadvantages
INSTIs Dolutegravir (DTG) Elvitegravir (EVG) Raltegravir (RTG)	Potential for rare systemic allergic reaction Hepatitis	Susceptibility of HIV to a new class of ARV Some available as a one tablet fixed combination Well tolerated	Limited data on pediatric dosing Drug–drug interactions (cobicistat)
NNRTIs Efavirenz (EFV) Etravirine (ETR) Nevirapine (NVP) Rilpivirine (RPV)	Rash (mild to severe)/hypersensitivity reaction (higher with NVP) Hepatitis and hepatotoxicity (highest with NVP) Drug–drug interactions Neuropsychiatric adverse events (EFV)	Long half-life Once daily dosing available Less dyslipidemia and fat maldistribution than PIs PI-sparing Lower pill burden	Low threshold for resistance Rilpivirine not recommended in patients with HIV VL >100,000 copies/ml
PIs Atazanavir/ritonavir (ATV/r) Atazanavir/cobicistat (ATV/cobi) Darunavir (DRV/r) Darunavir/cobicistat (DRV/cobi) Fosamprenavir (FVP) Indinavir (IDV) Lopinavir (LPV/r) Nelfinavir (NFV) Tipranavir /ritonavir (TPV/r) Saquinavir/ritonavir (SQV/r)	Hyperglucemia Hyperlipidemia Lipodystrophy Fat redistribution Increased transaminases Increased bleeding (TPV) Interactions with oral contraceptives Many drug interactions	NNRTI-sparing Clinical, virologic, and immunologic efficacy are well documented Resistance to PIs requires multiple mutations	Poor palatability of liquid formulations may affect adherence High pill burden Most PIs require ritonavir or cobicistat boosting resulting in associated drug interactions

(continued)

Table 2.3 (continued)

ARV class	Class side effects	Advantages	Disadvantages
NRTIs Abacavir (ABC) Didanosine (DDI) Emtricitabine (FTC) Lamivudine (3TC) Stavudine (d4T) Tenofovir (TDF) Tenofovir Alafenamide(TAF) Zidovudine (ZDV)	Lactic acidosis (higher risk with DDI, D4T) Hepatic steatosis Hypersensitivity reaction (HLA B5701) with abacavir Pancreatitis (DDI) Reduce renal function/proteinuria/glycosuria (TDF) Hematologic toxicity (ZDV, 3TC) Lipoatrophy (DZV) Neurotoxicity (DDI) Osteopenia (TDF)	Several options of combined NRTIs in single pill *Palatable liquid formulations* Some are available for daily dosing (TDF, TAF, FTC, delayed-release DDI)	Risk of ABC HSR; perform HLA-B5701 screening before initiation of ABC treatment Long-term use, increase risk of resistance in treatment-experienced patients
Fusion Inhibitors Enfuvirtide (ENF)	Local side effects Hepatitis	Has been used in salvage regimens when limited therapeutic options	Only injectable formulation affecting long-term adherence
CCR5 Inhibitors Maraviroc (MVC)	Same serious side effects had occurred in adults (angina, MI, cirrhosis, hepatotoxicity with allergic features) Drug–drug interactions	Novel mechanism of action	Requires tropism testing prior to its use to exclude CXCR4-using virus

Adapted from www.aidsinfo.nih.gov/guidelines

INSTIs integrase inhibitors; *PIs* protease inhibitors; *NNRTIs* non-nucleoside reverse transcriptase inhibitors; *NRTIs* nucleoside reverse transcriptase inhibitors

Adapted from panel on antiretroviral therapy and medical management of HIV-infected children. Guidelines for the use of antiretroviral agents in pediatric HIV infection. Available at http://aidsinfo.nih.gov/contentfiles/lvguidelines/pediatricguidelines.pdf. Accessed July 1, 2016 incidence and severity of IRIS; however, this possible advantage of delayed ART must be weighed against the potential benefit of earlier ART in improving immune function and preventing progression of HIV disease and mortality.

Adherence

Adherence to highly active antiretroviral therapy (HAART) is a major factor in therapeutic outcomes. Complete viral suppression has been shown in regimens with >95% adherence, although the degree of adherence may be decreased with continued virologic suppression. The pattern of medication non-adherence (treatment interruptions versus missed dosages), the individual drug therapies, and drug class may impact the degree of virologic failure. It is imperative for healthcare workers to discuss the importance of HAART medication adherence with patients and/or caregivers, whether they are newly diagnosed, or perinatally or behaviorally acquired cases. Challenges facing medication adherence are seen in most chronic illnesses, including HIV (Phan and Nahata 2013). Factors influencing medication adherence are usually multifaceted: some factors that may preclude optimal medication adherence include medication formulation, frequency of dosing, forgetting to administer the medication, the child's age, psychosocial, behavioral, or socioeconomic characteristics of the child and their caregivers, personal beliefs, concomitant illnesses, adverse effects of the medication, understanding of the disease and the medication, improper measurement of liquid medication, and more. Other barriers of medication adherence may include unwillingness to disclose HIV status to the child and other caregivers, or other family members that may care for the child. The household environment may also jeopardize medication adherence. Often, patients with HIV may be in an unstable living situation, parents or caregivers may have psychosocial or behavioral issues, or patients themselves may suffer from unstable mental or social status, which may affect compliance with medications (Panel on Antiretroviral Therapy and Medical Management of HIV-Infected Children n.d.).

Infants and young children in particular are only as adherent to their medication regimens as their caregivers will allow. Major factors of medication non-adherence in this subpopulation specifically include palatability of medication, caregiver capacity to understand and administer medications, and ability and willingness of the child to take the medication. Many antiretroviral medications used in children are either commercially available as liquid solutions or suspensions, or extemporaneously compounded to a suspension that may be unpalatable, posing difficulty for caregivers to administer medications.

Adolescents pose a particular challenge in medication adherence as they shift to become the primary advocate for their care. Caregivers often rely on their adolescent children to be responsible for and take ownership of their own healthcare; however, this shift may be difficult if the patient has not been an advocate for their health in prior years. Another layer of complexity is added if patients are unaware of their HIV status. The American Academy of Pediatrics (AAP) recommends that all adolescents should have their HIV status disclosed either by their physician or their caregiver by the time they reach adolescence (Wilfert et al. 1999). If patients are unaware of their status, they may be unwilling or refusing to take medications in which an indication is unknown. Adherence may also be challenging in the adolescent years when patients do not want to be different from their peers, and patients are unwilling to disclose their status to friends or family due to fear of being stigmatized. Older adolescents may be products of an unstable home life or may be homeless, posing difficulties with medication receipt or storage, as well as consistency of clinic visits. Although medications are refilled, this does not indicate adherence at home, so this should not be a sole tool in addressing compliance. Providers may also ask patients to bring their pill bottles to all appointments to conduct a pill count, which may be indicative of compliance. Other approaches may include pill packs or blister packages labeled by day and storing medications in pillboxes. Later innovative tools include mobile phone technologies with reminder applications, voice response systems, SMS text messaging reminders, or email reminders (Horvath et al. 2012).

Perinatal HIV Prevention

The decline of mother-to-child transmission of HIV infection is one of the successes in HIV care. Recommended mother-to-child HIV-1 transmission interventions have resulted in a ten times reduction in this risk, and complete elimination of mother-to-child HIV-1 transmission could be potentially feasible though gaps in testing and treatment availability remain an obstacle. Risk of perinatal transmission has declined from 25 to 40% in the early epidemic to less than 2%. HIV-1 transmission happens at a rate of 8.9 per 100 child-years of breastfeeding after the fourth week, with higher rates during the first four weeks. Mixed feeding doubles the risk of HIV-1 transmission compared with exclusive breastfeeding. Prolonged breastfeeding is the norm in most resource-poor settings, where the risk of transmitting HIV-1 to children reached about 40% without interventions leading to different and prolonged prophylactic strategies to reduce the risk of transmission. Antiretroviral therapy is the mainstay of prevention of mother-to-child HIV-1 transmission. Highly active antiretroviral therapy (HAART) is more effective at prevention of mother-to-child HIV-1 transmission than zidovudine plus one dose of nevirapine and has the additional advantages of reducing sexual HIV transmission and reducing HIV-associated morbidity and mortality. All pregnant women with HIV should receive HAART to prevent perinatal transmission regardless of plasma HIV RNA copy number or CD4 T lymphocyte count. The goal of HAART is to maintain a viral load below the limit of detection throughout pregnancy. Combined antepartum, intrapartum, and infant antiretroviral prophylaxis is recommended because antiretroviral drugs reduce perinatal transmission by several mechanisms, including lowering maternal antepartum viral load and providing infant pre- and post-exposure prophylaxis. In resource-limited settings, the reduction in infant HIV transmission by formula feeding is offset by a higher infant mortality, which shows the crucial role that breastfeeding has in child health. Most recent guidelines from the WHO recommend all pregnant and breastfeeding women living with HIV should initiate HAART, which should be maintained for at least the duration of mother-to-child transmission. Women meeting treatment eligibility criteria should receive HAART for life (CD4 <500 cells/mm^3). Depending on the programmatic infrastructure, particularly in generalized epidemics, WHO recommends that all pregnant and breastfeeding women living with HIV should start and maintain HAART as lifelong treatment. This strategy is known as option B+ (U.S. Preventive Services Task Force n.d.).

Access to antenatal care, HIV testing, and mother-to-child HIV-1 transmission interventions need to be substantially increased in regions with high HIV prevalence. In low-income and middle-income countries, many women present late for antenatal care or deliver without antenatal care; therefore, HIV transmission to infants will be higher. A further challenge to prevent transmission from breastfeeding is that antiretroviral therapy adherence postpartum has been found to be significantly lower than antepartum.

HIV infection should be identified prior to pregnancy or as early in pregnancy as possible. This provides the best opportunity to prevent infant HIV infection and to identify and start therapy as soon as possible in infants who become infected. Universal HIV counseling and voluntary HIV testing are recommended as the standard of care for all pregnant women in the US (U.S. Preventive Services Task Force 2013). All HIV testing should be performed in a manner consistent with state and local laws (http://nccc.ucsf.edu/clinical-resources/hiv-aids-resources/state-hiv-testing-laws/). The CDC recommends the "opt-out" approach, which involves notifying pregnant women that HIV testing will be performed as part of routine care unless they choose not to be tested for HIV. The "opt-out" approach during pregnancy is allowed in every jurisdiction in the US. HIV testing early in pregnancy is recommended as standard of care for all pregnant women in the US. Repeat HIV testing in the third trimester, before 36 weeks of gestation, should be considered for all pregnant women who are HIV seronegative and is recommended for pregnant women who are at high risk of HIV infection. Rapid or expedited HIV testing at the time of labor or delivery should be performed on women with undocumented HIV status; if results are positive, intrapartum and infant postnatal antiretroviral prophylaxis should be initiated immediately, pending results of the confirmatory HIV antibody test. In addition, women who have not been tested for HIV before or during labor should undergo rapid or expedited HIV antibody testing during the immediate postpartum period or their newborns should undergo rapid HIV antibody testing. If results in mother or infant are positive, infant antiretroviral prophylaxis should be initiated immediately and the mothers should not breastfeed unless confirmatory HIV antibody testing is negative. In infants with initial positive HIV viral tests (RNA, DNA), prophylaxis should be stopped and antiretroviral treatment initiated (American Academy of Pediatrics Committee on Pediatric AIDS 2008). When acute HIV infection is suspected during pregnancy, in the intrapartum period, or while breastfeeding, initial testing should be performed with an antigen/antibody combination immunoassay; if the initial testing was performed with an HIV antibody test or supplemental testing is negative, an additional virologic test (RNA, DNA) may be necessary to diagnose HIV infection. Current recommendations also include documentation of the maternal HIV status in the newborn's medical record and communicated to the newborn's primary care provider as well as to perform HIV testing for infants in foster care and adoptees for whom maternal HIV infection status is unknown.

Technological improvements have resulted in increased sensitivity for early infection and reduced performance time for laboratory-based assays, allowing completion in less than one hour. US guidelines recommend that HIV testing begins with a fourth-generation immunoassay capable of detecting HIV-1 and HIV-2 antibodies and HIV-1 p24 antigen (antigen/antibody combination assay). Individuals with a reactive antigen/antibody combination assay should be tested further with an HIV-1/HIV-2 antibody differentiation assay (supplemental testing). Individuals with a reactive antigen/antibody combination assay and a non-reactive differentiation test should be tested with a Food and Drug Administration-approved HIV nucleic acid test to establish diagnosis of acute HIV infection (Centers for Disease Control and Prevention n.d. b).

The fourth-generation immunoassay testing for both antigen and antibody is the test of choice and can be done quickly, but requires trained laboratory staff and therefore may not be available in some hospitals 24 h a day. If this test is unavailable, then initial testing should be performed by the most sensitive expedited or rapid test available. Every delivery unit needs to have access to an HIV test that can be done rapidly (<1 h) 24 h a day. If positive, testing for confirmation of infection should be done as soon as possible (as with all initial positive assays). HIV RNA and HIV DNA nucleic acid tests (NATs) are the recommended preferred virologic assays that must be used to diagnose HIV infection in infants younger than 18 months. Tests for antibodies to HIV do not establish the presence of HIV infection in infants because of transplacental transfer of maternal antibodies to HIV. Virologic diagnostic testing in infants with known perinatal HIV exposure is recommended at ages 14–21 days, 1–2 months (2–4 weeks after cessation of ARV prophylaxis for infants receiving combination of antiretroviral infant prophylaxis), and 4–6 months. Virologic testing at birth should be considered for newborns at high risk of perinatal HIV transmission, such as infants born to mothers with HIV who did not receive prenatal care or prenatal ARVs, who were diagnosed with acute HIV infection during pregnancy, or who had HIV viral loads >1000 copies/mL close to the time of delivery. As many as 30–40% of infants with HIV can be identified by age 48 h. Prompt diagnosis is critical to allow for discontinuing ARV prophylaxis and instituting early ARV therapy. Blood samples from the umbilical cord should not be used for diagnostic evaluations because of the potential for contamination with maternal blood. A positive virologic test should be confirmed as soon as possible by a repeat virologic test on a second specimen.

HIV DNA PCR is a sensitive technique used to detect specific HIV viral DNA in peripheral blood mononuclear cells. The specificity of the HIV DNA PCR is 99.8%

at birth and 100% at ages one, three, and six months. The sensitivity of the test performed at birth is 55% but increases to more than 90% by two to four weeks of age and to 100% at ages three months and six months (Burgard et al. 2012). Although the AMPLICOR® HIV-1 DNA test has been widely used for diagnosis of infants born to HIV-1-infected mothers since it was introduced in 1992, it is no longer commercially available in the US. The sensitivity and specificity of non-commercial HIV-1 DNA tests (using individual laboratory reagents) may differ from the sensitivity and specificity of the Food and Drug Administration (FDA)-approved commercial test. HIV quantitative RNA assays detect extracellular viral RNA in the plasma. Their specificity (for results $\geq$5000 copies/mL) is 100% at birth and at one, three, and six months of age and is comparable to HIV DNA PCR. Eight HIV RNA levels <5000 copies/mL may not be reproducible and should be repeated. The sensitivity of HIV RNA assays has been shown to be 25–58% during the first weeks of life, 89% at age one month, and 90–100% by age two to three months. HIV RNA assays were found to be as sensitive as HIV DNA PCR for early diagnosis of HIV infection in infants exposed to HIV regardless of receipt of infant zidovudine prophylaxis. An HIV RNA assay can be used as the supplemental test for infants who have an initial positive HIV DNA PCR test. HIV RNA assays may be more sensitive than HIV DNA PCR for detecting HIV non-subtype B.

The HIV qualitative RNA assay (APTIMA HIV-1 RNA Qualitative Assay) is an alternative diagnostic test that can be used for infant testing. It is the only qualitative RNA test that is FDA approved (U.S. Food and Drug Administration 2009). When evaluating an infant whose mother's HIV transmission risk is linked to an area endemic for non-subtype B HIV or Group O strains, such as Africa or Southeast Asia, real-time PCR assays or the qualitative RNA assays should be used as they are more sensitive for non-subtype B viruses.

HIV infection can be presumptively excluded in non-breastfed infants with two or more negative virologic tests (one at age $\geq$14 days and one at age $\geq$4 weeks) or one negative virologic test (i.e., negative NAT [RNA or DNA]) test at age $\geq$8 weeks, or one negative HIV antibody test at age $\geq$6 months. *Pneumocystis jirovecii* pneumonia (PCP) prophylaxis is recommended for infants with indeterminate HIV infection status starting at age four to six weeks until they are determined to be HIV uninfected or presumptively uninfected. Thus, initiation of PCP prophylaxis can be avoided or discontinued if an infant has negative virologic tests at ages 2 weeks and $\geq$4 weeks, or if virologic testing is negative at age $\geq$8 weeks.

Definitive exclusion of HIV infection in non-breastfed infants is based on two or more negative virologic tests, with one obtained at age $\geq$1 month and one at age $\geq$4 months, or two negative HIV antibody tests from separate specimens obtained at age $\geq$6 months. Some experts confirm the absence of HIV infection at 12–18 months of age in infants with prior negative virologic tests by performing an antibody test to document loss of maternal HIV antibodies. Children with perinatal HIV exposure aged 18–24 months may have residual maternal HIV antibodies (called late seroreverters). Definitive exclusion or confirmation of HIV infection in children in this age group who are HIV antibody positive should be based on a nucleic acid amplification tests (NATs). Diagnosis of HIV infection in children with non-perinatal exposure or children with perinatal exposure aged >24 months relies primarily on the use of HIV antibody tests. If acute HIV infection is suspected, testing with an HIV NAT should be considered to diagnose HIV infection (Havens and Mofenson 2009).

Infant Antiretroviral Prophylaxis

All infants exposed to HIV should receive postpartum antiretroviral (ARV) drugs to reduce perinatal transmission of HIV. In all situations, infant prophylaxis should be initiated as soon as possible after delivery. A six-week neonatal zidovudine prophylaxis regimen is recommended in the US for all neonates exposed to HIV to reduce perinatal transmission of HIV. Recent guidelines added an acceptable shorter four-week course of neonatal zidovudine prophylaxis for full-term infants when the mother has received standard combination antiretroviral therapy during pregnancy with consistent viral suppression and there are no concerns related to maternal adherence. Zidovudine, at gestational age-appropriate doses (see Table 2.4), should be initiated as close to the time of birth as possible, preferably within 6–12 h of delivery. Infants at higher risk of HIV acquisition, including those born to women with HIV who have received only intrapartum antiretroviral drugs or have not received antepartum or intrapartum antiretroviral drugs or have received antepartum antiretroviral drugs but have had suboptimal viral suppression (>1000 copies/mL) near delivery, should receive prophylaxis with zidovudine for six weeks combined with three doses of nevirapine in the first week of life (i.e., at birth, 48 h later, and 96 h after the second dose), begun as soon after birth as possible. Some experts recommend triple-antiretroviral prophylaxis for infants at higher risk of acquisition although there are no data demonstrating improved efficacy for a three-drug regimen over a two-drug regimen in prevention of transmission. A decision to administer triple-antiretroviral prophylaxis should be made only in consultation with a pediatric HIV specialist and accompanied by parental counseling on the potential risks (e.g., neonatal toxicity) and benefits (e.g., prevention of perinatal transmission) of this approach. For infants born to mothers with unknown HIV status, expedited HIV testing of mothers and/or infants is recommended as soon as possible, either during labor or after birth, with immediate initiation of infant antiretroviral prophylaxis if the initial expedited test is positive. If supplemental testing is negative, antiretroviral prophylaxis can be discontinued. In the US, the use of antiretroviral drugs other than zidovudine and nevirapine cannot be recommended in premature infants as prophylaxis to prevent transmission because of lack of dosing and safety data. In developing settings where breastfeeding is the norm, WHO recommends additional infant prophylaxis (World Health Organization 2016). As this field changes rapidly, the clinician should refer to their most recent local guidelines.

Table 2.4 Neonatal dosing for prevention of perinatal transmission of HIV

	Dosing	Duration
Zidovudine	**≥ 35 weeks of gestation**: 4 mg/kg/dose PO twice daily. If unable to tolerate PO, 3 mg/kg/dose IV every 12 h[a]	Birth through 4–6 weeks
Zidovudine	**≥ 30 to <35 weeks of gestation at birth**: 2 mg/kg/dose PO or (1.5 mg/kg/dose IV), advanced to 3 mg/kg/dose PO (or 2.3 mg/kg/dose IV) every 12 h at age 15 days[a]	Birth through 6 weeks
Zidovudine	**<30 weeks of gestation at birth**: 2 mg/kg body weight/dose PO (or 1.5 mg/kg/dose IV) advanced to 3 mg/kg/dose PO (or 2.3 mg/kg/dose IV) every 12 h after age 4 weeks[a]	Birth through 6 weeks
Additional antiretroviral prophylaxis for infants of women who had been exposed to HIV and received no antepartum antiretroviral prophylaxis or other high risk of transmission		
Nevirapine (in addition to zidovudine)	**Birth weight 1.5–2 kg**: 8 mg/dose PO **Birth weight >2 kg**: 12 mg/dose PO	Three doses in the first week of life: 1. Within 48 h of birth (birth–48 h) 2. 48 h after 1st 3. 96 h after 2nd

Adapted from panel on treatment of HIV-infected pregnant women and prevention of perinatal transmission. Recommendations for use of antiretroviral drugs in pregnant HIV-1-infected women for maternal health and interventions to reduce perinatal HIV transmission in the US. Available at http://aidsinfo.nih.gov/contentfiles/lvguidelines/PerinatalGL.pdf. Accessed June 2016
[a]Start as soon as possible after birth, preferable within 6–12 h

Future Directions

HIV Vaccines and Other Therapeutic and Preventive Approaches

Significant challenges face the development of an effective HIV vaccine, including the genetic diversity of HIV, uncertainty about what constitutes protective immunity, and difficulty in the development of antigens that are highly immunogenic. So far, an effective HIV vaccine remains elusive. The ability of HIV to mutate and evolve and the host inability to create a broadly neutralizing antibody responses against the conserved region of the envelope are some of the road blocks encountered during the development of an HIV vaccine. Several candidate vaccines have not shown efficacy. For example, the STEP trial of a prime-boost HIV vaccine strategy that used an adenovirus vector resulted in an increased rate of HIV infections in the active group in uncircumcised men and men who had pre-existing antibodies to the adenovirus vector serotype. The RV144 trial done in Thailand provided the only evidence to date that vaccine protection could be achieved with a 31% reduction in HIV acquisition. Immune correlates of protection from the RV144 trial, together with new vector approaches that improve the breadth of T cell responses and identify targets for broadly neutralizing antibodies, are being studied for the development of more effective vaccines (Haynes et al. 2012).

Recent advances in understanding the immunologic response of elite controllers as well as the results from the Thai vaccine trial have been encouraging. Elite controllers are able to suppress the virus to lower or undetectable level of viral replication without antiretroviral therapy. Elite controllers have an overrepresentation of specific HLA-B alleles and potent $CD8^+$ T cell-mediated suppressive immune responses. In addition to these controllers, the VISCONTI (viro-immunological sustained control after treatment interruption) study showed that individuals who had initiated ART in the acute phase of HIV infection subsequently controlled viral replication. These patients, who underwent three years of prolonged and continued therapy, could still control viral replication ten years on, even though treatment had been discontinued.

Other areas of investigation include the search for a "functional cure" (that is, permanently controlling HIV infection without completely eradicating it). The case of the so-called Mississippi baby shed light into the benefits of very early therapy to reduce the viral reservoir (Persaud et al. 2013). Very early treatment of perinatally infected infants limits exposure to HIV-1 replication and cell-associated HIV-1 DNA levels. Interestingly, some of these infants that become virologically suppressed rapidly post-infection may lose immunologic responses to HIV (McManus et al. 2016).

Another treatment and potential cure strategy focuses on eliminating the latent viruses. Several drugs are under investigation to include reactivation and potential reduction in the viral reservoir. The only "cure" documented so far is the so-called Berlin patient. This strategy used stem cell transplantation from a donor carrying a protective CCR5 mutation. The virus remained undetectable even following interruption of ARV therapy (Allers et al. 2011). Genetic modification of T cells is underway mimicking this experiment from nature where individuals with CCR5 delta 32 homozygous mutation are resistant to infection with HIV-1 CCR5 tropic viruses. Lastly, the use of ARV to prevent transmission through the use of pre-exposure prophylaxis (PrEP) and the use of other strategies such as microbicides and long-term ARV therapy are under study.

Conclusion

Advances in HIV diagnosis, perinatal prevention, antiretroviral therapy, and other strategies have significantly impacted the survival of children and youth infected with HIV and dramatically decreased the risk of perinatal transmission and transmission to others. The management of HIV infection in the pediatric and adolescent population is rapidly evolving and faces new challenges as HIV infection is no longer a fatal disease, but a chronic condition. New tools to facilitate adherence, simplified therapeutic combinations adapted for younger children, and limiting long-term toxicities are the goals of current research. Although scientific challenges remain, mainly in the development of an HIV vaccine and an HIV cure, global scale-up of current evidence-based interventions leads us one step closer to the end of HIV.

Annotated Bibliography

AIDSinfo|Information on HIV/AIDS Treatment, Prevention and Research. (n.d.). Retrieved August 16, 2016, from https://www.aidsinfo.nih.gov/

This website represents the current state of knowledge in HIV including guidelines for the use of antiretroviral therapy, treatment and prophylaxis for opportunistic infections, post-exposure prophylaxis, and perinatal guidelines. The site includes latest information on drugs, clinical trials, and can be used as a resource for patient friendly information.

Centers for Disease Control and Prevention. (2016). HIV/AIDS. Retrieved August 16, 2016, from http://www.cdc.gov/hiv/

This website, by the Centers for Disease Control and Prevention, contains updated information on multiple topics related to HIV disease including HIV testing, policy and law, guidelines and recommendations along with current statistics, information for the community, and areas of related research.

Gona, P., Van Dyke, R. B., Williams, P. L., Dankner, W. M., Chernoff, M. C., Nachman, S. A., et al. (2006). Incidence of opportunistic and other infections in HIV-infected children in the HAART era. *Jama, 296*(3), 292–300. doi:10.1001/jama.296.3.292

This study shows the impact of HAART in the decline of opportunistic infections and other related infections in comparison to the pre-HAART era.

Hazra, R., Siberry, G. K., & Mofenson, L. M. (2010). Growing up with HIV: Children, adolescents, and young adults with perinatally acquired HIV infection. *Annual Review of Medicine, 61*, 169–185. doi:10.1146/annurev.med.050108.151127

This review article describes the advances in the treatment of HIV in pediatrics, the effect on co-morbidities, the impact of long term complications, and the challenges ahead.

Violari, A., Cotton, M. F., Gibb, D. M., Babiker, A. G., Steyn, J., Madhi, S. A., … & McIntyre, J. A. (2008). Early antiretroviral therapy and mortality among HIV-infected infants. *New England Journal of Medicine, 359*(21), 2233–2244. doi:10.1056/NEJMoa0800971

This study investigated antiretroviral-treatment strategies in the Children with HIV Early Antiretroviral Therapy (CHER) trial and firmly established the benefits and the need for early treatment in infants with HIV. Early HIV diagnosis and early antiretroviral therapy reduced early infant mortality by 76% and HIV progression by 75%.

References

Abrams, E. J., Wiener, J., Carter, R., Kuhn, L., Palumbo, P., Nesheim, S., … & Bulterys, M. (2003). Maternal health factors and early pediatric antiretroviral therapy influence the rate of perinatal HIV-1 disease progression in children. *Aids, 17*(6), 867–877. doi:10.1097/00002030-200304110-00012

Allers, K., Hütter, G., Hofmann, J., Loddenkemper, C., Rieger, K., Thiel, E., et al. (2011). Evidence for the cure of HIV infection by CCR5Δ32/Δ32 stem cell transplantation. *Blood, 117* (10), 2791–2799. doi:10.1182/blood-2010-09-309591

American Academy of Pediatrics Committee on Pediatric AIDS. (2008). HIV testing and prophylaxis to prevent mother-to-child transmission in the United States. *Pediatrics, 122*(5), 1127. doi:10.1542/peds.2008-2175

Barre-Sinoussi, F., Chermann, J. C., Rey, F., Nugeyre, M. T., Chamaret, S., Gruest, J., et al. (2004). Isolation of T-lymphotropic retrovirus from a patient at risk for acquired immune deficiency syndrome (AIDS). *Revista de investigación clínica, 56*(2), 126–129.

Boyd, K., Dunn, D. T., Castro, H., Gibb, D. M., Duong, T., Aboulker, J. P., … & Giaquinto, C. (2010). Discordance between CD4 cell count and CD4 cell percentage: implications for when to start antiretroviral therapy in HIV-1 infected children. *AIDS (London, England), 24*(8), 1213–1217.

Brady, M. T., Oleske, J. M., Williams, P. L., Elgie, C., Mofenson, L. M., Dankner, W. M., et al. (2010). Declines in mortality rates and changes in causes of death in HIV-1-infected children during the HAART era. *Journal of Acquired Immune Deficiency Syndromes, 53*(1), 86. doi:10.1097/QAI.0b013e3181b9869f

Brenchley, J. M., Price, D. A., Schacker, T. W., Asher, T. E., Silvestri, G., Rao, S., et al. (2006). Microbial translocation is a cause of systemic immune activation in chronic HIV infection. *Nature Medicine, 12*(12), 1365–1371. doi:10.1038/nm1511

Burgard, M., Blanche, S., Jasseron, C., Descamps, P., Allemon, M. C., Ciraru-Vigneron, N., et al. (2012). Performance of HIV-1 DNA or HIV-1 RNA tests for early diagnosis of perinatal HIV-1 infection during anti-retroviral prophylaxis. *The Journal of pediatrics, 160*(1), 60–66. doi:10.1016/j.jpeds.2011.06.053

Byrne, L., Thorne, C., Foster, C., & Tookey, P. (2014). Pregnancy outcomes in women growing up with perinatally acquired HIV in the United Kingdom and Ireland. *Journal of the International AIDS Society, 17*(4Suppl 3). doi:10.7448/IAS.17.4.19693

Centers for Disease Control. (2014). Revised surveillance case definition for HIV infection—United States, 2014. *MMWR, 63*(3), 1–10

Centers for Disease Control and Prevention. (n.d. a). HIV among youth. Retrieved July 10, 2016 from http://www.cdc.gov/hiv/group/age/youth

Centers for Disease Control and Prevention. (n.d. b). Retrieved June 3, 2016, from http://www.cdc.gov/hiv/pdf/hivtestingalgorithmrecommendation-final.pdf#page=11

Church, J. A., Fitzgerald, F., Walker, A. S., Gibb, D. M., & Prendergast, A. J. (2015). The expanding role of co-trimoxazole in developing countries. *The Lancet Infectious Diseases, 15*(3), 327–339. doi:10.1016/S1473-3099(14)71011-4

Ciaranello, A., Lu, Z., Ayaya, S., Losina, E., Musick, B., Vreeman, R., et al. (2014). Incidence of World Health Organization stage 3 and 4 events, tuberculosis and mortality in untreated, HIV-infected children enrolling in care before 1 year of age: an IeDEA (international epidemiologic databases to evaluate AIDS) East Africa regional analysis. *The Pediatric Infectious Disease Journal, 33*(6), 623–629. doi:10.1097/INF.0000000000000223

Dunn, D. (2003). HIV paediatric prognostic markers collaborative study group: Short-term risk of disease progression in HIV-1-infected children receiving no antiretroviral therapy or zidovudine monotherapy: A metaanalysis. *Lancet, 362*(9396), 1605–1611. doi:10.1016/S0140-6736(03)14793-9

Feng, Y., Broder, C. C., Kennedy, P. E., & Berger, E. A. (2011). HIV-1 entry cofactor: Functional cDNA cloning of a seven-transmembrane, g protein–coupled receptor. *Journal of immunology (Baltimore, Md.: 1950), 186*(11), 6076.

Ferrand, R. A., Corbett, E. L., Wood, R., Hargrove, J., Ndhlovu, C. E., Cowan, F. M., … & Williams, B. G. (2009). AIDS among older children and adolescents in Southern Africa: Projecting the time course and magnitude of the epidemic. *AIDS (London, England), 23*(15), 2039. doi:10.1097/QAD.0b013e32833016ce

Fouda, G. G., Moody, M. A., & Permar, S. R. (2015). Antibodies for prevention of mother-to-child transmission of HIV-1. *Current Opinion in HIV and AIDS, 10*(3), 177–182. doi:10.1097/COH.0000000000000150

Galli, L., De Martino, M., Tovo, P. A., Gabiano, C., & Zappa, M. (2000). Predictive value of the HIV paediatric classification system for the long-term course of perinatally infected children. *International Journal of Epidemiology, 29*(3), 573–578. doi:10.1093/ije/29.3.573

Gaur, A. H., Dominguez, K. L., Kalish, M. L., Rivera-Hernandez, D., Donohoe, M., Brooks, J. T., et al. (2009). Practice of feeding premasticated food to infants: a potential risk factor for HIV transmission. *Pediatrics, 124*(2), 658–666. doi:10.1542/peds.2008-3614

Gona, P., Van Dyke, R. B., Williams, P. L., Dankner, W. M., Chernoff, M. C., Nachman, S. A., et al. (2006). Incidence of opportunistic and other infections in HIV-infected children in the HAART era. *JAMA, 296*(3), 292–300. doi:10.1001/jama.296.3.292

Gottlieb, I. M. S. (1984). Serological analysis of subgroup of human T-lymphotropic retroviruses (HTLV-III) associated with AIDS. *Leukemia, 8*, 4.

Gray, L., Newell, M. L., Thorne, C., Peckham, C., & Levy, J. (2001). Fluctuations in symptoms in human immunodeficiency virus-infected children: the first 10 years of life. *Pediatrics, 108*(1), 116–122. doi:10.1542/peds.108.1.116

Havens, P. L., & Mofenson, L. M. (2009). Evaluation and management of the infant exposed to HIV-1 in the United States. *Pediatrics, 123*(1), 175–187. doi:10.1542/peds.2008-3076

Haynes, B. F., Gilbert, P. B., McElrath, M. J., Zolla-Pazner, S., Tomaras, G. D., Alam, S. M., et al. (2012). Immune-correlates analysis of an HIV-1 vaccine efficacy trial. *New England Journal of Medicine, 366*(14), 1275–1286. doi:10.1056/NEJMoa1113425

Hazra, R., Siberry, G. K., & Mofenson, L. M. (2010). Growing up with HIV: Children, adolescents, and young adults with perinatally acquired HIV infection. *Annual Review of Medicine, 61*, 169–185. doi:10.1146/annurev.med.050108.151127

Hemelaar, J., Gouws, E., Ghys, P. D., & Osmanov, S. (2011). Global trends in molecular epidemiology of HIV-1 during 2000–2007. *AIDS (London, England), 25*(5), 679. doi:10.1097/QAD.0b013e328342ff93

HIV, P. P. M. C. S. (2006). Predictive value of absolute CD4 cell count for disease progression in untreated HIV-1-infected children. *AIDS (London, England), 20*(9), 1289. doi:10.1097/01.aids.0000232237.20792.68

Horvath, T., Azman, H., Kennedy, G. E., & Rutherford, G. W. (2012). Mobile phone text messaging for promoting adherence to antiretroviral therapy in patients with HIV infection. *The Cochrane Library*,. doi:10.1002/14651858.cd009756

Hütter, G., Nowak, D., Mossner, M., Ganepola, S., Müßig, A., Allers, K., et al. (2009). Long-term control of HIV by CCR5 Delta32/Delta32 stem-cell transplantation. *New England Journal of Medicine, 360*(7), 692–698. doi:10.1056/NEJMoa0802905

Judd, A., Sohn, A. H., & Collins, I. J. (2016). Interventions to improve treatment, retention and survival outcomes for adolescents with perinatal HIV-1 transitioning to adult care: Moving on up. *Current opinion in HIV and AIDS*,. doi:10.1097/COH.0000000000000302

Kapogiannis, B. G., Soe, M. M., Nesheim, S. R., Abrams, E. J., Carter, R. J., Farley, J., et al. (2011). Mortality trends in the US perinatal AIDS collaborative transmission study (1986–2004). *Clinical Infectious Diseases, 53*(10), 1024–1034. doi:10.1093/cid/cir641

Lambert, G., Thea, D. M., Pliner, V., Steketee, R. W., Abrams, E. J., Matheson, P., et al. (1997). Effect of maternal CD4+ cell count, acquired immunodeficiency syndrome, and viral load on disease progression in infants with perinatally acquired human immunodeficiency virus type 1 infection. *The Journal of pediatrics, 130*(6), 890–897. doi:10.1016/S0022-3476(97)70274-9

Liu, R., Paxton, W. A., Choe, S., Ceradini, D., Martin, S. R., Horuk, R., et al. (1996). Homozygous defect in HIV-1 coreceptor accounts for resistance of some multiply-exposed individuals to HIV-1 infection. *Cell, 86*(3), 367–377. doi:10.1016/S0092-8674(00)80110-5

McManus, M., Mick, E., Hudson, R., Mofenson, L. M., Sullivan, J. L., Somasundaran, M., … & PACTG 356 Investigators. (2016). Early combination antiretroviral therapy limits exposure to HIV-1 replication and cell-associated HIV-1 DNA levels in infants. *PloS one, 11*(4), e0154391. doi:10.1371/journal.pone.0154391

Mofenson, L. M., Korelitz, J., Meyer, W. A., Bethel, J., Rich, K., Pahwa, S., et al. (1997). The relationship between serum human immunodeficiency virus type 1 (HIV-1) RNA level, CD4 lymphocyte percent, and long-term mortality risk in HIV-1—infected children. *Journal of Infectious Diseases, 175*(5), 1029–1038. doi:10.1086/516441

Ofori-Mante, J. A., Kaul, A., Rigaud, M., Fidelia, A., Rochford, G., Krasinski, K., et al. (2007). Natural history of HIV infected pediatric long-term or slow progressor population after the first decade of life. *The Pediatric Infectious Disease Journal, 26*(3), 217–220. doi:10.1097/01.inf.0000254413.11246.e1

Panel on Antiretroviral Therapy and Medical Management of HIV-Infected Children. (n.d.). Guidelines for the use of antiretroviral agents in pediatric HIV infection. Retrieved August 2015, from AIDSInfo: http://aidsinfo.nih.gov/contentfiles/lvguidelines/pediatricguidelines.pdf

Penazzato, M., Prendergast, A. J., Muhe, L. M., Tindyebwa, D., & Abrams, E. (2014). Optimisation of antiretroviral therapy in HIV-infected children under 3 years of age. *The Cochrane Library*. doi:10.1002/14651858.cd004772.pub4

Persaud, D., Gay, H., Ziemniak, C., Chen, Y. H., Piatak, M., Jr., Chun, T. W., et al. (2013). Absence of detectable HIV-1 viremia after treatment cessation in an infant. *New England Journal of Medicine, 369*(19), 1828–1835. doi:10.1056/NEJMoa1302976

Phan, H., & Nahata, M. C. (2013). Introduction to pediatrics. In S. Benavides & M. C. Nahata (Eds.), *Pediatric pharmacotherapy* (1st ed., pp. 3–17). Lenexa, KS, USA: American College of Clinical Pharmacy.

Philbin, M. M., Tanner, A. E., DuVal, A., Ellen, J. M., Xu, J., Kapogiannis, B., et al. (2016). HIV testing, care referral, and linkage to care intervals affect time to engagement in care for newly diagnosed HIV-infected adolescents in 15 adolescent medicine clinics in the United States. *JAIDS Journal of Acquired Immune Deficiency Syndromes, 72*(2), 222–229. doi:10.1097/QAI.0000000000000958

Popovic, M., Sarngadharan, M. G., Read, E., & Gallo, R. C. (1984). Detection, isolation, and continuous production of cytopathic retroviruses (HTLV-III) from patients with AIDS and pre-AIDS. *Science, 224*(4648), 497–500. doi:10.1126/science.6200935

Prendergast, A., Tudor-Williams, G., Jeena, P., Burchett, S., & Goulder, P. (2007). International perspectives, progress, and future challenges of paediatric HIV infection. *The Lancet, 370* (9581), 68–80. doi:10.1016/S0140-6736(07)61051-4

Samson, M., Libert, F., Doranz, B. J., Rucker, J., Liesnard, C., Farber, C. M., et al. (1996). Resistance to HIV-1 infection in caucasian individuals bearing mutant alleles of the CCR-5 chemokine receptor gene. *Nature, 382*(6593), 722–725. doi:10.1038/382722a0

Sharp, P. M., & Hahn, B. H. (2011). Origins of HIV and the AIDS pandemic. *Cold Spring Harbor Perspectives in Medicine, 1*(1), a006841. doi:10.1101/cshperspect.a006841

Siberry, G. K., Patel, K., Bellini, W. J., Karalius, B., Purswani, M. U., Burchett, S. K., … & Yogev, R. (2015). Immunity to measles, mumps, and rubella in US children with Perinatal HIV infection or perinatal HIV exposure without infection. *Clinical Infectious Diseases*, civ440. doi:10.1093/cid/civ440

Simpson, B. J., Shapiro, E. D., & Andiman, W. A. (2000). Prospective cohort study of children born to human immunodeficiency virus-infected mothers, 1985 through 1997: Trends in the risk of vertical transmission, mortality and acquired immunodeficiency syndrome indicator diseases in the era before highly active antiretroviral therapy. *The Pediatric Infectious Disease Journal, 19*(7), 618–624. doi:10.1097/00006454-200007000-00007

Spira, R., Lepage, P., Msellati, P., Van de Perre, P., Leroy, V., Simonon, A., et al. (1999). Natural history of human immunodefiency virus type 1 infection in children: a five-year prospective study in Rwanda. *Pediatrics, 104*(5), e56–e56. doi:10.1542/peds.104.5.e56

Sutcliffe, C. G., & Moss, W. J. (2010). Do children infected with HIV receiving HAART need to be revaccinated? *The Lancet Infectious Diseases, 10*(9), 630–642. doi:10.1016/S1473-3099(10)70116-X

Tebas, P., Stein, D., Tang, W. W., Frank, I., Wang, S. Q., Lee, G., et al. (2014). Gene editing of CCR5 in autologous CD4 T cells of persons infected with HIV. *New England Journal of Medicine, 370*(10), 901–910. doi:10.1056/NEJMoa1300662

Thea, D. M., St. Louis, M. E., Atido, U., Kanjinga, K., Kembo, B., Matondo, M., … & Rand, W. M. (1993). A prospective study of diarrhea and HIV-1 infection among 429 Zairian infants. *New England Journal of Medicine, 329*(23), 1696–1702. doi:10.1056/NEJM199312023292304

U.S. Food and Drug Administration. (2009). APTIMA HIV-1 RNA qualitative assay. Retrieved from http://www.fda.gov/BiologicsBloodVaccines/BloodBloodProducts/ApprovedProducts/LicensedProductsBLAs/BloodDonorScreening/InfectiousDisease/ucm149922.htm

U.S. Preventive Services Task Force. (2013, April). Screening for HIV: Recommendation statement. Retrieved March 2016, from U.S. Preventive services task force: http://www.uspreventiveservicestaskforce.org/uspstf/uspshivi.htm

U.S. Preventive Services Task Force. (n.d.). Consolidated guidelines on HIV prevention, diagnosis, treatment, and care for key populations—2016 update. Retrieved March 2016, from http://www.uspreventiveservicestaskforce.org/uspstf/uspshivi.htm

Violari, A., Cotton, M. F., Gibb, D. M., Babiker, A. G., Steyn, J., Madhi, S. A., et al. (2008). Early antiretroviral therapy and mortality among HIV-infected infants. *New England Journal of Medicine, 359*(21), 2233–2244. doi:10.1056/NEJMoa0800971

Wallet, M. A., Rodriguez, C. A., Yin, L., Saporta, S., Chinratanapisit, S., Hou, W., … & Goodenow, M. M. (2010). Microbial translocation induces persistent macrophage activation unrelated to HIV-1 levels or T cell activation following therapy. *AIDS (London, England), 24* (9), 1281. doi:10.1097/QAD.0b013e328339e228

Warszawski, J., Lechenadec, J., Faye, A., Dollfus, C., Firtion, G., Meyer, L., et al. (2007). Long-term nonprogression of HIV infection in children: evaluation of the ANRS prospective French Pediatric Cohort. *Clinical Infectious Diseases, 45*(6), 785–794. doi:10.1086/521165

Weintrob, A. C., Giner, J., Menezes, P., Patrick, E., Benjamin, D. K., Lennox, J., et al. (2003). Infrequent diagnosis of primary human immunodeficiency virus infection: missed opportunities in acute care settings. *Archives of Internal Medicine, 163*(17), 2097–2100. doi:10.1001/archinte.163.17.2097

Wilfert, C., Beck, D. T., Fleischman, A. R., Mofenson, L. M., Pantell, R. H., Schonberg, S. K., et al. (1999). Disclosure of illness status to children and adolescents with HIV infection. *Pediatrics, 103*(1), 164–166. doi:10.1542/peds.103.1.164

Williams, S. F., Keane-Tarchichi, M. H., Bettica, L., Dieudonne, A., & Bardeguez, A. D. (2009). Pregnancy outcomes in young women with perinatally acquired human immunodeficiency virus-1. *American Journal of Obstetrics and Gynecology, 200*(2), 149-e1. doi:10.1016/j.ajog.2008.08.020

World Health Organization. (2016). In *Consolidated guidelines on the use of antiretroviral drugs for treating and preventing HIV infection: Recommendations for a public health approach*, 2nd ed. Retrieved from http://apps.who.int/iris/bitstream/10665/208825/1/9789241549684_eng.pdf?ua=1

Yin, D. E., Warshaw, M. G., Miller, W. C., Castro, H., Fiscus, S. A., Harper, L. M., et al. (2014). Using CD4 percentage and age to optimize pediatric antiretroviral therapy initiation. *Pediatrics, 134*(4), e1104–e1116. doi:10.1542/peds.2014-0527

Chapter 3
Developmental Considerations for Children and Youth with HIV

Sharon Nichols

Over the more than three decades since human immunodeficiency virus (HIV) and acquired immunodeficiency syndrome (AIDS) were first recognized in adults and children, developmental and neurological concerns have been prominent. During the early years of the epidemic, significant neurological and developmental sequelae were common in advanced HIV disease. As advances in antiretroviral therapy (ART) have transformed HIV into a chronic disease and now prevent the most severe central nervous system (CNS) complications, relevant issues have shifted to long-term cognitive and behavioral outcomes, prevention of CNS and developmental morbidity, ongoing subtle cognitive dysfunction, CNS toxicity of antiretroviral regimens, and the role of cognitive functioning in transition to independent adulthood.

Because HIV acquired during the fetal or neonatal period may affect the CNS system differently than HIV acquired later during childhood or adolescence, children with perinatally acquired HIV (PHIV) will be discussed separately from those with HIV acquired behaviorally during adolescence.

Developmental and CNS Impact of HIV

Perinatally Acquired HIV

Cognitive and Neurological Sequelae: Historical Perspective

In the absence of ART, HIV acquired before or during birth can have devastating developmental consequences. Prior to effective ART being widely used in children with PHIV, several patterns of HIV-associated encephalopathy occurred, with prevalence estimates ranging up to 90% of children (Mintz et al. 2012). In general,

S. Nichols (✉)
University of California, San Diego, La Jolla, CA, USA
e-mail: slnichols@ucsd.edu

T. Chenneville (ed.), *A Clinical Guide to Pediatric HIV*,
DOI 10.1007/978-3-319-49704-4_3

encephalopathy was more common in children than in adults. Progressive encephalopathy (PE) was defined by three features: impaired brain growth or atrophy, motor sequelae such as abnormal muscle tone, and loss of developmental milestones or cognitive abilities (Belman 2008; Mintz et al. 2012). Although PE could develop at any point during childhood, the most virulent form was a rapidly progressive encephalopathy seen in the first two years of life in the context of rapid disease progression. Babies with this form of encephalopathy typically died within 24 months following diagnosis (Shanbhag et al. 2005). A second, "plateau," pattern consisted of slowed acquisition rather than loss of skills or milestones so that the child's functioning gradually diverged more and more from the typical developmental trajectory. Although usually seen in the context of other AIDS-defining symptoms or opportunistic infections, PE could also appear as the first manifestation of AIDS. Cerebral atrophy, white matter abnormalities, and calcifications of the basal ganglia were seen on magnetic resonance imaging (MRI) or computed tomographic (CT) scans for some infants and children (Allison et al. 2009). Appearance of imaging, motor or focal neurological abnormalities, slowing of head growth or milestone acquisition, or frank loss of milestones or abilities were used as indicators of disease progression in the CNS and treatment failure in the early days of ART. Although uncommon in the era of combination ART, PE is still a possibility where ART is unavailable or not used for some other reason.

"Static encephalopathy" was a term used to describe a developmental trajectory similar in rate to that of typically developing children but shifted downward; in other words, children had stable impairments in cognitive or motor functioning relative to their age peers, but could develop PE as their disease progressed. Static encephalopathy could be related to other neurological risks and events other than HIV, such as prematurity. Opportunistic infections in the CNS could also occur in children with advanced immune suppression, although less commonly than in adults, and if resolved, contribute to stable deficits.

Since the introduction of highly active antiretroviral therapy (HAART) in 1996, and particularly following the introduction of protease inhibitors, HIV-related encephalopathy has become much less common in both children and adults (Chiriboga et al. 2005; Patel et al. 2009). However, a subset of children with past diagnoses of AIDS and subsequent viral suppression show stable cognitive impairment relative to typical development. Neurodevelopmental patterns observed in the current context of ART will be discussed following a brief introduction to neuropathogenesis of HIV.

Neuropathogenesis

HIV is thought to enter the CNS within days or weeks of infection (Crowell et al. 2014). Although it does not infect neurons directly, it is able to affect CNS functioning through exposure of the neurons to HIV proteins and through infection of other cells such as perivascular macrophages, microglia, and astrocytes, with resulting production of cytokines and other neurotoxins as well as alteration of the blood–brain barrier (Gannon et al. 2011). Studies in adults suggest that continued trafficking of HIV into the CNS is facilitated by an ongoing state of systemic inflammation and immune activation established soon after infection and maintained by changes in other body compartments such as the gut (Ancuta et al. 2008). This state may continue despite ART (Garvey et al. 2014) and result in the production of activated, infected macrophages that are able to cross the blood–brain barrier. Although the blood–brain barrier is designed to prevent toxins from entering the CNS, it also prevents some medications from entering. The resulting sequestration of the virus in the brain may allow it to replicate and evolve separately from that in the body and permit the brain to serve as a reservoir of virus (Crowell et al. 2014).

Associations of neurocognitive outcomes with biomarkers of ongoing inflammation and immune activation in children with PHIV support the importance of these factors in children as well as adults (Kapetanovic et al. 2010, 2014). Although similar in basic mechanisms, however, the neuropathogenesis of infection in utero or perinatally may differ from later infection in some respects, such as due to immaturity of the blood–brain barrier, the ability of HIV to infect neural progenitor cells, and greater susceptibility of the developing brain to the toxic effects of chemokines and HIV proteins (see Crowell et al. 2014, for review). In adults, neuroimaging and autopsy studies have shown cortical atrophy and white matter changes in the brain, with particular susceptibility of frontal regions, hippocampus, and subcortical structures such as the basal ganglia (Tate et al. 2010). Neuroimaging studies in children have shown a similar pattern of subcortical and frontostriatal atrophy and white matter abnormalities in addition to poor brain growth and calcifications in the basal ganglia in those with early disease progression (Sharer 2005). Children with long-term control of HIV nevertheless show lower brain volumes, poorer white matter integrity and increased diffusion (Cohen et al. 2016; Hoare et al. 2014), and white matter alterations associated with past disease severity appear to be related to cognitive performance (e.g., working memory; Uban et al. 2015). Recent studies using functional MRI have demonstrated that youth with PHIV show altered patterns of functional connectivity that correlate with processing speed, suggesting potential reorganization of brain networks (Herting et al. 2015).

Developmental Functioning in the Era of Antiretroviral Therapy

Several reviews have summarized studies of cognitive functioning in children with PHIV (Laughton et al. 2013; Le Doare et al. 2012; Smith and Wilkins 2015). Key and updated findings for global and specific cognitive functions will be presented.

Global Functioning

In the current era, transmission of HIV from mother to infant is rare in high-resource countries such as the US. Studies of infants and young children in the US and Europe prior to therapy for prevention of mother-to-child HIV transmission found that infants with PHIV had neurodevelopmental scores below those of population means, and infants with greater disease severity were more likely to have scores indicative of moderate-to-severe delays (Le Doare et al. 2012). Infants with infection that was thought to have occurred in utero, rather than at the time of birth, had worse functioning (Smith et al. 2000). More recent research conducted in settings with continuing high rates of infant infection, such as sub-Saharan Africa, have demonstrated developmental deficits, particularly in motor skills but also in mental and language development, among infants with PHIV (Abubakar et al. 2008; McGrath et al. 2006; Van Rie et al. 2009) in comparison with babies with perinatal HIV exposure but uninfected (PHEU) and unexposed babies. As expected, HIV disease severity, as well as other risk factors such as low weight for age, has been associated with outcomes (Abubakar et al. 2009).

The prospect of survival to adulthood brought by advancements in ART has magnified concerns about long-term cognitive functioning for youth with PHIV. Studies of older children with PHIV (Martin et al. 2006; Smith et al. 2012; Wood et al. 2009) have on the whole found that, when viewed as a homogeneous group, they have global functioning in the low average to average range, with scores that differ from population norms but generally not from PHEU children. When children not exposed to HIV prenatally are included as a comparison group, some studies have shown differences between them and children with PHIV (Brahmbhatt et al. 2014; Puthanakit et al. 2010, 2013) while others have not found differences on global measures (Bagenda 2006). Ruel et al. (2012) compared a group of relatively healthy children with PHIV to uninfected community controls in Uganda and found significantly lower motor and cognitive scores in the PHIV group, taking differences in demographic variables such as socioeconomic status into account (although note that other psychosocial impacts of living in a family impacted by HIV may account at least in part for these differences). In a study of young children also in Uganda, Brahmbhatt et al. (2014) observed that young children with PHIV differed from both unexposed and PHEU groups, but with different patterns.

Subsets of children with PHIV are at risk for lower functioning compared to PHEU, and studies have begun to clarify factors that are associated with long-term developmental issues. In particular, those with a past episode of immune suppression and HIV-related illness sufficient to qualify for a Centers for Disease Control (CDC) Class C (AIDS) diagnosis (Centers for Disease Control 1994) have significantly lower scores on measures of global cognitive functioning, particularly if they had a diagnosis of encephalopathy (Smith et al. 2012; Wood et al. 2009). This is true even if subsequent viral control and immune reconstitution were achieved. This pattern is similar to that observed in adults, where the individual's lowest ever immune functioning (CD4+ nadir) predicts cognitive outcomes regardless of current immune status (Ellis et al. 2011). Children with other indicators of CNS impact, such as abnormalities noted on CT scans, are also more likely to have lower scores (S.C. Martin et al. 2006). In children, diagnosis with AIDS prior to the age of three appears to increase the risk of cognitive impairments (Smith et al. 2006; Wood et al. 2009). This may suggest a reduced ability of the CNS to recover similar to that seen in other early, non-focal CNS impacts. In general, studies demonstrating the deleterious effects of early severe disease and the benefits of initiating treatment before AIDS diagnosis (Lazarus et al. 2015) support current recommendations to initiate ART in infancy (*Guideline on When to Start Antiretroviral Therapy and on Pre-Exposure Prophylaxis for HIV* 2015).

Findings regarding associations of global cognitive functioning with measures of ongoing disease severity vary. Studies have shown cognitive impairment, albeit subtle, in adults with well-controlled HIV (Heaton et al. 2010) and the disconnect between systemic viral load and CNS functioning may be linked in part to viral "escape," indicated by virus appearing in the cerebrospinal fluid but not plasma (Crowell et al. 2014). Other factors, such as toxicity of ART regimens or ART-resistant inflammation, may also contribute to observed impairments in the absence of systemic disease. Some studies in children have shown associations of cognitive functioning with current plasma viral load or other indicators of HIV activity and immune functioning in children (Nichols et al. 2016; Ruel et al. 2012) and imaging studies reviewed above suggest subtle brain changes even in children with good immune functioning. In addition, associations of cognitive outcomes with measures of inflammation and immune activation or with lymphocyte and monocyte cell subsets are beginning to emerge and may provide additional clues to neuropathogenesis and treatment (Ananworanich et al. 2014; Kapetanovic et al. 2010, 2014; Mekmullica et al. 2009).

Cognitive Domains

Interest in implications for functional outcomes and intervention, as well as studies demonstrating differential susceptibility of cognitive domains to HIV in adults, have inspired a research literature focusing on domain-specific differences in PHIV. The domains that have generated the most research are executive functions, language, processing speed, and to some extent learning and memory.

Executive Functioning

Executive functioning (EF) is a broad domain that includes a variety of skills involved in performing goal-directed behaviors, such as monitoring of the self and environment, inhibition, cognitive flexibility, shifting of behavior and mental focus, problem-solving, and fluency of memory retrieval and response generation (Strauss et al. 2006). In adults with HIV, EF has proven to be a cognitive domain at particular risk for impairment (Heaton et al. 2011), and it has been linked to multiple functional outcomes such as medication management (Thames et al. 2013), sexual risk behaviors (Golub et al. 2012), and occupational (Heaton et al. 2004) and educational (Jacobson and Mahone 2012) outcomes. As youth with PHIV become more independent, the role of EF in their daily lives may play an increasing role.

A number of studies have examined EF in cohorts of children with PHIV (Nichols 2012). Several studies have found differences between PHIV and PHEU children in EF (Hoare et al. 2012; Koekkoek et al. 2008; Martin et al. 2006) and noted that EF was particularly sensitive to differences between PHIV and uninfected children (Koekkoek et al. 2008). However, others have failed to find differences (Llorente et al. 2014; Nagarajan et al. 2012). Llorente et al. (2014), using both objective and questionnaire measures of EF, observed differences between children with PHIV and PHEU age 8–12 that disappeared when controlling for other variables such as exposure to prenatal drugs or receiving special services in school. Similarly, Nichols and colleagues compared children with PHIV and PHEU in a similar age range using objective and caregiver- and self-report measures of EF and found no impairments in the PHIV group, compared to PHEU, on objective or questionnaire measures of behavioral regulation; however, both groups showed more problems than would be expected based on normative databases for the measures used (Nichols et al. 2015). In addition, youth with PHIV and past encephalopathy endorsed more everyday problems with metacognition (e.g., cognitive regulation). These youth also showed slower processing speed, a finding noted in other studies of EF as well (Nagarajan et al. 2012). Thus, EF may be an example of differences in the cognitive effects of HIV between adults and children; however, self-perceived problems in some aspects of EF, and other cognitive impairments that may complicate long-term acquisition of EF skills, indicate the need for further research as youth age into adolescence and adulthood.

Language and Hearing

Prior to availability of ART, language deficits were reported in children with PHIV (Wolters et al. 1997). Impairment or loss of milestones in expressive language, in particular, were viewed as part of an overall deficit in expressive behavior associated with PE and appearing in young children as reduced vocalization and emotional expression and, in the end stages, muteness (Moss et al. 1996). In the era of ART, language has continued to be of interest because of its central role in academic achievement and other aspects of daily life that are critical as youth with PHIV mature, such as social functioning and communication with health providers. Although studies continue to demonstrate a relatively high rate of language impairments in children and youth with PHIV (Brackis-Cott et al. 2009b; Rice et al. 2012), associations with demographic variables and inconsistent differences from children who are PHEU suggest that HIV may not be a primary driver of these impairments. Rice et al. (2012) examined both primary language impairment and language impairment observed in conjunction with cognitive or hearing deficits (LI-Con), and documented higher levels of both in children with PHIV and PHEU, with no differences between the groups. Children with PHIV and greater disease severity had higher levels of LI-Con, suggesting that language deficits in this group can appear as part of a more global impact of HIV on neurodevelopment. It should be noted, in examining language development, that children with PHIV, particularly those with a Class C diagnosis, are also at higher risk for hearing deficits than the general population (Torre et al. 2012) and hearing assessment should be a standard part of their care.

Processing Speed

Processing speed is known to be sensitive to the impact of HIV on the CNS in adults (Heaton et al. 2010), and consequently, measures of processing speed are commonly included in cognitive batteries for adults with HIV. Numerous studies have demonstrated that children are similarly vulnerable to effects of HIV on processing speed (Koekkoek et al. 2008; Martin et al. 2006; Nachman et al. 2012; Nichols et al. 2015; Ruel et al. 2012; Smith et al. 2012). Processing speed, more than other cognitive domains, shows significant associations not only with past severe disease (Smith et al. 2012), but with markers of ongoing disease processes such as brain metabolites (Nagarajan et al. 2012), functional connectivity using functional MRI (Herting et al. 2015), and biomarkers of vascular functioning (Kapetanovic et al. 2014).

Learning and Memory

Memory is known to be an area commonly affected in adults with HIV (Heaton et al. 2011) and important for functional outcomes such as medication adherence and activities of daily living in that population (Thames et al. 2013). Furthermore, learning is a primary developmental task during childhood and adolescence. A limited literature suggests poorer performance on measures of verbal and visual recall in children with PHIV compared to non-infected youth or normative data (Koekkoek et al. 2008; Nichols et al. 2016). One study of children with PHIV, using magnetic resonance spectroscopy, found relationships between choline concentrations and spatial memory (Keller et al. 2004). A recent study (Nichols et al. 2016) found that youth with PHIV achieved lower scores on measures of verbal learning and delayed visual memory than youth who were PHEU and that, among the PHIV group, performance on some measures was associated with current CD4% and past Class C diagnosis. Children with PHIV had particular difficulty with verbal learning, which is consistent with their increased risk for learning disorders (Wood et al. 2009). Although adjusting for socioeconomic variables affected results concerning verbal memory, lower performance on delayed visual memory persisted, suggesting that youth with PHIV are at risk for inefficient encoding and forgetting of visual information. Whether or not these patterns are caused by HIV, their potential to contribute to poor academic and occupational outcomes indicates the need for additional research. Another area where studies of youth with PHIV are needed as they approach adulthood is prospective memory, or remembering to carry out future intentions. Deficits in this domain, which relies on both EF and retrospective memory, are seen in adults with HIV (Carey et al. 2006;

Martin et al. 2007), for whom they are a strong predictor of problems with medication management and other outcomes (Martin et al. 2007; Woods et al. 2008a, b).

Other Developmental Risks for Children with PHIV

Sociodemographic and Psychosocial Risks

Determining the impact of HIV on the developing child is complicated by the high prevalence of other developmental risks in the population of children likely to acquire HIV perinatally. Several categories of risk affect this group of children. Environmental risks include poverty and associated problems such as high levels of chronic stress, exposure to violence, lack of access to health care, educational disadvantages, greater likelihood of exposure to toxins such as lead, and fewer enrichment opportunities. Because of potential impacts of poverty on development and the brain (Hair et al. 2015; Shonkoff and Garner 2012), socioeconomic status is usually taken into consideration in research on PHIV. Familial learning and language disorders, as well as psychiatric disorders with potential impact on neurocognitive development such as attention-deficit/hyperactivity disorder, must be considered when examining patterns of cognitive abilities in children with PHIV. Among children with PHIV, cognitive outcomes have been shown to be affected by caregiver identity (e.g., biological parent versus other individual), mental health, education, overall health, and cognitive functioning, and by family income (Smith et al. 2012). Nutrition and weight for age impact neurodevelopment in this population particularly in lower-resource settings (Horacio et al. 2015). Among the most significant developmental risks other than HIV facing these children are pre- and perinatal exposures and events, such as low birth weight, prenatal exposure to alcohol and drugs of abuse, and other congenital infections such as cytomegalovirus.

A comprehensive review of psychosocial and mental health issues related to PHIV is covered in a separate chapter (see Albright et al. 2017) and, therefore, will not be included here. However, within the context of thinking about neurodevelopment in children with PHIV, it is important to consider this population is at increased risk for mental health concerns (Mellins and Malee 2013) through genetic routes and through the impacts of parental mental illness, living with a chronic, stigmatizing illness and attendant issues of disclosure, pain, treatment side effects, and worry about the future including the possibility of death. Mental health issues such as attention-deficit/hyperactivity disorder, depression, and stress are important potential contributors to cognitive impairment that must be taken into account. As young people with PHIV age up through adolescence and into adulthood, they are also likely to face increased risk for substance use (Alperen et al. 2014), which has the potential to impact cognitive performance.

Prenatal Exposure to HIV and ART

Because of the relatively unique constellation of developmental risks faced by children born to mothers with HIV, research on the effects of PHIV commonly uses as a comparison group children who were PHEU. In recent years, however, concern has grown that in utero exposure to HIV and to antiretroviral agents can themselves impact neurodevelopment adversely, particularly in the context of interest in long-term effects of maternal infections in general and greater recognition of epigenetic and other mechanisms by which such effects can occur. Although studies comparing test scores of children who were PHEU with published norms have shown low average global functioning, few studies have compared children who were PHEU to controls matched for their sociodemographic and other risks. Studies from Africa have shown impairments in language, cognitive and motor functioning in children who were PHEU compared to those who were unexposed (McGrath et al. 2006; Van Rie et al. 2008) and a Thai cohort demonstrated lower performance on measures of verbal IQ and memory (Kerr et al. 2014); however, a recent neuroimaging study in Thailand found no differences between children who were PHEU and those who were unexposed (Jahanshad et al. 2015). Children who were PHEU in lower-resource countries show increased mortality, possibly as a result of reduced breastfeeding and caregiving (Filteau 2009), illustrating the magnitude of other risks faced by this population in some settings. Further concerns have centered on the developmental impact of prenatal exposure to ART, particularly with research suggesting potential mitochondrial toxicities, increased risk of preterm birth, and cardiac and other effects related to individual drugs (Guerra et al. 2016; Heidari et al. 2011). However, a study comparing Kenyan infants exposed to ART in utero and during one year of breastfeeding with non-exposed children found no adverse effects on cognitive and language development (Ngoma et al. 2014). Given the undisputed benefits of prevention via ART of mother-to-child transmission of HIV during pregnancy, recent studies in high-resource settings have focused on comparative safety of different regimens. In general, large-scale studies comparing different regimens have supported the safety of prenatal ART exposure with respect to neurodevelopment (Nozyce et al. 2014; Sirois et al. 2013; Williams et al. 2010).

Behaviorally Acquired HIV (BHIV)

Adolescents and young adults ("youth") have the highest rates of HIV infection of any age group in the US (Centers for Disease Control and Prevention 2015). Since brain development continues into the 20s (Blakemore and Choudhury 2006), it is reasonable to assume that HIV acquired during this period, and possible neurotoxic effects of ART, may impact the CNS differently than in adults. Furthermore, this age group may have a different profile than adults of other risk factors affecting neurocognition, such as substance use. Limitations in cognitive functioning may impact youths' ability to acquire academic, social, and practical skills needed for successful independent functioning in adulthood, and may affect tasks critical for long-term survival and prevention of HIV transmission, such as medication adherence and avoiding sexual risk behaviors. Despite this, few studies of HIV and neurocognitive functioning have focused on youth.

The limited existing literature regarding neurocognitive functioning in the context of HIV acquired during adolescence suggests cause for concern. A study of factors affecting medication adherence of youth with HIV (Hosek et al. 2005) indicated that almost 70% of 42 participants exhibited concrete reasoning, suggesting delays in the development of abstract reasoning, and their vocabulary scores fell in the borderline range. A recent study of cognitive functioning and risk behavior (Baker et al. 2014) in 23 young adults with HIV and 21 uninfected controls age 18–24 found that youth with HIV demonstrated lower verbal fluency; however, it should be noted that there were significant demographic differences between the groups.

A study of the neurocognitive impact of the timing of ART initiation (Nichols et al. 2013; Nichols et al. 2016) used a broad battery of tests similar to those used to diagnose HIV-Associated Neurocognitive Disorder (HAND) in adults (Antinori et al. 2007). Among the 220 ART-naïve participants with BHIV age 18–24, more than two-thirds qualified for a diagnosis of HAND, primarily in the category of Asymptomatic Neurocognitive Impairment. This category is used when cognitive impairments in multiple domains are observed but without declines in daily functioning; for youth with fairly recent HIV infection (more than half diagnosed less than 12 months previously) and possibly ongoing support for daily tasks, declines of this sort may be unlikely. The most striking impairments were on tests of learning and memory, both verbal and nonverbal, with 18–39% of scores in this domain falling more than two standard deviations below population norms. Measures of fine and gross motor functioning also showed high rates of impairment. Test performance was associated with some indicators of HIV severity; for example, lower CD4 counts were associated with poorer performance in executive functions and higher likelihood of HAND, whereas longer time since HIV diagnosis was significantly associated with lower full scale IQ. Because the youth were relatively healthy at the time of the assessment, this raises concern regarding the impact of subclinical neuroimmune events. However, as anticipated, performance was also associated with other risk factors, such as alcohol use, education level and history of academic problems (repeating a grade in school, for example), emotional distress, comorbid conditions, and demographic factors such as race and income. As with youth with PHIV, the importance of taking other risk factors into account when attempting to interpret HIV effects cannot be overstated, particularly since cognitive impairments may result in part from other modifiable factors that are common in this population, such as depression, chronic and traumatic stress, and substance use. In general, the degree to which neurocognitive impairments in this population are related to their HIV infection remains an unresolved issue requiring further research. Potential long-term CNS effects, such as decreased cognitive reserve leading to greater risk for later cognitive decline (Basso and Bornstein 2000), and interactions with cardiovascular and other risks over time are also a concern.

Functional Impact of Child and Adolescent HIV

Academic Outcomes

Academic learning is a major task of childhood and adolescence, and critical for optimizing adult outcomes. Its importance for youth with HIV is magnified by links between academic achievement and health outcomes in general, through multiple routes such as greater occupational achievement and resulting availability of healthcare and health insurance, for example (Freudenberg and Ruglis 2007; Ruglis and Freudenberg 2010). In addition, limited health literacy (LHL), which is linked to literacy in general, increases risk of suboptimal health outcomes, including poor health status, more hospitalizations, non-adherence to prescribed medications, and higher mortality (Berkman et al. 2011). Patients with LHL are more likely to experience disparities in health and healthcare access and have lower rates of screening and preventive services. Among adults with HIV, patients with LHL are more likely to have poorer knowledge about their disease, medication regimens and methods for managing their disease (Valenti 2007), worse medication adherence (Colbert et al. 2013), and greater difficulty evaluating the quality of online health information (Chesser et al. 2016; Kalichman et al. 2006). Relationships between health literacy, general literacy, and HIV management may differ for youth and adults with HIV (Murphy et al. 2010; Navarra et al. 2014). A recent review of health literacy and HIV points out the urgent need for studies on special populations such as adolescents (Wawrzyniak et al. 2013). Despite these potential links to poor long-term outcomes in adulthood, health literacy has not been evaluated among youth with HIV.

A small literature suggests that children with PHIV show poor academic achievement and a high rate of receiving special education in school (Brackis-Cott et al. 2009b; Souza et al. 2010). However, results are mixed concerning whether their performance is lower than expected given socioeconomic and other risks (Brackis-Cott et al. 2009a, b). In a study comparing 295 children and adolescents with PHIV to 167 children who were PHEU, Garvie et al. (2014) used an academic screening measure and found that both groups had low performance based on normative standards. Although the two groups differed in total achievement and math performance, these differences did not remain following adjustment for sociodemographic variables such as income, race, and caregiver IQ. However, children with PHIV and a history of encephalopathy had lower achievement overall, and a greater discrepancy between actual achievement and that predicted by their global cognitive functioning. This suggests that all youth exposed to HIV would benefit from structural changes to address school disparities, but that in addition a subset of youth with PHIV should be monitored closely for school failure. Among youth with BHIV, more than a fifth had a history of school problems indicated by receiving special services or repeating a grade (Nichols et al. 2013) and 34% had scores more than one standard deviation below age norms on a test of word reading; however, significant demographic risks for school failure exist in this population as well and increased rates of preexisting learning problems are possible. Regardless of their origin, academic and health literacy issues need to be addressed in research and in preparing youth for transition to adulthood.

Medication Management

Of all functional outcomes, medication adherence has received the most attention in research on HIV in both adults and children. With advances in ART, individuals born with HIV or acquiring it before adulthood via other risks have the potential to live into adulthood, possibly reaching a normal life span. However, this potential is realized only with adherence adequate to maintain suppression of HIV. Medication adherence can be impacted by multiple factors, including some that are magnified among youth such as motivational issues, depression and other problems with mental health, substance use, structural factors such as homelessness, and desires for independence and resistance to authority in general (MacDonell et al. 2015). Adherence is difficult for youth with chronic illnesses in general, and those with HIV face additional obstacles such as side effects of ART, stigma of HIV, and fears that others will see them taking their medications. Caregiver factors and relationships with caregivers are important as youth gain increased responsibility for adherence (Naar-King et al. 2013). The importance of adherence for youth is in some respects even greater than for adults for two reasons. First, they face the prospect of living for many decades with HIV and the likelihood that immune compromise could lead not only to short-term problems, but also to poorer long-term outcomes including higher risk of age-associated cardiovascular and cognitive decline. Second, they are more likely to engage in sexual risk behaviors, and viral suppression is critical to prevent secondary transmission of HIV to sexual partners; furthermore, poor adherence can lead to viral resistance to ART and resistant virus can be transmitted to others. Estimates that only 6% of youth with HIV age 13–29 achieve viral suppression emphasize the importance of improving all levels of care, including medication adherence (Zanoni and Mayer 2014).

Among adults with HIV, neurocognitive impairment is an additional risk factor for poor adherence, and a vicious cycle has been hypothesized whereby cognitive impairment contributes to poor adherence, which in turn contributes to lack of viral control and subsequently worsening of cognitive functioning (Ettenhofer et al. 2010). However, among children and youth, few studies have examined relationships of adherence with cognitive functioning and findings generally do not support a link despite children and adolescents with both PHIV and BHIV reporting forgetfulness as a reason for non-adherence (Buchanan et al. 2012; Chandwani et al. 2012). In a study of almost 1500 children age 3–18 (Malee et al. 2009), global cognitive functioning was not associated with adherence overall, although youth with borderline IQ (70–84) were less adherent to one class of medications, protease inhibitors. This finding may suggest that youth with mild cognitive problems require additional adherence support that is not recognized as readily as for youth with more severe impairment. This possibility is supported by a follow-up study with a subset of that cohort (Nichols et al. 2012) which found better adherence in children with lower scores on measures of verbal memory and reading. However, little is known yet regarding contributions of cognitive functioning to adherence in adolescents and young adults with perinatally or behaviorally acquired HIV despite the associations of cognitive functioning and adherence seen in adults and the need for effective adherence interventions.

Adaptive and Daily Functioning

The ability to acquire life skills needed to meet social, self-care, and ultimately occupational demands has vital importance for youth with PHIV who now face possibilities and responsibilities associated with adulthood. Although few studies have been conducted with older youth with PHIV as yet, one study conducted in the US with children and younger adolescents showed adaptive functioning measured using caregiver questionnaires in the average to low average range and comparable to that of children who were PHEU (Smith et al. 2012). Among children with a past CDC Class C diagnosis, adaptive behavior was higher than global cognitive functioning; this suggests that adaptive behavior may be an area of resilience, although the different assessment methodologies make comparison difficult. In contrast, a study of older youth with PHIV (age 13–24) found lower ratings for daily living skills by both caregivers and youth, and for self-care by caregivers, compared to youth who were PHEU (Pearlstein et al. 2014). The groups were comparable with regard to ratings of social skills. This study suggests that interventions to increase life skills may be indicated prior to transition to adulthood. It should be noted that agreement between caregiver and youth ratings was low. Although not an unexpected finding, this emphasizes the need for multiple informants and for incorporation of performance-based measures of life skills such as have been used to demonstrate the impact of HAND in adults on such areas as medication management (Thames et al. 2011), driving (Thames et al. 2013), and other functional outcomes (Heaton et al. 2004).

Substance Use and Risk Behaviors

As youth with PHIV have aged into adolescence, studies have begun to examine their participation in risk behaviors such as substance use and engaging in unprotected sexual activity. Alcohol and other substance use is common in adolescents in the population as a whole (Johnston et al. 2012), and recently published data from the Pediatric HIV/AIDS Cohort Study suggest that youth with PHIV follow similar substance use trajectories (Alperen et al. 2014) and are comparable to youth who were PHEU. Risk behaviors of all kinds, including substance use, among youth with BHIV are high (Fernandez et al. 2015). Despite evidence indicating that cognitive patterns or impairments may increase likelihood of risk behaviors among adults with HIV (Shrestha and Copenhaver 2016; Thames et al. 2012) these associations have not yet been examined among youth with HIV.

An additional potential connection between substance use and neurocognition among youth with HIV lies in the developing literature suggesting that alcohol and marijuana use can lead to negative brain changes, and that these changes are greater if substance use is initiated during adolescence when neuronal connections are not yet finalized (Squeglia et al. 2009). In the population of youth as a whole, substance abuse and dependence are associated in some studies with alterations in neural activity and reduced cognitive performance (Squeglia et al. 2012; Thoma et al. 2011), and cannabis in particular with decrements in learning, memory, and working memory (Schweinsburg et al. 2008). Among adults with HIV, neurocognitive deficits are associated with use of alcohol and methamphetamine, and potentially with cannabis, where the literature is more limited (Levine et al. 2012; Rosenbloom et al. 2010). A study of neurocognitive functioning in youth with BHIV found high levels of substance use and a significant effect of alcohol risk (self-reported frequency and consequences of use) on cognition (Nichols et al. 2013). Furthermore, substances of abuse can be related to systemic inflammatory and immune system changes (Costello et al. 2013) that may have the potential to affect cognitive outcomes in youth with HIV. For these reasons, studies examining the interactive effects of HIV and substance use on the brain among youth with HIV are needed.

Transition to Adult HIV Care

For youth with chronic illnesses in general, transition to adult care systems is difficult (Irwin 2010; Weissberg-Benchell et al. 2007) and illness management may deteriorate following transition (MacDonell et al. 2010), with decreased adherence, increased health problems and costs (Bonnie et al. 2014). After transition, typically recommended in their early to mid-20s (Transitioning HIV-infected youth into adult health care 2013), youth with HIV have high risk of loss to care and they experience increases in mortality (Zanoni and Mayer 2014). Youth with HIV who are cared for in adult clinics are more likely to discontinue ART than those followed in adolescent clinics (Agwu et al. 2012) and have lower rates of virologic suppression than older adults in the same clinics (Ryscavage et al. 2011). Young people are expected to assume independent management of their own health care and medication in an adult healthcare model at a developmental point characterized by skill development, knowledge acquisition, exploration (Bonnie et al. 2014), and reductions in support, all of which may contribute to transition difficulty (*The Future of Disability in America* 2007). For youth in their teens and early 20s, a need for developmentally appropriate care is widely recognized (IAPAC Guidelines for Optimizing the HIV Care Continuum for Adults and Adolescents 2015); they are typically cared for in youth-friendly adolescent clinics with monitoring and assistance for critical tasks like medication adherence from staff as well as caregivers at home (Tanner et al. 2014). Youth cognitive and literacy challenges may play a minor role due to the support provided. Thus, the need for additional assistance to acquire healthcare management skills and knowledge may go unrecognized before transition to an adult healthcare system where independence is expected. Because transition to adult care is typically triggered by age, rather than developmental maturity, youth may not be ready to assume the required responsibility for their own healthcare self-management.

The potential for the cognitive impairments described above for youth with both PHIV and BHIV to affect their ability to retain and follow recommendations conveyed by healthcare professionals and to impede acquisition of skills needed to manage HIV is a concern. This concern is supported by evidence of the impact of cognitive impairments and low health literacy on medication and healthcare management in adults with HIV (Thames et al. 2011, 2013; Waldrop-Valverde et al. 2010). Models of self-management of chronic diseases typically recognize the important role of cognitive processes such as problem-solving, decision-making, and self-monitoring (Lorig and Holman 2003; Rotheram-Borus et al. 2012; Swendeman et al. 2009), and published transition guidelines (Davison et al. 2006; New York State Department of Health AIDS Institute 2011) identify low youth health literacy and poor knowledge of their own healthcare condition as obstacles to transition. The American Academy of Pediatrics suggests assessment of developmental readiness as part of preparing to transition adolescents with HIV to adult care (Transitioning HIV-infected youth into adult health care, 2013). Currently, there is a lack of literature concerning the role of youth developmental functioning in transition to guide intervention efforts. Until our lack of knowledge in this area is addressed, it is reasonable to assume that assessment of youth cognitive development may be helpful for both adolescent clinics preparing youth for transition and the adult clinics receiving them.

Prevention and Intervention for Neurodevelopmental Complications of HIV

Antiretroviral Therapy

By far, the most significant impact on developmental functioning in children and youth with HIV has come from the development of effective ART using combinations of medications (Chiriboga et al. 2005). The progressive encephalopathy, in children, and HIV-associated dementia, in adults, once common and feared for individuals with HIV can now, in most instances, be prevented with ART.

Encephalopathy in children can be not only prevented, but in some cases reversed by ART (Crowell et al. 2014). In addition, the ability to prevent mother-to-child transmission of HIV through ART may someday mean that concerns about developmental effects of HIV will be relevant for an increasingly rare population. At this point, however, perinatal HIV infection continues to occur globally, and significant challenges related to preventing and treating CNS effects of HIV remain for children as well as adults. Despite our ability to prevent severe CNS effects, subtle developmental and cognitive impacts may still occur for children, as described above, and for adults (Heaton et al. 2010, 2011) and, most likely, youth with BHIV. In fact, mild neurocognitive impairment may be more common now in adults as people live longer with HIV, and the cognitive domains most affected have shifted to a pattern characterized more by deficits in learning, memory, and executive functions (Heaton et al. 2011). The literature on the effect of ART on developmental and neurocognitive functioning in the context of less severe disease has some inconsistencies, however. In adults, ART has robust albeit modest positive effects on HIV-associated cognitive dysfunction (Al-Khindi et al. 2011); however, in a study of youth with BHIV followed for three years after initiating ART, no effects on neurocognitive functioning were observed (Nichols et al. 2016).

Given variable impact of ART, and the current lack of CNS-targeted medications (McGuire et al. 2014), optimizing the effectiveness of ART through timing of initiation and characteristics of drug regimens have received focus for the prevention of CNS effects of HIV. In 2015, previous recommendations to initiate ART at the time of HIV diagnosis for adults and adolescents were strengthened based on a preponderance of data suggesting reduced mortality and morbidity when immune suppression is prevented as well as reduction in HIV transmission (Panel on Antiretroviral Guidelines for Adults and Adolescents 2016). Although the studies on which the updated recommendations were based did not address adolescence, the guidelines were extrapolated to that population, while recognizing that adherence requires special attention for adolescents. Studies demonstrating that both metabolic and structural changes in the brain can occur in the first year of infection in some individuals (Lentz et al. 2011; Peluso et al. 2013; Ragin et al. 2012) as well as other evidence suggests that early ART initiation may be neuroprotective. Although starting ART with CD4 counts above and below the previously used threshold of 350 did not affect neurocognitive outcomes in a study of adolescents (Nichols et al. 2016), it could be that youth in that study were already past the point where ART was likely to prevent inflammatory and other changes with the potential to affect cognitive outcomes. Unknown interactions of ART, including potential toxicities, with brain development during adolescence call for additional research with this population to maximize gains and minimize the potential for side effects.

Pediatric guidelines call for immediate initiation of ART in infants under 12 months of age due to the potential for rapid disease progression and evidence indicating reduction of mortality with immediate treatment (Panel on Antiretroviral Therapy and Medical Management of HIV-Infected Children 2015). For children over 12 months of age, recommendations differ from those of adults due to concerns about development of resistance, adherence, and long-term toxicities;

guidelines recommend that treatment should be initiated in children who are symptomatic, and considered for those who are asymptomatic. The guidelines point out that ART initiation before 12 months of age, versus waiting until immunosuppression occurs, likely prevents neurological complications; however, the impact of early versus later treatment initiation on neurodevelopment in children over 12 months of age is not entirely clear. Evidence from the Pediatric HIV/AIDS Cohort Study suggests that initiation during infancy or early childhood is associated with better cognitive outcomes (Crowell et al. 2015). The PREDICT study in Thailand found no difference in neurodevelopment in children over one year of age who did or did not wait to initiate ART until clinical indicators developed (Puthanakit et al. 2013); both groups showed developmental impairments, possibly further supporting recommendations to begin treatment before age one. Additional support for early treatment comes from a study of children age 0–6 in Uganda, showing that duration of ART treatment was associated with better neurodevelopment (Brahmbhatt et al. 2014).

In a recent review, Crowell et al. (2014) discuss potential reasons for the continuing incidence of neurocognitive impairments in children with PHIV despite ART. In addition to demographic and other psychosocial risks, CNS impacts prior to the initiation of ART, and the failure of ART to address ongoing inflammation, which are presented above, they discuss several factors associated with the ART regimens themselves. One characteristic that varies across medications is the ability of the drug to penetrate the blood–brain barrier and enter the brain. Ideally, it would seem reasonable that higher blood–brain barrier penetration would be desirable, although it must be balanced against greater potential for toxicity and long-term side effects (Gannon et al. 2011). Systems of ranking the CNS penetration effectiveness (CPE) of regimens based on comparisons of plasma and cerebrospinal fluid drug levels have been developed (Letendre et al. 2008), although they are based on adults. However, studies comparing the effects of regimens with higher and lower CPE scores on neurocognitive outcomes in adults have had mixed results, with some indicating improved outcomes (Carvalhal et al. 2015; Smurzynski et al. 2011) and others indicating continued neurocognitive decline even with high CPE or no relationship (Baker et al. 2015; Marra et al. 2009). The few studies that have examined CPE in children have not found effects on neurocognitive functioning (Crowell et al. 2015; Patel et al. 2009). Currently, alternative methods for examining the effect of antiretroviral medications on the CNS are being developed.

Finally, ART regimens vary in their potential for neurotoxicity. One drug with known neurological side effects is efavirenz, which can be associated with headache, dizziness, confusion, hallucinations, and sleep disturbances including vivid dreams. Although these side effects typically resolve, efavirenz may be associated with reduced neurocognitive functioning (Ciccarelli et al. 2011). Other mechanisms for neurotoxicity including mitochondrial toxicity, metabolic, and cardiovascular effects (Crowell et al. 2014) increase concern for children for whom length of treatment may magnify such risks.

Interventions for Developmental Delay and Impairment

A variety of interventions that may be applicable for individuals with HIV have been developed to address problems with cognitive functioning throughout the life span, including, for example, early interventions for young children with or at risk for developmental delay, specialized programs for children with learning disabilities or ADHD, and cognitive rehabilitation for adults with traumatic brain injury or older adults with dementia. Furthermore, lifestyle changes that have the potential to improve cognitive functioning in general may be relevant to youth with HIV, including avoiding substance use, increasing physical activity, and getting adequate sleep and nutrition. Although individual children and youth with HIV may receive services based on clinical or academic indications, very few controlled studies of cognitive interventions have been performed with this population (Sherr et al. 2014). Two intervention studies have been conducted in Africa with children with PHIV. In the first, 122 South African children with PHIV less than 2.5 years of age were randomized to standard care or to a home stimulation intervention. The investigators found greater positive change in mental and motor development for children in the intervention group, although their scores still indicated delay (Potterton et al. 2010). In the second, 60 children with PHIV in Uganda were randomly assigned to a computerized cognitive intervention or no intervention (Boivin et al. 2010). The intervention involved exercises designed to enhance attention, conceptual/memory, visual motor, and logic skills. Findings from this pilot study demonstrated significantly better performance on two subtests of a computerized cognitive measure in the intervention group. These studies suggest that studies of interventions to prevent developmental delay and enhance cognitive functioning in children with PHIV are warranted.

Best Practices

Prevention of developmental and cognitive sequelae of HIV is a primary goal. Initiation of ART prior to the development of immune compromise and encephalopathy has been clearly shown to reduce the likelihood of long-term CNS impact in children and adults alike. Early ART initiation may prevent the development of more subtle neurocognitive sequelae as well, although at this time further research is required for children and adolescents. In addition, children and youth have non-HIV risk factors for cognitive and developmental problems that could impact their quality of life and ability to manage their lives and health care independently. Healthcare providers, educators, and others who provide services to this population need to be aware of these risks and provide appropriate preventive and intervention services, including developmental and neuropsychological evaluations, cognitively based interventions for adherence (e.g., memory or EF-based strategies), and assistance with accessing and utilizing resources, particularly for those with low literacy. Cognitive difficulties should be considered when working with youth on such issues as reduction of risk behaviors, preparation for disclosure of HIV status to others, participation in mental health interventions, and transition to adult care. In turn, cognitive issues (e.g., slowing, distractibility) may be indicative of treatable mental health disorders such as attention-deficit disorder or depression. Finally, maintenance of brain health through viral suppression and lifestyle modifications (e.g., avoiding substance use; increasing physical activity) should be discussed with young people preventively.

Future Directions

Despite decades of research, much remains unknown about HIV and the CNS among children and youth. With severe neurological sequelae preventable through effective viral suppression using ART, focus has shifted to understanding and preventing more subtle impacts on the CNS and their interaction with other risk factors such as substance use; elucidating the role of inflammation and immune activation as well as other mechanisms of neuropathogenesis; addressing issues of neurotoxicity; CNS sequestration and viral escape despite suppression; and exploring amelioration through adjunctive means such increasing physical activity. Development and validation of sensitive indicators of CNS effects using neuroimaging, blood and CSF markers, and sensitive cognitive paradigms is critical for these lines of research.

As children and youth with HIV approach and proceed through adulthood, an understanding of their developmental and cognitive functioning may be critical for maximizing their quality of life and ability to function as citizens, employees or employers, and parents, and for preventing future cognitive problems. Research is urgently needed on the relationships of cognitive impairments, whatever their origin, to substance use, risk behaviors, mental health outcomes, self- and health-care management, and independent functioning in general among youth and young adults with HIV.

Conclusion

Although the most devastating CNS sequelae of HIV can now be prevented in most cases, the developmental and neurocognitive impacts of HIV continue to be important. Significant CNS effects remain a possibility due to the unavailability of ART in some settings and the numerous issues that interfere with consistent medication adherence among youth. More subtle effects may occur even with good viral control; in addition, other neurocognitive, academic, and functional risks are prevalent among children and youth with HIV. Thus, monitoring developmental and neurocognitive outcomes continues to be indicated for this population, particularly as youth are required to learn the skills needed for successful adult independence and management of their own health care.

Annotated Bibliography

Crowell, C. S., Malee, K. M., Yogev, R., & Muller, W. J. (2014). Neurologic disease in HIV-infected children and the impact of combination antiretroviral therapy. *Reviews in Medical Virology, 24*(5), 316–331. doi:10.1002/rmv.1793

A concise summary of the neuropathogenesis of HIV in children and current issues.

Gendelman, H. E., Gelbard, H. A., Grant, I., Lipton, S. A., Everall, I. P., Fox, H. S., et al. (Eds.). (2012). *The neurology of AIDS* (3rd ed.). New York, NY: Oxford University Press.

A comprehensive volume with chapters covering all aspects of the biology and immunology of HIV infection, the impact of HIV and antiretroviral therapies on the central nervous system in adults and children, and cognitive and psychiatric outcomes.

Mellins, C. A., & Malee, K. M. (2013). Understanding the mental health of youth living with perinatal HIV infection: lessons learned and current challenges. *Journal of the International AIDS Society, 16*, 18593. doi:10.7448/IAS.16.1.18593

A review of research concerning mental health in adolescents with perinatal HIV infection, risk and protective factors, and intervention needs.

Nichols, S. L., Bethel, J., Garvie, P. A., Patton, D. E., Thornton, S., Kapogiannis, B. G., … Woods, S. P. (2013). Neurocognitive functioning in antiretroviral therapy-naive youth with behaviorally acquired human immunodeficiency virus. *Journal of Adolescent Health, 53*(6), 763–771. doi:10.1016/j.jadohealth.2013.07.006

The largest study to date of neurocognitive functioning in youth with behaviorally acquired HIV along with sociodemographic and psychiatric risk factors.

Smith, R., & Wilkins, M. (2015). Perinatally acquired HIV infection: Long-term neuropsychological consequences and challenges ahead. *Child Neuropsychology, 21*(2), 234–268. doi:10.1080/09297049.2014.898744

A comprehensive review of neurologic and neuropsychological consequences of perinatally acquired HIV.

References

Abubakar, A., Holding, P., Newton, C. R., van Baar, A., & van de Vijver, F. J. (2009). The role of weight for age and disease stage in poor psychomotor outcome of HIV-infected children in Kilifi, Kenya. *Developmental Medicine and Child Neurology, 51*(12), 968–973. doi:10.1111/j.1469-8749.2009.03333.x

Abubakar, A., Van Baar, A., Van de Vijver, F. J. R., Holding, P., & Newton, C. R. (2008). Paediatric HIV and neurodevelopment in sub-Saharan Africa: A systematic review. *Tropical Medicine & International Health, 13*(7), 880–887. doi:10.1111/j.1365-3156.2008.02079.x

Agwu, A. L., Siberry, G. K., Ellen, J., Fleishman, J. A., Rutstein, R., Gaur, A. H., … Gebo, K. A. (2012). Predictors of highly active antiretroviral therapy utilization for behaviorally HIV-1-infected youth: impact of adult versus pediatric clinical care site. *Journal of Adolescent Health, 50*(5), 471–477. doi:10.1016/j.jadohealth.2011.09.001

Albright, J. N., Fair, C. D., & Newman, C. (2017). Psychosocial considerations for children and adolescents with HIV. In T. Chenneville (Ed), *A Clinical Guide to Pediatric HIV*, 73–94. Dordrecht: Springer.

Al-Khindi, T., Zakzanis, K. K., & van Gorp, W. G. (2011). Does antiretroviral therapy improve HIV-associated cognitive impairment? A quantitative review of the literature. *Journal of the International Neuropsychological Society, 17*(6), 956–969. doi:10.1017/s1355617711000968

Allison, S., Wolters, P., & Brouwers, P. (2009). Youth with HIV/AIDS: Neurobehavioral consequences. In R. H. Paul, N. Sacktor, V. Valcour & K. T. Tashima (Eds.), *HIV and the Brain: New challenges in the modern era* (pp. 187–211). New York: Humana Press. doi:10.1007/978-1-59745-434-6_9

Alperen, J., Brummel, S., Tassiopoulos, K., Mellins, C. A., Kacanek, D., Smith, R., … Moscicki, A. B. (2014). Prevalence of and risk factors for substance use among perinatally human immunodeficiency virus-infected and perinatally exposed but uninfected youth. *Journal of Adolescent Health*. doi:10.1016/j.jadohealth.2013.09.003

Ananworanich, J., Bunupuradah, T., Apornpong, T., Kosalaraksa, P., Hansudewechakul, R., Kanjanavanit, S., … Puthanakit, T. (2014). Association between lymphocyte and monocyte subsets and cognition in children with HIV. *AIDS Research and Therapy, 11*(1), 7. doi:10.1186/1742-6405-11-7

Ancuta, P., Kamat, A., Kunstman, K. J., Kim, E. Y., Autissier, P., Wurcel, A., … Gabuzda, D. (2008). Microbial translocation is associated with increased monocyte activation and dementia in AIDS patients. *PLoS One, 3*(6), e2516. doi:10.1371/journal.pone.0002516

Antinori, A., Arendt, G., Becker, J. T., Brew, B. J., Byrd, D. A., Cherner, M., … Wojna, V. E. (2007). Updated research nosology for HIV-associated neurocognitive disorders. *Neurology, 69*(18), 1789–1799. doi:10.1212/01.WNL.0000287431.88658.8b

Bagenda, D. (2006). Health, neurologic, and cognitive status of HIV-infected, long-surviving, and antiretroviral-naive Ugandan children. *Pediatrics, 117*(3), 729–740. doi:10.1542/peds.2004-2699

Baker, L. M., Paul, R. H., Heaps, J. M., Westerhaus, E., Chang, J. Y., Williams, S., … Ances, B. M. (2014). Impact of human immunodeficiency virus on neurocognition and risky behaviors in young adults. *Journal of NeuroVirology, 20*(5), 466–473. doi:10.1007/s13365-014-0264-4

Baker, L. M., Paul, R. H., Heaps-Woodruff, J. M., Chang, J. Y., Ortega, M., Margolin, Z., … Ances, B. M. (2015). The effect of central nervous system penetration effectiveness of highly active antiretroviral therapy on neuropsychological performance and neuroimaging in HIV infected individuals. *Journal of NeuroImmune Pharmacology, 10*(3), 487–492. doi:10.1007/s11481-015-9610-4

Basso, M. R., & Bornstein, R. A. (2000). Estimated premorbid intelligence mediates neurobehavioral change in individuals infected with HIV across 12 months. *Journal of Clinical and Experimental Neuropsychology, 22*(2), 208–218. doi:10.1076/1380-3395(200004)22:2;1-1;ft208

Belman, A. (2008). Pediatric neuro-AIDS. In K. Goodkin, P. Shapshak, & A. Verma (Eds.), *The spectrum of neuro-AIDS disorders: Pathophysiology, diagnosis, and treatment* (pp. 455–471). Washington, DC: ASM Press.

Berkman, N. D., Sheridan, S. L., Donahue, K. E., Halpern, D. J., & Crotty, K. (2011). Low health literacy and health outcomes: An updated systematic review. *Annals of Internal Medicine, 155*, 97–107. doi:10.7326/0003-4819-155-2-201107190-00005

Blakemore, S. J., & Choudhury, S. (2006). Development of the adolescent brain: implications for executive function and social cognition. *Journal of Child Psychology and Psychiatry, 47*(3–4), 296–312. doi:10.1111/j.1469-7610.2006.01611.x

Boivin, M. J., Busman, R. A., Parikh, S. M., Bangirana, P., Page, C. F., Opoka, R. O., et al. (2010). A pilot study of the neuropsychological benefits of computerized cognitive rehabilitation in Ugandan children with HIV. *Neuropsychology, 24*(5), 667–673. doi:10.1037/a0019312

Bonnie, R. J., Stroud, C., Breiner, H., Committee on Improving the Health, Safety, and Well-Being of Young Adults, Board on Children, Youth, and Families, Institute of Medicine, & National Research Council (Eds.). (2014). *Investing in the health and well-being of young adults*. The National Academies Press.

Brackis-Cott, E., Kang, E., Dolezal, C., Abrams, E. J., & Mellins, C. A. (2009a). Brief report: language ability and school functioning of youth perinatally infected with HIV. *Journal of Pediatric Health Care, 23*(3), 158–164. doi:10.1016/j.pedhc.2008.02.005

Brackis-Cott, E., Kang, E., Dolezal, C., Abrams, E. J., & Mellins, C. A. (2009b). The impact of perinatal HIV infection on older school-aged children's and adolescents' receptive language and word recognition skills. *AIDS Patient Care and STDs, 23*(6), 415–421. doi:10.1089/apc.2008.0197

Brahmbhatt, H., Boivin, M., Ssempijja, V., Kigozi, G., Kagaayi, J., Serwadda, D., et al. (2014). Neurodevelopmental benefits of antiretroviral therapy in Ugandan children aged 0–6 years with HIV. *Journal of Acquired Immune Deficiency Syndromes, 67*(3), 316–322. doi:10.1097/qai.0000000000000295

Buchanan, A. L., Montepiedra, G., Sirois, P. A., Kammerer, B., Garvie, P. A., Storm, D. S., et al. (2012). Barriers to medication adherence in HIV-infected children and youth based on self- and caregiver report. *Pediatrics, 129*(5), e1244–e1251. doi:10.1542/peds.2011-1740

Carey, C. L., Woods, S. P., Rippeth, J. D., Heaton, R. K., & Grant, I. (2006). Prospective memory in HIV-1 infection. *Journal of Clinical and Experimental Neuropsychology, 28*(4), 536–548. doi:10.1080/13803390590949494

Carvalhal, A., Gill, M. J., Letendre, S. L., Rachlis, A., Bekele, T., Raboud, J., … Rourke, S. B. (2015). Central nervous system penetration effectiveness of antiretroviral drugs and neuropsychological impairment in the Ontario HIV Treatment Network Cohort Study. *Journal of NeuroVirology*. doi:10.1007/s13365-015-0404-5

Centers for Disease Control. (1994). Revised classification system for human immunodeficiency virus infection in children less than 13 years of age. *Morbidity and Mortality Weekly Report, 43*(1–12).

Centers for Disease Control and Prevention. (2015). HIV Surveillance Report, 2014 (Vol. 26).

Chandwani, S., Koenig, L. J., Sill, A. M., Abramowitz, S., Conner, L. C., & D'Angelo, L. (2012). Predictors of antiretroviral medication adherence among a diverse cohort of adolescents with HIV. *Journal of Adolescent Health, 51*(3), 242–251. doi:10.1016/j.jadohealth.2011.12.013

Chesser, A., Burke, A., Reyes, J., & Rohrberg, T. (2016). Navigating the digital divide: A systematic review of eHealth literacy in underserved populations in the United States. *Informatics for Health and Social Care, 41*(1), 1–19. doi:10.3109/17538157.2014.948171

Chiriboga, C. A., Fleishman, S., Champion, S., Gaye-Robinson, L., & Abrams, E. J. (2005). Incidence and prevalence of HIV encephalopathy in children with HIV infection receiving highly active anti-retroviral therapy (HAART). *The Journal of Pediatrics, 146*(3), 402–407. doi:10.1016/j.jpeds.2004.10.021

Ciccarelli, N., Fabbiani, M., Di Giambenedetto, S., Fanti, I., Baldonero, E., Bracciale, L., … Silveri, M. C. (2011). Efavirenz associated with cognitive disorders in otherwise asymptomatic HIV-infected patients. *Neurology, 76*(16), 1403–1409. doi:10.1212/WNL.0b013e31821670fb

Cohen, S., Caan, M. W., Mutsaerts, H. J., Scherpbier, H. J., Kuijpers, T. W., Reiss, P., … Pajkrt, D. (2016). Cerebral injury in perinatally HIV-infected children compared to matched healthy controls. *Neurology, 86*(1), 19–27. doi:10.1212/wnl.0000000000002209

Colbert, A. M., Sereika, S. M., & Erlen, J. A. (2013). Functional health literacy, medication-taking self-efficacy and adherence to antiretroviral therapy. *Journal of Advances in Nursing, 69*, 295–304. doi:10.1111/j.1365-2648.2012.06007.x

Costello, E. J., Copeland, W. E., Shanahan, L., Worthman, C. M., & Angold, A. (2013). C-reactive protein and substance use disorders in adolescence and early adulthood: A prospective analysis. *Drug and Alcohol Dependence, 133*(2), 712–717. doi:10.1016/j.drugalcdep.2013.08.027

Crowell, C. S., Huo, Y., Tassiopoulos, K., Malee, K. M., Yogev, R., Hazra, R., … Muller, W. J. (2015). Early viral suppression improves neurocognitive outcomes in HIV-infected children. *AIDS, 29*, 295–304. doi:10.1097/QAD.0000000000000528

Crowell, C. S., Malee, K. M., Yogev, R., & Muller, W. J. (2014). Neurologic disease in HIV-infected children and the impact of combination antiretroviral therapy. *Reviews in Medical Virology, 24*(5), 316–331. doi:10.1002/rmv.1793

Davison, C., Donovan, M., Donohoe, M., Vanneman, M., Lyle, M., Robinson, P., & Cavalier, Y. (2006). Adolescent transition workbook, from http://aidsetc.org/resource/adolescent-transition-workbook

Ellis, R., Badiee, J., Vaida, F., Letendre, S., Heaton, R., Clifford, D., … Charter Group. (2011). CD4 nadir is a predictor of HIV neurocognitive impairment in the era of combination antiretroviral therapy. *AIDS, 25*(14), 1747–1751. doi:10.1097/QAD.0b013e32834a40cd

Ettenhofer, M. L., Foley, J., Castellon, S. A., & Hinkin, C. H. (2010). Reciprocal prediction of medication adherence and neurocognition in HIV/AIDS. *Neurology, 74*(15), 1217–1222. doi:10.1212/WNL.0b013e3181d8c1ca

Fernandez, M. I., Huszti, H. C., Wilson, P. A., Kahana, S., Nichols, S., Gonin, R., ... Kapogiannis, B. G. (2015). Profiles of risk among HIV-infected youth in clinic settings. *AIDS and Behavior, 19*(5), 918–930. doi:10.1007/s10461-014-0876-y

Filteau, S. (2009). The HIV-exposed, uninfected African child. *Tropical Medicine & International Health, 14*(3), 276–287. doi:10.1111/j.1365-3156.2009.02220.x

Freudenberg, N., & Ruglis, J. (2007). Reframing school dropout as a public health issue. *Preventing Chronic Disease, 4*(4), A107.

Gannon, P., Khan, M. Z., & Kolson, D. L. (2011). Current understanding of HIV-associated neurocognitive disorders pathogenesis. *Current Opinion in Neurology, 24*(3), 275–283. doi:10.1097/WCO.0b013e32834695fb

Garvey, L. J., Pavese, N., Politis, M., Ramlackhansingh, A., Brooks, D. J., Taylor-Robinson, S. D., et al. (2014). Increased microglia activation in neurologically asymptomatic HIV-infected patients receiving effective ART. *AIDS, 28*(1), 67–72. doi:10.1097/01.aids.0000432467.54003.f7

Garvie, P. A., Zeldow, B., Malee, K., Nichols, S. L., Smith, R. A., Wilkins, M. L., Williams, P. L., for the Pediatric HIV/AIDS Cohort Study (PHACS). (2014). *Discordance of cognitive and academic achievement outcomes in youth with perinatal HIV exposure. Pediatric Infectious Disease Journal, 33*(9), 232–238.

Golub, S. A., Starks, T. J., Kowalczyk, W. J., Thompson, L. I., & Parsons, J. T. (2012). Profiles of executive functioning: associations with substance dependence and risky sexual behavior. *Psychology of Addictive Behaviors, 26*(4), 895–905. doi:10.1037/a0029034

Guerra, V. C., Leister, E. C., Williams, P. L., Starc, T. J., Lipshultz, S. E., Wilkinson, J., ... Colan, S. (2016). Long-term effects of in utero antiretroviral exposure: systolic and diastolic function in HIV-exposed uninfected youth. *AIDS Research and Human Retroviruses*. doi:10.1089/aid.2015.0281

Guideline on When to Start Antiretroviral Therapy and on Pre-Exposure Prophylaxis for HIV. (2015). Geneva: World Health Organization 2015.

Hair, N. L., Hanson, J. L., Wolfe, B. L., & Pollak, S. D. (2015). Association of child poverty, brain development, and academic achievement. *JAMA Pediatrics, 169*(9), 822–829. doi:10.1001/jamapediatrics.2015.1475

Heaton, R., Marcotte, T., Mindt, M., Sadek, J., Moore, D., Bentley, H., ... & The HNRC Group. (2004). The impact of HIV-associated neuropsychological impairment on everyday functioning. *Journal of the International Neuropsychological Society, 10*(3), 317–331. doi:10.1017/S1355617704102130

Heaton, R. K., Clifford, D. B., Franklin, D. R., Jr., Woods, S. P., Ake, C., Vaida, F., ... Grant, I. (2010). HIV-associated neurocognitive disorders persist in the era of potent antiretroviral therapy: CHARTER study. *Neurology, 75*(23), 2087–2096. doi:10.1212/WNL.0b013e318200d727

Heaton, R. K., Franklin, D. R., Ellis, R. J., McCutchan, J. A., Letendre, S. L., Leblanc, S., ... Grant, I. (2011). HIV-associated neurocognitive disorders before and during the era of combination antiretroviral therapy: differences in rates, nature, and predictors. *Journal of NeuroVirology, 17*(1), 3–16. doi:10.1007/s13365-010-0006-1

Heidari, S., Mofenson, L., Cotton, M. F., Marlink, R., Cahn, P., & Katabira, E. (2011). Antiretroviral drugs for preventing mother-to-child transmission of HIV: A review of potential effects on HIV-exposed but uninfected children. *Journal of Acquired Immune Deficiency Syndromes,*. doi:10.1097/QAI.0b013e318221c56a

Herting, M. M., Uban, K. A., Williams, P. L., Gautam, P., Huo, Y., Malee, K., ... Sowell, E. R. (2015). Default mode connectivity in youth with perinatally acquired HIV. *Medicine (Baltimore), 94*(37), e1417. doi:10.1097/md.0000000000001417

Hoare, J., Ransford, G. L., Phillips, N., Amos, T., Donald, K., & Stein, D. J. (2014). Systematic review of neuroimaging studies in vertically transmitted HIV positive children and adolescents. *Metabolic Brain Disease, 29*(2), 221–229. doi:10.1007/s11011-013-9456-5

Hoare, J., Westgarth-Taylor, J., Fouche, J. P., Spottiswoode, B., Paul, R., Thomas, K., … Joska, J. (2012). A diffusion tensor imaging and neuropsychological study of prospective memory impairment in South African HIV positive individuals. *Metabolic Brain Disease, 27*(3), 289–297. doi:10.1007/s11011-012-9311-0

Horacio, R. E., Itziar, F. L., Alla, S., Nikita, J., Noelline, N., Robert, O., … Michael, B. (2015). Nutritional and immunological correlates of memory and neurocognitive development among HIV infected children living in Kayunga, Uganda. *Journal of Acquired Immune Deficiency Syndromes*. doi:10.1097/qai.0000000000000905

Hosek, S. G., Harper, G. W., & Domanico, R. (2005). Predictors of medication adherence among HIV-infected youth. *Psychology, Health & Medicine, 10*(2), 166–179. doi:10.1080/13543500420003265 84

IAPAC Guidelines for Optimizing the HIV Care Continuum for Adults and Adolescents. (2015). *Journal of the International Association of Providers of AIDS Care, 14*(Suppl. 1), S3–S34. doi:10.1177/2325957415613442

Irwin, C. E. (2010). Young adults are worse off than adolescents. *Journal of Adolescent Health, 46*, 405–406. doi:10.1016/j.jadohealth.2010.03.001

Jacobson, L. A., & Mahone, E. M. (2012). Educational implications of executive dysfunction. In S. J. Hunter & E. P. Sparrow (Eds.), *Executive function and dysfunction* (pp. 232–246). New York, NY: Cambridge University Press. doi:10.1017/CBO9780511977954.021

Jahanshad, N., Couture, M. C., Prasitsuebsai, W., Nir, T. M., Aurpibul, L., Thompson, P. M., … Valcour, V. G. (2015). Brain imaging and neurodevelopment in HIV-uninfected Thai children born to HIV-infected mothers. *Pediatr Infect Dis J, 34*(9), e211–216. doi:10.1097/inf.0000000000000774

Johnston, L. D., O'Malley, P. M., Bachman, J. G., & Schulenberg, J. E. (2012). *Monitoring the future: national results on adolescent drug use: Overview of key findings, 2011*. Ann Arbor: Institute for Social Research, The University of Michigan.

Kalichman, S. C., Cherry, C., Cain, D., Weinhardt, L. S., Benotsch, E., Pope, H., et al. (2006). Health information on the Internet and people living with HIV/AIDS: information evaluation and coping styles. *Health Psychology, 25*(2), 205–210. doi:10.1037/0278-6133.25.2.205

Kapetanovic, S., Griner, R., Zeldow, B., Nichols, S., Leister, E., Gelbard, H. A., … Williams, P. L. (2014). Biomarkers and neurodevelopment in perinatally HIV-infected or exposed youth: a structural equation model analysis. *AIDS, 28*(3), 355–364. doi:10.1097/qad.0000000000000072

Kapetanovic, S., Leister, E., Nichols, S., Miller, T., Tassiopoulos, K., Hazra, R., … Williams, P. L. (2010). Relationships between markers of vascular dysfunction and neurodevelopmental outcomes in perinatally HIV-infected youth. *AIDS, 24*(10), 1481–1491. doi:10.1097/QAD.0b013e32833a241b

Keller, M. A., Venkatraman, T. N., Thomas, A., Deveikis, A., LoPresti, C., Hayes, J., … Chang, L. (2004). Altered neurometabolite development in HIV-infected children: correlation with neuropsychological tests. *Neurology, 62*(10), 1810–1817. doi:10.1212/01.WNL.0000125492.57419.25

Kerr, S. J., Puthanakit, T., Vibol, U., Aurpibul, L., Vonthanak, S., Kosalaraksa, P., … Valcour, V. (2014). Neurodevelopmental outcomes in HIV-exposed-uninfected children versus those not exposed to HIV. *AIDS Care, 26*(11), 1327–1335. doi:10.1080/09540121.2014.920949

Koekkoek, S., de Sonneville, L. M., Wolfs, T. F., Licht, R., & Geelen, S. P. (2008). Neurocognitive function profile in HIV-infected school-age children. *European Journal of Paediatric Neurology, 12*(4), 290–297. doi:10.1016/j.ejpn.2007.09.002

Laughton, B., Cornell, M., Boivin, M., & Van Rie, A. (2013). Neurodevelopment in perinatally HIV-infected children: A concern for adolescence. *Journal of the International AIDS Society, 16*, 18603. doi:10.7448/IAS.16.1.18603

Lazarus, J. R., Rutstein, R. M., & Lowenthal, E. D. (2015). Treatment initiation factors and cognitive outcome in youth with perinatally acquired HIV infection. *HIV Medications, 16*(6), 355–361. doi:10.1111/hiv.12220

Le Doare, K., Bland, R., & Newell, M. L. (2012). Neurodevelopment in children born to HIV-infected mothers by infection and treatment status. *Pediatrics, 130*(5), e1326–e1344. doi:10.1542/peds.2012-0405

Lentz, M. R., Kim, W. K., Kim, H., Soulas, C., Lee, V., Venna, N., … Gonzalez, R. G. (2011). Alterations in brain metabolism during the first year of HIV infection. *Journal of NeuroVirology, 17*(3), 220–229. doi:10.1007/s13365-011-0030-9

Letendre, S., Marquie-Beck, J., Capparelli, E., Best, B., Clifford, D., Collier, A. C., … Ellis, R. J. (2008). Validation of the CNS Penetration-Effectiveness rank for quantifying antiretroviral penetration into the central nervous system. *Archives of Neurology, 65*(1), 65–70. doi:10.1001/archneurol.2007.31

Levine, A. J., Gonzalez, R., & Martin, E. M. (2012). Neurocognition in HIV and substance use disorders. In H. E. Gendelman, I. Grant, I. P. Everall, H. S. Fox, H. A. Gelbard, S. A. Lipton, & S. Swindells (Eds.), *The neurology of AIDS* (3rd ed., pp. 1034–1044). New York, NY: Oxford University Press.

Llorente, A. M., Brouwers, P., Leighty, R., Malee, K., Smith, R., Harris, L., et al. (2014). An analysis of select emerging executive skills in perinatally HIV-1-infected children. *Applied Neuropsychology: Child, 3*(1), 10–25. doi:10.1080/21622965.2012.686853

Lorig, K. R., & Holman, H. (2003). Self-management education: History, definition, outcomes, and mechanisms. *Annals of Behavioral Medicine, 26*(1), 1–7. doi:10.1207/S15324796ABM2601_01

MacDonell, K., Jacques-Tiura, A., Naar, S., & Fernandez, I. (2015). Predictors of self-reported adherence to antiretroviral medication in a multisite study of ethnic and racial minority HIV-positive youth. *Journal of Pediatric Psychology,*. doi:10.1093/jpepsy/jsv097

MacDonell, K. E., Naar-King, S., Murphy, D. A., Parsons, J. T., & Harper, G. W. (2010). Predictors of medication adherence in high risk youth of color living with HIV. *Journal of Pediatric Psychology, 35*(6), 593–601. doi:10.1093/jpepsy/jsp080

Malee, K., Williams, P. L., Montepiedra, G., Nichols, S., Sirois, P. A., Storm, D., … Kammerer, B. (2009). The role of cognitive functioning in medication adherence of children and adolescents with HIV infection. *Journal of Pediatric Psychology, 34*(2), 164–175. doi:10.1093/jpepsy/jsn068

Marra, C. M., Zhao, Y., Clifford, D. B., Letendre, S., Evans, S., Henry, K., … Robertson, K. (2009). Impact of combination antiretroviral therapy on cerebrospinal fluid HIV RNA and neurocognitive performance. *AIDS, 23*(11), 1359–1366. doi:10.1097/QAD.0b013e32832c4152

Martin, E. M., Nixon, H., Pitrak, D. L., Weddington, W., Rains, N. A., Nunnally, G., … Bechara, A. (2007). Characteristics of prospective memory deficits in HIV-seropositive substance-dependent individuals: preliminary observations. *Journal of Clinical and Experimental Neuropsychology, 29*(5), 496–504. doi:10.1080/13803390600800970

Martin, S. C., Wolters, P. L., Toledo-Tamula, M. A., Zeichner, S. L., Hazra, R., & Civitello, L. (2006). Cognitive functioning in school-aged children with vertically acquired HIV infection being treated with highly active antiretroviral therapy (HAART). *Developmental Neuropsychology, 30*(2), 633–657. doi:10.1207/s15326942dn3002_1

McGrath, N., Fawzi, W. W., Bellinger, D., Robins, J., Msamanga, G. I., Manji, K., et al. (2006). The timing of mother-to-child transmission of human immunodeficiency virus infection and the neurodevelopment of children in Tanzania. *Pediatric Infectious Disease Journal, 25*(1), 47–52. doi:10.1097/01.inf.0000195638.80578.e0

McGuire, J. L., Barrett, J. S., Vezina, H. E., Spitsin, S., & Douglas, S. D. (2014). Adjuvant therapies for HIV-associated neurocognitive disorders. *Annals of Clinical and Translational Neurology, 1*(11), 938–952. doi:10.1002/acn3.131

Mekmullica, J., Brouwers, P., Charurat, M., Paul, M., Shearer, W., Mendez, H., … McIntosh, K. (2009). Early immunological predictors of neurodevelopmental outcomes in HIV-infected children. *Clinical Infectious Diseases, 48*(3), 338–346. doi:10.1086/595885

Mellins, C. A., & Malee, K. M. (2013). Understanding the mental health of youth living with perinatal HIV infection: lessons learned and current challenges. *Journal of the International AIDS Society, 16*, 18593. doi:10.7448/IAS.16.1.18593

Mintz, M., Sharer, L. R., & Civitello, L. (2012). Clinical and pathological features of HIV-1 encephalopathy in children and adolescents. In H. E. Gendelman, H. A. Gelbard, I. Grant, S. A. Lipton, I. P. Everall, H. S. Fox, & S. Swindells (Eds.), *The neurology of AIDS* (3rd ed.). New York, NY: Oxford University Press.

Moss, H. A., Wolters, P. L., Brouwers, P., Hendricks, M. L., & Pizzo, P. A. (1996). Impairment of expressive behavior in pediatric HIV-infected patients with evidence of CNS disease. *Journal of Pediatric Psychology, 21*(3), 379–400. doi:10.1093/jpepsy/21.3.379

Murphy, D. A., Lam, P., Naar-King, S., Robert Harris, D., Parsons, J. T., Muenz, L. R., et al. (2010). Health literacy and antiretroviral adherence among HIV-infected adolescents. *Patient Education and Counseling, 79*(1), 25–29. doi:10.1016/j.pec.2009.07.014

Naar-King, S., Montepiedra, G., Garvie, P., Kammerer, B., Malee, K., Sirois, P. A., … Nichols, S. L. (2013). Social ecological predictors of longitudinal HIV treatment adherence in youth with perinatally acquired HIV. *Journal of Pediatric Psychology, 38*(6), 664–674. doi:10.1093/jpepsy/jst017

Nachman, S., Chernoff, M., Williams, P., Hodge, J., Heston, J., & Gadow, K. D. (2012). Human immunodeficiency virus disease severity, psychiatric symptoms, and functional outcomes in perinatally infected youth. *Archives of Pediatrics and Adolescent Medicine, 166*(6), 528–535. doi:10.1001/archpediatrics.2011.1785

Nagarajan, R., Sarma, M. K., Thomas, M. A., Chang, L., Natha, U., Wright, M., … Keller, M. A. (2012). Neuropsychological function and cerebral metabolites in HIV-infected youth. *Journal of NeuroImmune Pharmacology, 7*(4), 981–990. doi:10.1007/s11481-012-9407-7

Navarra, A. M., Neu, N., Toussi, S., Nelson, J., & Larson, E. L. (2014). Health literacy and adherence to antiretroviral therapy among HIV-infected youth. *Journal of the Association of Nurses in AIDS Care, 25*(3), 203–213. doi:10.1016/j.jana.2012.11.003

New York State Department of Health AIDS Institute. (2011). Transitioning HIV-infected adolescents into adult care, from www.hivguidelines.org

Ngoma, M. S., Hunter, J. A., Harper, J. A., Church, P. T., Mumba, S., Chandwe, M., … Silverman, M. S. (2014). Cognitive and language outcomes in HIV-uninfected infants exposed to combined antiretroviral therapy in utero and through extended breast-feeding. *AIDS, 28* (Suppl. 3), S323–330. doi:10.1097/qad.0000000000000357

Nichols, S. L. (2012). Executive functions in HIV. In S. J. Hunter & E. P. Sparrow (Eds.), *Executive function and dysfunction* (pp. 168–173). New York, NY: Cambridge University Press. doi:10.1017/CBO9780511977954.016

Nichols, S. L., Bethel, J., Garvie, P. A., Patton, D. E., Thornton, S., Kapogiannis, B. G., … Woods, S. P. (2013). Neurocognitive functioning in antiretroviral therapy-naive youth with behaviorally acquired human immunodeficiency virus. *Journal of Adolescent Health, 53*(6), 763–771. doi:10.1016/j.jadohealth.2013.07.006

Nichols, S. L., Bethel, J., Kapogiannis, B. G., Li, T., Woods, S. P., Patton, E. D., … Garvie, P. A. (2016). Antiretroviral treatment initiation does not differentially alter neurocognitive functioning over time in youth with behaviorally acquired HIV. *Journal of NeuroVirology, 22*(2), 218–230. doi:10.1007/s13365-015-0389-0

Nichols, S. L., Brummel, S. S., Smith, R. A., Garvie, P. A., Hunter, S. J., Malee, K. M., … Mellins, C. A. (2015). Executive functioning in children and adolescents with perinatal HIV infection. *The Pediatric Infectious Disease Journal, 34*(9), 969–975. doi:10.1097/inf.0000000000000809

Nichols, S. L., Chernoff, M. C., Malee, K., Sirois, P. A., Williams, P. L., Figueroa, V., & Woods, S. P. (2016). Learning and memory in children and adolescents with perinatal HIV infection and perinatal HIV exposure. *The Pediatric Infectious Disease Journal, 35*(6), 649–654. doi:10.1097/inf.0000000000001131

Nichols, S. L., Montepiedra, G., Farley, J. J., Sirois, P. A., Malee, K., Kammerer, B., … Naar-King, S. (2012). Cognitive, academic, and behavioral correlates of medication adherence in children and adolescents with perinatally acquired HIV infection. *Journal of Developmental & Behavioral Pediatrics*, *33*(4), 298–308. doi:10.1097/DBP.0b013e31824bef47

Nozyce, M. L., Huo, Y., Williams, P. L., Kapetanovic, S., Hazra, R., Nichols, S., … Sirois, P. A. (2014). Safety of in utero and neonatal antiretroviral exposure: cognitive and academic outcomes in HIV-exposed, uninfected children 5–13 years of age. *The Pediatric Infectious Disease Journal*, *33*(11), 1128-1133. doi:10.1097/inf.0000000000000410

Panel on Antiretroviral Guidelines for Adults and Adolescents. (2016). *Guidelines for the use of antiretroviral agents in HIV-1-infected adults and adolescents*. Retrieved from http://www.aidsinfo.nih.gov/ContentFiles/AdultandAdolescentGL.pdf

Panel on Antiretroviral Therapy and Medical Management of HIV-Infected Children. (2015). Guidelines for the use of antiretroviral agents in pediatric HIV infection.

Patel, K., Ming, X., Williams, P. L., Robertson, K. R., Oleske, J. M., & Seage, G. R., 3rd. (2009). Impact of HAART and CNS-penetrating antiretroviral regimens on HIV encephalopathy among perinatally infected children and adolescents. *AIDS, 23*(14), 1893–1901. doi:10.1097/QAD.0b013e32832dc041

Pearlstein, S. L., Mellins, C. A., Dolezal, C., Elkington, K. S., Santamaria, E. K., Leu, C. S., … Abrams, E. J. (2014). Youth in transition: life skills among perinatally HIV-infected and HIV-exposed adolescents. *Journal of Pediatric Psychology*, *39*(3), 294–305. doi:10.1093/jpepsy/jst077

Peluso, M. J., Meyerhoff, D. J., Price, R. W., Peterson, J., Lee, E., Young, A. C., … Spudich, S. (2013). Cerebrospinal fluid and neuroimaging biomarker abnormalities suggest early neurological injury in a subset of individuals during primary HIV infection. *The Journal of Infectious Diseases*, *207*(11), 1703–1712. doi:10.1093/infdis/jit088

Potterton, J., Stewart, A., Cooper, P., & Becker, P. (2010). The effect of a basic home stimulation programme on the development of young children infected with HIV. *Developmental Medicine and Child Neurology, 52*(6), 547–551. doi:10.1111/j.1469-8749.2009.03534.x

Puthanakit, T., Ananworanich, J., Vonthanak, S., Kosalaraksa, P., Hansudewechakul, R., van der Lugt, J., … Ruxrungtham, K. (2013). Cognitive function and neurodevelopmental outcomes in HIV-infected children older than 1 year of age randomized to early versus deferred antiretroviral therapy: the PREDICT neurodevelopmental study. *The Pediatric Infectious Disease Journal*, *32*(5), 501–508. doi:10.1097/INF.0b013e31827fb19d

Puthanakit, T., Aurpibul, L., Louthrenoo, O., Tapanya, P., Nadsasarn, R., Insee-ard, S., et al. (2010). Poor cognitive functioning of school-aged children in thailand with perinatally acquired HIV infection taking antiretroviral therapy *AIDS Patient Care STDS, 24*(3), 141–146. doi:10.1089/apc.2009.0314

Ragin, A. B., Du, H., Ochs, R., Wu, Y., Sammet, C. L., Shoukry, A., et al. (2012). Structural brain alterations can be detected early in HIV infection. *Neurology, 79*(24), 2328–2334. doi:10.1212/WNL.0b013e318278b5b4

Rice, M. L., Buchanan, A. L., Siberry, G. K., Malee, K. M., Zeldow, B., Frederick, T., … Williams, P. L. (2012). Language impairment in children perinatally infected with HIV compared to children who were HIV-exposed and uninfected. *Journal of Developmental & Behavioral Pediatrics*, *33*(2), 112–123. doi:10.1097/DBP.0b013e318241ed23

Rosenbloom, M. J., Sullivan, E. V., & Pfefferbaum, A. (2010). Focus on the brain: HIV infection and alcoholism: comorbidity effects on brain structure and function. *Alcohol Research & Health, 33*(3), 247–257.

Rotheram-Borus, M. J., Ingram, B. L., Swendeman, D., & Lee, A. (2012). Adoption of self-management interventions for prevention and care. *Primary Care, 39*(4), 649–660. doi:10.1016/j.pop.2012.08.006

Ruel, T. D., Boivin, M. J., Boal, H. E., Bangirana, P., Charlebois, E., Havlir, D. V., … Wong, J. K. (2012). Neurocognitive and motor deficits in HIV-infected Ugandan children with high CD4 cell counts. *Clinical Infectious Diseases*, *54*(7), 1001–1009. doi:10.1093/cid/cir1037

Ruglis, J., & Freudenberg, N. (2010). Toward a healthy high schools movement: strategies for mobilizing public health for educational reform. *American Journal of Public Health, 100*(9), 1565–1571. doi:10.2105/ajph.2009.186619

Ryscavage, P., Anderson, E. J., Sutton, S. H., Reddy, S., & Taiwo, B. (2011). Clinical outcomes of adolescents and young adults in adult HIV care. *Journal of Acquired Immune Deficiency Syndromes, 58*(2), 193–197. doi:10.1097/QAI.0b013e31822d7564

Schweinsburg, A. D., Brown, S. A., & Tapert, S. F. (2008). The influence of marijuana use on neurocognitive functioning in adolescents. *Current Drug Abuse Reviews, 1*, 99–111. doi:10.2174/1874473710801010099

Shanbhag, M. C., Rutstein, R. M., Zaoutis, T., Zhao, H., Chao, D., & Radcliffe, J. (2005). Neurocognitive functioning in pediatric human immunodeficiency virus infection: Effects of combined therapy. *Archives of Pediatrics and Adolescent Medicine, 159*(7), 651–656. doi:10.1001/archpedi.159.7.651

Sharer, L. R. (2005). Neuropathological aspects of HIV-1 infection in children. In H. E. Gendelman, I. Grant, I. P. Everall, S. A. Lipton, & S. Swindells (Eds.), *The neurology of AIDS* (2nd ed.). Oxford: Oxford University Press.

Sherr, L., Croome, N., Bradshaw, K., & Parra Castaneda, K. (2014). A systematic review examining whether interventions are effective in reducing cognitive delay in children infected and affected with HIV. *AIDS Care, 26*(Suppl. 1), S70–S77. doi:10.1080/09540121.2014.906560

Shonkoff, J. P., & Garner, A. S. (2012). The lifelong effects of early childhood adversity and toxic stress. *Pediatrics, 129*(1), e232–e246. doi:10.1542/peds.2011-2663

Shrestha, R., & Copenhaver, M. (2016). The influence of neurocognitive impairment on HIV risk behaviors and intervention outcomes among high-risk substance users: A systematic review. *Frontiers in Public Health, 4*, 16. doi:10.3389/fpubh.2016.00016

Sirois, P. A., Huo, Y., Williams, P. L., Malee, K., Garvie, P. A., Kammerer, B., … Nozyce, M. L. (2013). Safety of perinatal exposure to antiretroviral medications: developmental outcomes in infants. *The Pediatric Infectious Disease Journal, 32*(6), 648–655. doi:10.1097/INF.0b013e318284129a

Smith, R., Chernoff, M., Williams, P. L., Malee, K. M., Sirois, P. A., Kammerer, B., … Rutstein, R. (2012). Impact of HIV severity on cognitive and adaptive functioning during childhood and adolescence. *The Pediatric Infectious Disease Journal, 31*(6), 592–598. doi:10.1097/INF.0b013e318253844b

Smith, R., Malee, K., Charurat, M., Magder, L., Mellins, C., Macmillan, C., … Moye, J. (2000). Timing of perinatal human immunodeficiency virus type 1 infection and rate of neurodevelopment. The Women and Infant Transmission Study Group. *The Pediatric Infectious Disease Journal, 19*(9), 862–871.

Smith, R., Malee, K., Leighty, R., Brouwers, P., Mellins, C., Hittelman, J., … Blasini, I. (2006). Effects of perinatal HIV infection and associated risk factors on cognitive development among young children. *Pediatrics, 117*(3), 851–862. doi:10.1542/peds.2005-0804

Smith, R., & Wilkins, M. (2015). Perinatally acquired HIV infection: Long-term neuropsychological consequences and challenges ahead. *Child Neuropsychology, 21*(2), 234–268. doi:10.1080/09297049.2014.898744

Smurzynski, M., Wu, K., Letendre, S., Robertson, K., Bosch, R. J., Clifford, D. B., … Ellis, R. (2011). Effects of central nervous system antiretroviral penetration on cognitive functioning in the ALLRT cohort. *AIDS, 25*(3), 357–365. doi:10.1097/QAD.0b013e32834171f8

Souza, E., Santos, N., Valentini, S., Silva, G., & Falbo, A. (2010). Long-term follow-up outcomes of perinatally HIV-infected adolescents: infection control but school failure. *Journal of Tropical Pediatrics, 56*(6), 421–426. doi:10.1093/tropej/fmq008

Squeglia, L. M., Jacobus, J., & Tapert, S. F. (2009). The influence of substance use on adolescent brain development. *Clinical EEG and Neuroscience, 40*(1), 31–38. doi:10.1177/155005940904000110

Squeglia, L. M., Pulido, C., Wetherill, R. R., Jacobus, J., Brown, G. G., & Tapert, S. F. (2012). Brain response to working memory over three years of adolescence: Influence of initiating heavy drinking. *Journal of Studies on Alcohol and Drugs, 73*(5), 749–760. doi:10.15288/jsad.2012.73.749

Strauss, E., Sherman, E. M. S., & Spreen, O. (2006). *A compendium of neuropsychological tests: Administration, norms, and commentary*. New York, NY: Oxford University Press.

Swendeman, D., Ingram, B. L., & Rotheram-Borus, M. J. (2009). Common elements in self-management of HIV and other chronic illnesses: An integrative framework. *AIDS Care, 21* (10), 1321–1334. doi:10.1080/09540120902803158

Tanner, A. E., Philbin, M. M., Duval, A., Ellen, J., Kapogiannis, B., & Fortenberry, J. D. (2014). "Youth friendly" clinics: considerations for linking and engaging HIV-infected adolescents into care. *AIDS Care, 26*(2), 199–205. doi:10.1080/09540121.2013.808800

Tate, D. F., Conley, J., Paul, R. H., Coop, K., Zhang, S., Zhou, W., … Tashima, K. (2010). Quantitative diffusion tensor imaging tractography metrics are associated with cognitive performance among HIV-infected patients. *Brain Imaging and Behavior, 4*(1), 68–79. doi:10.1007/s11682-009-9086-z

Thames, A. D., Arentoft, A., Rivera-Mindt, M., & Hinkin, C. H. (2013). Functional disability in medication management and driving among individuals with HIV: A 1-year follow-up study. *Journal of Clinical and Experimental Neuropsychology, 35*(1), 49–58. doi:10.1080/13803395.2012.747596

Thames, A. D., Kim, M. S., Becker, B. W., Foley, J. M., Hines, L. J., Singer, E. J., … Hinkin, C. H. (2011). Medication and finance management among HIV-infected adults: the impact of age and cognition. *Journal of Clinical and Experimental Neuropsychology, 33*(2), 200–209. doi:10.1080/13803395.2010.499357

Thames, A. D., Streiff, V., Patel, S. M., Panos, S. E., Castellon, S. A., & Hinkin, C. H. (2012). The role of HIV infection, cognition, and depression in risky decision-making. *Journal of Neuropsychiatry and Clinical Neurosciences, 24*(3), 340–348. doi:10.1176/appi.neuropsych.11110340

The Future of Disability in America. (2007). Washington, DC: National Academy of Sciences.

Thoma, R. J., Monnig, M. A., Lysne, P. A., Ruhl, D. A., Pommy, J. A., Bogenschutz, M., … Yeo, R. A. (2011). Adolescent substance abuse: The effects of alcohol and marijuana on neuropsychological performance. *Alcoholism: Clinical and Experimental Research, 35*(1), 39–46. doi:10.1111/j.1530-0277.2010.01320.x

Torre, P., 3rd, Zeldow, B., Hoffman, H. J., Buchanan, A., Siberry, G. K., Rice, M., … Williams, P. L. (2012). Hearing loss in perinatally HIV-infected and HIV-exposed but uninfected children and adolescents. *The Pediatric Infectious Disease Journal, 31*(8), 835–841. doi:10.1097/INF.0b013e31825b9524

Transitioning HIV-infected youth into adult health care. (2013). *Pediatrics, 132*(1), 192–197. doi:10.1542/peds.2013-1073

Uban, K. A., Herting, M. M., Williams, P. L., Ajmera, T., Gautam, P., Huo, Y., … Sowell, E. R. (2015). White matter microstructure among youth with perinatally acquired HIV is associated with disease severity. *AIDS, 29*(9), 1035–1044. doi:10.1097/qad.0000000000000648

Valenti, W. M. (2007). Health literacy, HIV and outcomes. *AIDS Read, 17*(3), 124–126, 128.

Van Rie, A., Dow, A., Mupuala, A., & Stewart, P. (2009). Neurodevelopmental trajectory of HIV-infected children accessing care in Kinshasa, Democratic Republic of Congo. *Journal of Acquired Immune Deficiency Syndromes, 52*(5), 636–642. doi:10.1097/QAI.0b013e3181b32646

Van Rie, A., Mupuala, A., & Dow, A. (2008). Impact of the HIV/AIDS epidemic on the neurodevelopment of preschool-aged children in Kinshasa, Democratic Republic of the Congo. Pediatrics, *122*(1), e123–e128. doi:10.1542/peds.2007-2558

Waldrop-Valverde, D., Jones, D. L., Gould, F., Kumar, M., & Ownby, R. L. (2010). Neurocognition, health-related reading literacy, and numeracy in medication management for HIV infection. *AIDS Patient Care and STDs, 24*(8), 477–484. doi:10.1089/apc.2009.0300

Wawrzyniak, A. J., Ownby, R. L., McCoy, K., & Waldrop-Valverde, D. (2013). Health literacy: Impact on the health of HIV-infected individuals. *Current HIV/AIDS Reports, 10*(4), 295–304. doi:10.1007/s11904-013-0178-4

Weissberg-Benchell, J., Wolpert, H., & Anderson, B. J. (2007). Transitioning from pediatric to adult care: A new approach to the post-adolescent young person with type 1 diabetes. *Diabetes Care, 30*, 2441–2446. doi:10.2337/dc07-1249

Williams, P. L., Marino, M., Malee, K., Brogly, S., Hughes, M. D., & Mofenson, L. M. (2010). Neurodevelopment and in utero antiretroviral exposure of HIV-exposed uninfected infants. *Pediatrics, 125*(2), e250–e260. doi:10.1542/peds.2009-1112

Wolters, P. L., Brouwers, P., Civitello, L., & Moss, H. A. (1997). Receptive and expressive language function of children with symptomatic HIV infection and relationship with disease parameters: a longitudinal 24-month follow-up study. *AIDS, 11*(9), 1135–1144. doi:10.1097/00002030-199709000-00009

Wood, S. M., Shah, S. S., Steenhoff, A. P., & Rutstein, R. M. (2009). The impact of AIDS diagnosis on long-term neurocognitive and psychiatric outcomes of surviving adolescents with perinatally acquired HIV. *AIDS, 23*, 1859–1865. doi:10.1037/0894-4105.22.1.110

Woods, S. P., Iudicello, J. E., Moran, L. M., Carey, C. L., Dawson, M. S., & Grant, I. (2008a). HIV-associated prospective memory impairment increases risk of dependence in everyday-functioning. *Neuropsychology, 22*(1), 110–117. doi:10.1037/0894-4105.22.1.110

Woods, S. P., Moran, L. M., Carey, C. L., Dawson, M. S., Iudicello, J. E., Gibson, S., … Atkinson, J. H. (2008b). Prospective memory in HIV infection: is "remembering to remember" a unique predictor of self-reported medication management? *Archives of Clinical Neuropsychology, 23*(3), 257–270. doi:10.1016/j.acn.2007.12.006

Zanoni, B. C., & Mayer, K. H. (2014). The adolescent and young adult HIV cascade of care in the United States: exaggerated health disparities. *AIDS Patient Care and STDs, 28*(3), 128–135. doi:10.1089/apc.2013.0345

Chapter 4
Psychosocial Considerations for Children and Adolescents with HIV

Jamie N. Albright, Cynthia D. Fair and Christy Newman

Background

Children and young people growing up with HIV face considerable challenges. Whether HIV was acquired perinatally or behaviorally, distinctive features characterize the experience of learning to make sense of and live with a communicable and highly stigmatized infection during childhood and adolescence. In addition to the potential for HIV and antiretroviral therapy to have effects on neurocognitive development, some children with HIV have experienced significant grief and trauma as a result of the death of loved ones, family stress resulting from poverty, migration, or substance dependence, and/or instability in care and housing. Despite the very great differences in life circumstances and trajectories in children and adolescents growing up with HIV around the world, the social stigma attached to HIV is internationally pervasive and is believed to underpin many of the social, cultural, and psychological barriers to mental and emotional well-being in this population. As a consequence of stigma, disclosure of HIV status to children can be delayed due to fear that the family secret of HIV will be inadvertently shared with others. Learning how to keep and share that secret appropriately, protecting the self in school and friendship networks, and also taking on responsibility for protecting family members, can be a significant burden to carry. Living with an infectious

J.N. Albright (✉)
University of Virginia, Charlottesville, VA, USA
e-mail: jna2db@virginia.edu

C.D. Fair
Elon University, Elon, NC, USA
e-mail: cfair@elon.edu

C. Newman
National Centre in HIV Social Research, University of New South Wales, Sydney, Australia
e-mail: c.newman@unsw.edu.au

T. Chenneville (ed.), *A Clinical Guide to Pediatric HIV*,
DOI 10.1007/978-3-319-49704-4_4

disease also requires the child or adolescent to take responsibility for a range of practices that would be largely unfamiliar to their HIV-negative peers: taking medicines, visiting doctors, monitoring health, taking caution with injuries, and for older adolescents, building literacy and skills in negotiating safer sexual practices. These are considerable pressures for children and adolescents already facing all of the usual challenges of navigating the complexities of their social and educational worlds as they grow up.

The transition from pediatric to adult HIV care settings, particularly in high-income settings, has become a key focus in the literature because of the specific risks for young people in moving out of highly supportive care environments into health service settings that expect users to be independent, self-directed, and responsible. Given the implications that disengagement with care and treatment can have for the health of this population at this vulnerable point in their lives, concerns about their potential to be "lost" to the system are grounded in justifiable fears (Newman et al. 2015). However, we must also recognize that there is a tendency in the research literature to be overly preoccupied with the vulnerabilities and problems associated with pediatric and adolescent HIV. Far less attention is—in general—paid to the strengths, assets, and capabilities of young people growing up with HIV, many of whom are doing exceptionally well (Persson and Newman 2012).

We know that at least some, but potentially many, children and adolescents are learning how to manage a lifelong, socially stigmatized infection successfully, albeit with substantial support from caregivers and clinicians, particularly during their younger years. Children and adolescents deserve recognition for their achievements in learning how to navigate complex social and clinical challenges in growing up and into young adult life with HIV. Careful attention needs to be paid to the framing of this population in the research that examines their mental and emotional health. Different answers may be found if research seeks to understand what supports young people in surviving and thriving with HIV in diverse contexts, as opposed to assuming that what matters most is to focus only on the challenges and problems they face. Nonetheless, these challenges and problems are undoubtedly real and also deserve deep appreciation.

This chapter is aimed at reviewing what is known about the mental health and well-being of children and adolescents living with HIV, and proposes a range of future directions in moving forward with this area of research. This chapter will also include clinical implications. There is a focus on the literature from the US, as that is where most of the research on this population has been conducted. This means that there may well be issues related to the limited transferability of key insights to other settings. The following sections explore the elements of HIV disease which can affect the mental health of children and adolescents living with HIV, with special attention to individual, family, and broader social factors. We then examine the relationship between the mode of transmission and well-being and the challenges of transitioning to adult care. Finally, we note the considerable resilience displayed by this population and describe empirically tested interventions aimed at supporting those living with pediatric HIV. We hope through this chapter to demonstrate both what is known about psychosocial considerations for children and adolescents with HIV, and also what could be achieved through a more deliberately positive reframing of the research on this population.

Current Status of Mental Health

Children and adolescents living with HIV can be particularly susceptible to psychosocial challenges, as they can face not only developmental vulnerabilities but also HIV-related stressors. Adolescence is considered a high-risk time for all young people regarding the emergence of mental health concerns and for psychological distress, both of which are predictive of poorer mental health later in life (Patel et al. 2007; Clark et al. 2007). Young people with HIV face additional issues, including persistent stigma, fear of disclosure, loss of parents or other family members, physical health problems, and the added burden of managing a chronic illness throughout early life. Moreover, children and adolescents living with HIV in developed countries are more likely to be members of racial/ethnic minority groups, lower socioeconomic status (SES), and have family members with mental health or drug/alcohol problems, all of which are associated with higher rates of mental illness (Mellins et al. 2003). Researchers estimate that the rate of internalizing emotional and behavioral problems to be approximately 20%, with externalizing problems displayed by nearly 30% of youth with HIV (Orban et al. 2010). Rates of mental illness and negative psychosocial sequelae have been compared to the general population and appear higher in this group; however, results are mixed. It appears that the constellation of co-occurring demographic features and shared life experiences (e.g., parental loss, poverty) in the population of children and adolescents with HIV may be more predictive of psychological distress than HIV alone. Nonetheless, the social implications of HIV infection are profound, and regardless of directionality, HIV is a considerable risk factor for mental health problems.

Health-Related Considerations

A number of HIV-specific risk factors for mental health concerns are important for clinicians and social service providers to keep in mind while working with this unique population. First, the iatrogenic artifacts of HIV treatment can contribute to poorer psychological functioning, including physical distress and managing physical discomfort. Further, neurocognitive deficits resulting from treatment or HIV disease itself can contribute to poorer mental health and later ability to adhere to medication regimens (Salama et al. 2013). These medication-related barriers to mental health maintenance can be particularly difficult for adolescents to manage, as they also serve as a constant reminder of being different from their HIV-negative peers. The complex relationship that many youth have with medication use and adherence can intersect in challenging ways with emotional well-being (Newman et al. 2015). It appears that medication adherence is associated with increased psychological distress and substance use; however, this may indicate that individuals with higher distress have more difficulty adhering to their medication regimen due to symptom interference (Reisner et al. 2009; Azzopardi et al. 2014). See Thurston et al. (2017) chapter on antiretroviral adherence and disease management for further details regarding the issues surrounding treatment adherence.

In light of the intersectional and multifaceted relationship between medication adherence and both physical and mental health, it is critical that clinicians acknowledge treatment compliance as a protective factor for youth development above and beyond physical health maintenance. Identifying psychological factors that contribute to non-adherence holds promise in ultimately improving physical and mental health (Naar-King et al. 2006). Periodic assessments of mental health status and its potential role in youths' adherence or non-adherence is one way for clinicians to best support patients. Further, directly acknowledging the potential for symptoms and treatment to cause psychological distress is an important aspect of working with youth with HIV—non-adherence must be treated with empathy rather than punitiveness. Thus, providing youth and caregivers with strategies to cope with physical discomfort is another potential point of intervention for children and adolescents with HIV.

Social Considerations

The social implications of HIV infection are often considered the most challenging part of the illness. Stigmatization of HIV remains, even into its third decade, and poor understanding of disease etiology abounds in the general population.

Family Context Many children and adolescents with perinatal HIV in higher-resource countries comprise a doubly marginalized group. Most are racial/ethnic minorities or from lower SES backgrounds, many have an incarcerated or drug-addicted parent (Mellins et al. 2003), and all have at least one biological parent with HIV. The mental health issues associated with one's primary marginalized status (e.g., race or sexuality) are compounded by resulting family stressors. For example, in the context of the US medical system, youth with HIV from lower SES backgrounds are often un- or underinsured, which limits the ability to access appropriate mental health support services.

Children and youth living with their HIV-positive parents face unique challenges as their parents age and are increasingly faced with health problems stemming from disease progression. Youth may be required to take on a caregiving role—caring for siblings, parents, or contributing financially—which presents challenges to engaging in the normative behaviors of childhood and adolescence, as well as considerable psychological strain (Cluver et al. 2008). Increasing medical complications can result in family financial stress, loss of employment, and isolation from previous social supports (Cluver and Orkin 2009).

Bereavement Many children and adolescents with HIV have lost one or both parents to HIV, and issues of bereavement remain salient. Bereavement is a normal response to loss, albeit an incredibly taxing part of life. However, youth are considered to be at heightened risk for complex grief or prolonged bereavement due to developmental disadvantages (i.e., difficulties with cognitive processing of loss), emotional immaturity, and dependency on caregivers (Worden and Silverman 1996). The loss of a parent, in general, is considered one of the most stressful events that a child can experience, one that is associated with less peer support, more difficulty with academics, fewer future-oriented goals, and increased risk for poverty in adulthood (Brent et al. 2012; Beegle et al. 2006). Youth who have lost a parent to HIV may be at increased risk for depression later in life, which may in part be due to residual symptoms of bereavement (Battles and Wiener 2002). Parental HIV-related deaths are often preceded by increased caregiving requirements from children, a disrupted social life, secrecy around the nature of the parent's illness, and considerable financial strain (Bernays et al. 2014). The aftermath of parental loss entails further disruption, particularly if the deceased parent was the primary caregiver. Youth may be required to move in with other family members, or sometimes, into foster care (Li et al. 2008). Moreover, the loss of a parent to HIV can make one's own HIV status more salient in terms of stigma and the possibility of serious illness in the future. Taken together, it is clear that parental loss due to HIV brings with it a host of psychological challenges beyond "normal" bereavement. As noted previously, children and adolescents with HIV are more likely to have neurocognitive deficits, difficulties with emotion regulation (i.e., externalizing or internalizing behaviors), fewer social resources, and less financial support to ensure stability after the loss of a parent.

Stigma and Social Relationships Research has demonstrated considerable internalized stigma related to HIV status among children, adolescents, and young adults living with HIV. Youth have described HIV as their "deep, dark secret" (e.g., Albright and Fair 2014). Unsurprisingly, these internalizations can contribute to poor self-concept to the detriment of psychological well-being. Stigmatization contributes to one of the most salient concerns for youth living with HIV: disclosure of HIV status. Stigmatization is well documented as one of the most detrimental aspects of living with a marginalized identity, and these effects are compounded by dual membership with another marginalized group (e.g., being Black and gay). However, stigma among youth who acquire HIV perinatally or during adolescence may also be viewed and experienced differently than for those who acquire HIV as adults and may therefore require different approaches to psychosocial support (Persson et al. in press). See Stangl (2017) chapter on HIV-related stigma for more information about the implications of stigma for child and youth development.

Individuals with HIV often find disclosure to be one of the most difficult aspects of living with the disease. Normative tasks of adolescence include establishing autonomy by increasingly relying on non-parent relationships (i.e., friends) and pursuing or entering romantic relationships. However, HIV presents a challenge to both of these developmental tasks. Many young people have not disclosed their HIV status to anyone outside of their immediate family. Non-disclosure to friends limits the ability to seek support for HIV-related stressors from non-familial others, who they may otherwise be relying upon more than parent/caregivers. Peers provide unique support to adolescents, owing to their more immediate understanding of what youth are "going through." Feelings of isolation stemming from HIV stigma can contribute to psychological distress, particularly for adolescents, who are susceptible to heightened worry about others' perceptions. An HIV diagnosis adds to marginalization by conferring a burden of secrecy. While HIV rates have drastically decreased and treatments have improved, stigma remains. However, the literature has documented mixed outcomes of youth disclosure to friends. Unfortunately, the reality of HIV is such that stigma abounds, and there is no guarantee that disclosure experiences will be positive. Indeed, negative experiences with disclosure are associated with poorer mental health. Lam et al. (2007, pp. 27) explain:

> The quality of the family's and friend's response to the disclosure (and their subsequent social support) is more important than the disclosure itself. [...] It should not be assumed that disclosure will automatically benefit youth, and the decision to disclose should be made on a case-by-case basis.

Romantic and Sexual Relationships Establishing romantic and sexual relationships is a normative part of development, and this aspect of adolescence is not absent from the lives of young people with HIV. However, youth living with HIV experience myriad challenges to establishing healthy romantic and sexual relationships due to stigma, requirements to disclose, and transmission risk. Moreover, research has documented that negative self-concept is common among youth living with HIV, who, as noted previously, may see themselves as "damaged" or "contaminated" by their illness. The normative task of exploring sexuality is of particular relevance to clinicians working with children and adolescents with HIV. First, sexual development is an important topic for clinicians to broach with patients early in puberty in order to familiarize patients with conversations about sexuality and diffuse discomfort around this sensitive topic. Clinicians are uniquely positioned to offer informed and sensitive support related to sexual development for children, adolescents, and young adults. Often, pediatric HIV providers have long-term relationships with patients and are non-parent figures with whom youth may be more comfortable discussing their sexual and romantic relationship concerns. Clinicians can offer medically informed advice about safe sex in the context of HIV, which is often not a component of traditional sex education, but some research suggests the provision of this information is limited in clinical settings (Albright and Fair 2014). The lack of accurate knowledge among youth with HIV has been documented in extant literature (e.g., Fair and Albright in press; Wiener et al. 2007; Ezeanolue et al. 2006). In addition to posing a risk to public health, this lack of knowledge can exacerbate difficulties in establishing healthy romantic and sexual relationships. Youth with limited knowledge of sexual transmission may avoid romantic relationships or may avoid disclosure to sexual partners (Fair and Albright 2012; Fernet et al. 2007). Distress related to establishing romantic relationships can contribute to worsening self-esteem to the detriment of psychosocial functioning. Conversely, healthy romantic relationships are associated with higher perceived social support and better emotional functioning in the general population of adolescents and thus, if supported, may be beneficial for youth in the short and long term (Raley et al. 2007; Collins 2003).

Mode of Transmission

Differences in psychological functioning related to the mode of acquisition have important implications for pediatric care settings as perinatal HIV becomes less common in developed countries, and youth with behaviorally acquired HIV (BHIV) comprise a larger proportion of people living with HIV. Similarly to youth born with HIV, most adolescents and young adults infected with HIV behaviorally are part of more than one marginalized group. Youth with BHIV face distinct challenges related to their acquisition of HIV—many are lesbian, gay, bisexual, transgender, or queer (LGBTQ)—and are rejected from their family as a result of their sexual identity. Adolescents with behaviorally acquired HIV appear to engage in substance abuse behaviors at higher rates than their counterparts who acquired HIV perinatally (Conner et al. 2013), and may experience greater psychological distress (Brown et al. 2015). Some researchers posit that youth with BHIV present with more psychosocial problems than their peers with perinatally acquired HIV (PHIV) because of the demographic composition of the group as opposed to the HIV diagnosis itself.

Youth with BHIV are often from lower socioeconomic status backgrounds, LGBTQ, and/or are racial/ethnic minorities. An HIV diagnosis can be a cause for many to be rejected from their romantic partners, peer group, or parents/caregivers. These risk factors culminate in a significant emotional burden, particularly for adolescents from lower-resource backgrounds or for those who are isolated from their family or peer group due to their sexuality or HIV status. Minority sexual orientation appears to be associated with poorer mental health—a group in which many youth with BHIV are members—as a result of lower social support (Lam et al. 2007). The effects of multiple marginalized identities are the key factor for clinicians to consider when seeking to support this population. Just as addressing the contextual challenges faced by those with pediatric HIV is a point of intervention, so too is holistic care (i.e., psychosocial support), a way in which clinicians can promote physical, emotional, and social functioning.

Transition from Pediatric to Adult Care

In addition to the medical challenges posed to mental health maintenance among this population, adolescents who age out of pediatric care are faced with the significant challenges of transitioning from pediatric to adult-centered care. This transition, which coincides with the developmental challenges of emerging adulthood, is a critical health-related and emotional juncture in the lives of young adults living with HIV which can have far-reaching consequences. Researchers have documented increased morbidity among young people with HIV who transitioned to adult care as well as significantly higher viral loads and more missed appointments among newly established patients in adult care (Foster et al. 2009; Ryscavage et al. 2011). Research has also documented low knowledge of HIV-related disease markers (e.g., viral load, CD4 count) as well as transmission risk factors which may adversely influence an adolescent's transition to adult care and post-transition health (Fair et al. 2014). Adult providers may make assumptions about the level of disease and transmission knowledge of their patients who are transitioning from pediatric care.

Poor understanding of the transition process and lack of preparation appear to be important factors in the observed negative outcomes of transition to adult care. Adolescents with PHIV may lack the ability to identify benefits or concerns about the transition to adult care and may be apprehensive about their readiness (Fair et al. 2012; Sharma et al. 2014). Further, their guardians may take a somewhat passive role to transition preparation, relying upon their child to let them know when the transition should occur and experiencing doubt related to their child's transition readiness. Indicators of readiness include the ability of youth with HIV to manage their complex medication regimes, navigate the new adult-oriented health system, and manage their own schedules (Newman et al. 2014). The comprehensive support offered by pediatric staff appears to be a "blessing and a curse" as it relates to adolescents transitioning into adult care. Given the wide variety of psychosocial concerns and medically complex aspects of HIV, the support offered by pediatric staff is seen as vital. However, leaving the often smaller, more attentive environment of pediatric care may exacerbate the difficulty of entering adult care, as adult settings are less often equipped with such extensive support for social and emotional functioning.

Because adolescents with PHIV have likely been engaged in care for most of their lives, they may develop particularly meaningful relationships with their pediatric care team. In fact, one of the most notable challenges to transition to adult care includes the loss of relationships with pediatric staff. Adolescents with HIV and their guardians have expressed sadness and apprehension about leaving the "safety" of the pediatric clinic (Fair et al. 2012; Dowshen and D'Angelo 2011; Wiener et al. 2011; Gilliam et al. 2011; Miles et al. 2004). As well, some youth with BHIV may have forged close and supportive relationships with their care providers in the absence of such relationships in their family as a result of contracting HIV or due to identifying as LGBTQ (Valenzuela et al. 2011). Thus, the warm and close

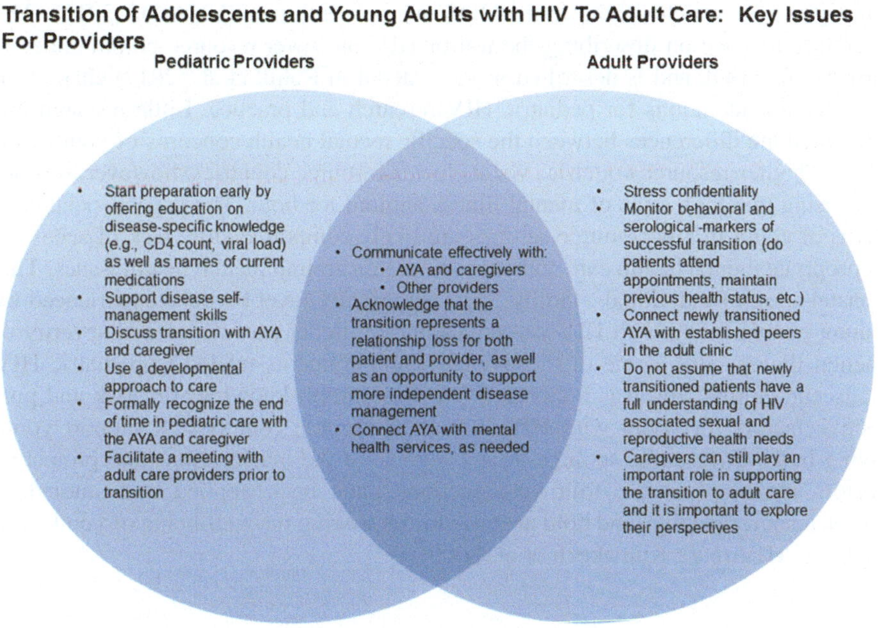

Fig. 4.1 Recommendations for providers supporting transition to adult care

relationships forged in pediatric and adolescent care may be beneficial to youths' overall physical and emotional well-being, but it may also make the transition to adult care particularly difficult. Adolescents and their guardians are not alone in their close connection with providers. Pediatric medical and social service providers, too, are hesitant to relinquish care to other providers (Vijayan et al. 2009) as they find fulfillment in offering care to this population (Newman et al. 2014).

In sum, it is clear that the transition from pediatric to adult care settings is fraught for youth living with HIV and is worthy of considerable attention from social service and medical providers alike. While pediatric providers must acknowledge their and their patients' complex feelings surrounding transition in order to adequately prepare their patients, adult providers must recognize just how stark the differences in pediatric and adult care settings can be (Newman et al. 2015). Figure 4.1 outlines researchers' recommendations for social service and medical providers who work with emerging adults with HIV.

International and Low-Resource Settings

Globally, access to effective care and treatment remains low for children and adolescents with HIV, with only one in four children under the age of 15 receiving antiretroviral treatment, and adolescents aged 10–15 years now recognized as the only group in which deaths from AIDS are not declining (UNAIDS 2015). The literature focused on describing the toll of HIV on lower-resource communities is broad and varied, and is described in more detail in Rahill et al. (2017) chapter on cultural considerations for pediatric HIV research and practice. Little research has identified the differences between the specific mental health concerns of youth with HIV in higher-resource countries versus lower-resource countries; however, it is not surprising that high rates of mental illness abound for both. The psychosocial concerns of youth in low-resource settings are likely compounded by lack of access to appropriate mental health care and/or more stigma around mental health issues. This constellation of individual-, family-, and community-level burdens experienced by young people living with HIV can contribute to higher prevalence and severity of mental illness. Still, some of the mental health concerns related to pediatric HIV transcend culture, and it is important to utilize current knowledge of risk and protective factors for youth with HIV in higher-resource countries to support youth living in lower-resource settings. Many aspects of the interventions and protective factors identified in the following sections have been applied and studied in lower-resource settings and hold promise for improving the well-being of youth with pediatric HIV (e.g., Kumakech et al. 2009).

Resilience and Protective Factors

Even though children, adolescents, and young adults living with HIV can face a range of challenges related to their illness, they can also display remarkable strengths and resilience (Betancourt et al. 2013; Persson and Newman 2012). Although rates of mental illness may be high among youth with HIV in comparison with the general population, many youth with HIV maintain psychological health, and some studies have found no significant differences between the psychological health of youth with and without HIV (Elkington et al. 2011). Thus, a number of protective factors are important to note in order for clinicians and social service providers to capitalize upon patients' existing resources.

Social support is an often overlooked resource for health promotion, even though it is a critical protective and promotive factor for those undergoing life transitions or challenges. Social relationships not only improve mental health but also improve physical health. In fact, social support is associated with lower viral load, higher CD4 counts, and fewer physical symptoms among people with HIV. Protective factors for children and youth with HIV can also include their positive relationships with their medical providers—some consider their providers as "part of the family." Even though this can pose a barrier to transition to adult care, it is nonetheless a significant resource to acknowledge and encourage youth and their families to draw upon (Persson et al. 2014). As this group is particularly at risk for social isolation, it is of utmost importance that healthcare providers monitor youths' social development and support their ability to forge healthy friendships—whether through disclosure guidance (e.g., how and when to disclose) or helping youth to build social skills.

While family relationships among this population can be complex and involve loss or tension due to parental HIV status, they can nonetheless be an important protective factor for youth living with HIV. In particular, family relationships often do not require explicit disclosure on the part of the youth. Family members (e.g., siblings or aunts/uncles) may already be aware of the child's HIV status and may thus offer a less stressful relationship in which youth do not bear the burden of secrecy experienced in their other relationships. Clinicians who aim to encourage positive social relationships among their patients may find that turning attention toward these family relationships is beneficial and less stressful for youth. Further, family members who are aware and supportive of a young person's HIV status may serve to model the potential for acceptance outside of the family context.

Treatment Recommendations and Interventions

A holistic approach to care is critical in supporting children, adolescents, and young adults living with HIV. Holistic approaches to care attend to psychological, social, and family functioning, in order to capitalize upon all aspects of potential health-promoting assets in youths' lives. In light of the well-documented association between mental and physical health, it is of utmost importance for clinicians to monitor the mental health of their young patients with HIV.

As noted previously, psychological functioning is associated with an array of health outcomes and should not be overlooked as a point of intervention for youth who are struggling to maintain physical health. Key factors in youth resilience include healthy coping, self-esteem, strong parental relationships, and social support (Betancourt et al. 2013). Fortunately, clinicians are well positioned to promote resilience by helping youth to improve coping strategies and self-concept, encourage better family communication, and increase youth self-efficacy in social relationships (Persson et al. 2014). The significant obstacles to healthy psychosocial development among children and adolescents with HIV have been mitigated by some therapeutic interventions. Interventions used with this population include individual, group, and family therapy, as well as art therapy and technology-based interventions (see Table 4.1).

Clinicians can also take an intervention-oriented approach in their interactions with clients by identifying personal strengths and social assets. For example, spirituality has been documented as a protective factor for people living with chronic illnesses, and this appears to hold true for some youth living with HIV. Although the relationship between religiosity and psychological well-being is complex for those living with HIV (e.g., viewing illness as punishment is associated with poorer outcomes), many take refuge in spiritual beliefs and experience mental health benefits as a result (Betancourt et al. 2011). Some youth report that religiosity provides a source of comfort and increases motivation to reach goals despite HIV

Table 4.1 Evidence-based interventions for youth with HIV

Author	Type	Population	Target outcome	Intervention	Outcome
Fair et al. (2014)	Individualized social work interventions	YLH (N = 37) 13 males and 24 females in initial examination, but the intervention focused on 15 participants ranging in age from 10 to 21 (MA = 14.8)	Improve medication adherence for at-risk patients, offer more intensive treatment, increase referrals for supportive family services	Interventions included daily phone communication between the patient and social worker. Developmentally appropriate disease and adherence education for parents and adolescents was also offered. Home visits took place and a reward system for improved laboratory work was implemented	Analyses indicated that CD4 counts were significantly higher and viral loads were significantly lower at the most recent clinic visit compared to baseline levels. Home-based services and referrals to social services agencies increased dramatically
Belzer et al. (2015)	Phone call reminders	YLH (N = 56, 37 enrolled, 19 assigned to intervention) ages 15–24 years (M = 20.43), with a history of non-adherence to ART. 54% had acquired HIV sexually and 46% perinatally	ART adherence	Participants in the intervention were contacted by cell phone on weekdays at a prearranged time by case managers, corresponding to the time and frequency of their taking ART. Callers reviewed medication, barriers to taking medications, and offered problem-solving support and relevant referrals	For participants on a once-daily regimen, the most common reasons participants did not take ART prior to the first call were forgetting to take medication (n = 23, 21.5%), change in schedule or routine (n = 17, 15.9%), sleeping through their designated time to take medication (n = 7, 6.5%), not having medication on hand (n = 6, 5.6%) and feeling ill (n = 5, 4.7%). The most common reasons named (by participants on a twice-daily regimen) for not taking ART prior to the second call was lapse in insurance coverage (n = 21, 52.5%), or that they were busy with other things (n = 5, 12.5%). However, only 12 of 19 participants were able to complete the 24-week intervention
Chandwani et al. (2011)	Adolescent impact, a multimodal behavioral intervention	YLH (N = 166, 83 in treatment and 83 in control group) 52.7% were females, mean age 16.8	Adherence and risk behavior	7 structured group sessions covered HIV knowledge, motivation, and skills related to medication adherence, availability of support resources, coping, risk reduction strategies, STIs, and disclosure. Material was presented didactically, via graphic software, video, and through interactive experiences. 5 one-to-one sessions with a counselor reinforced group sessions	79.5% of participants attended at least half of the 12 intervention sessions. Results indicate that a heterogeneous group of HIV-positive adolescents can be recruited and retained in a behavioral intervention program. An incentive structure that rewarded both regular and maximal attendance may have partially contributed to the intervention's high attendance rates

(continued)

Table 4.1 (continued)

Author	Type	Population	Target outcome	Intervention	Outcome
Chen et al. (2011)	MI-based program Healthy Choice	YLH (N = 142, 71 in therapy, 71 in control group) 16-24 years old with 2 or more risk behaviors	Decrease sexual risk behaviors, increase condom use, promoting adherence	Healthy Choices included 4 sessions delivered to individual clients in a clinic setting by mental health clinicians using MI where the participant identified one risk behavior to address	Receiving the intervention was associated with reductions in number of times of unprotected sexual intercourse over the trial period for participants in all groups. The level of unprotected sex was maintained at low levels throughout the trial period compared with the control subjects who reported higher levels of unprotected sex. YLH with different risk trajectories responded differently to Healthy Choices intervention
Dowshen et al. (2012)	Text message reminders to take medications	Participants (N = 25) ages 14–29 years (M = 23), 92% (n = 23) males, 60% (n = 15) black, and 84% (n = 21) infected through unprotected sex.	Adherence to Antiretroviral Therapy (ART)	Patients worked with the study coordinator to design their own personalized SMS reminder messages, which were programmed through a website to be delivered daily at the time(s) specified. Participants also designed a personalized follow-up message 1 h later assessing whether they took the medication	Improvements in adherence measures were seen as early as 6 weeks and sustained throughout the 24-week study period. However, there was no significant difference in CD4 cell count or viral load between baseline and the 12- or 24-week follow-ups. 81% of participants who completed the study said they would like to continue to receive text messages after the end of the study, and 20 of 21 (95%) participants indicated that the text messages helped them "very much" to miss fewer doses of medication
Fair et al. (2014)	Creative writing group	YLH (N = 7) ages 13–20 (MA = 16)	Improve communication skills, decrease isolation, increase peer support, lessen the burden of stigma	Teens Out Loud writing groups met for 4 h once a month for 8 months. Participants discussed disclosure, silencing, explored and responded to poetry and literature, as well as engaged in free writing and art making. Many of the writing projects focused on expressing personal experience with HIV to various audiences	Group members identified four benefits associated with participating in the group: increased confidence, better communication skills, increased support, and a desire to share their experiences with others. Adolescents unanimously reported increased confidence levels that were evident within the confines of the group, as well as in their everyday interactions. Guardians observed improved self-expression, behavior, and writing skills in their adolescent. All guardians described better communication between themselves and their child in the home

(continued)

Table 4.1 (continued)

Author	Type	Population	Target outcome	Intervention	Outcome
Foster et al. (2014)	Incentive Scheme aka Financial incentives (FIs)	Perinatally infected YLH ($N = 11$) ages 16–25 years, each with CD4 count ≤ 200, who had been off ART despite multiple attempts.	Adherence to ART	Intervention used an "Incentive Scheme (IS)" in conjunction with established multidisciplinary adherence support. The IS combined financial incentives linked to HIV viral load results and attendance for MI with a trained mental health provider	6/10 patients had an undetectable viral load 24 months post enrollment, 3 had viral loads >1000 copies/mL, 2 of whom had stopped ART, a third patient with ongoing poor adherence. Total FI expenditure was £1350 for the 11 patients
Funck-Brentano et al. (2005)	Peer support group	Youth ($N = 48$) ages 12–18	Perception (and acceptance) of self and HIV	Participants were assigned to one of 3 groups: two controls and a group therapy, which met for a 90-min session once every 6 weeks for 26 months. The open-ended format aimed to foster trust and enable the sharing of struggles and goals	After intervention, the percentage of adolescents with an undetectable viral load had increased in group 1 (the group therapy group) from 30 to 80% ($P = 0.063$) but was unchanged in groups 2 and 3. This pilot study suggests that the peer support group had a beneficial effect on the adolescents' acceptance and perceptions of their HIV infection
Hosek et al. (2011)	Project ACCEPT (Adolescents Coping, Connecting, Empowering, and Protecting Together)	Young adults ($N = 50$, 28 males and 22 females) mean age 19.24. 97% of males identified as gay or bisexual. 5% of females identified as bisexual	Increase HIV knowledge, decrease symptoms of depression, increase social support, improve coping	A 12-session behavioral intervention (based on the disability-stress-coping model) in which participants attended a combination of individual and group sessions. Each session was co-facilitated by a mental health provider and a peer facilitator (age ranges 18–26) living with HIV	Feasibility and acceptability data demonstrated high rates of participation and high levels of satisfaction with the intervention program. Exploratory outcome data demonstrated improved levels of HIV knowledge that were sustained over time and improvements in peer and formal social support
Kaihin et al. (2015)	Empowerment Intervention	Compared two groups of YLH ($N = 46$, 23 per group) ages 15–24 years who receive ART in Thailand, but were non-adherent	Adherence to ART	The experimental groups attended five sessions that empowered them to take control of their own health. The control group received standard of care	Participants in the experimental group were significantly more likely to be adherent to ART than those in the control group

(continued)

Table 4.1 (continued)

Author	Type	Population	Target outcome	Intervention	Outcome
Murphy et al. (2010)	MI-based program Healthy Choice	YLH (N = 143, 68 randomly assigned to the intervention group and 75 to the control group)	Decrease alcohol and marijuana use, promote adherence	Healthy Choices consisted of four sessions delivered to individual clients in a clinic setting by mental health clinicians using MI where the participant identified one risk behavior to address throughout the project	At the 15-month follow-up, self-reported rates of past-week alcohol use was significantly lower for the intervention youth than for the control youth; however, the differences in marijuana use were not significantly different
Naar-King et al. (2013)	Motivational Enhancement System for Adherence (MESA) intervention	Youth (N = 76) ages 16–24 years 11 months who had been newly prescribed ART	ART adherence	MESA intervention is delivered via a web-based server that uses realistic, personalized interactions with a two-dimensional animated character that delivered personalized health feedback, ART information, activities to promote motivation and confidence	Intervention group showed a greater drop than controls in viral load from baseline to 6 months (Cohen's d = 0.39 at 3 months; d = 0.19 at 6 months), and had more had an undetectable viral load by 6 months (d = 0.28)
Naar-King et al. (2010)	Motivational Interviewing (MI)	Youth (N = 186) ages 16–24 identified for one of the following reasons: sexual risk, substance use, or poor medication adherence	Reduction of non-compliance, substance use, and sexual risk-taking	46-minute MI therapy sessions. Youth worked on two of three possible problem behaviors: substance use, sexual risk, or medication adherence	Those who completed the intervention experienced significant improvements in depression, and improved motivational readiness compared to controls
Parsons et al. (2006)	Hospitalization	YLH (N = 19, mean age = 12.6) receiving treatment at an Intensive Primary Care Clinic who were failing HAART adherence	HAART adherence, decreased viral load	Admitted patients were managed by an interdisciplinary team that included medicine, nursing, nutrition, social work, behavioral psychology, neuropsychology, physical therapy, occupational therapy, education, and child life/therapeutic recreation. The average length of stay for hospitalization was 40 days	The value of this multidisciplinary intervention is highlighted by the sustainability of viral load reduction. More than half of the patients maintained significant decrease in viral load 6 months after discharge. More than one-third of patients in the study attained an undetectable viral load by 6 months after discharge. This intervention may produce a lasting difference in viral load in a challenging group of patients for whom outpatient efforts have failed. Hospitalization can confirm non-adherence or resistance

(continued)

Table 4.1 (continued)

Author	Type	Population	Target outcome	Intervention	Outcome
Puccio et al. (2006)	Phone call reminders	HAART patients (N = 8) ages 16–24, 7 males 1 female	HAART Adherence	Participants received free cell phones and were contacted for each medication dose every day for the first four weeks, then tapered off in frequency	Subjects that did not experience major chaotic life changes had improved adherence and significant decrease in viral load. Patients indicated that the calls were helpful, and used them to ask questions, such as when to make appointments or what to do about a personal problem

infection (Martinez et al. 2012). As well, involvement in a religious community opens the door to a supportive social community in the face of an often isolating illness. Clinicians can capitalize upon this potential resilience-promoting factor by inquiring about religiosity and, when appropriate, reinforcing its benefits to youth.

Considering the far-reaching benefits of social support and the paucity of opportunities for youth with HIV to engage with HIV-positive peers, clinicians who are able to organize support groups for their patients may observe significant improvements in patients' health. Few youth with HIV have opportunities to establish friendships with other people with HIV. Therefore, their ability to seek support from friends with a shared experience is limited or non-existent. Some research indicates that adolescents desire HIV-positive peer friendships and also benefit when they are able to forge such relationships (Travers and Paoletti 1999; Persson et al. in press). Participatory approaches such as digital storytelling and emotional maps (Alonso et al. 2013) offer innovative ways to harness the capacities and insights of children and adolescents regarding their mental and emotional well-being, and can feed into the design and delivery of services and programs in order to ensure they are appropriate, effective, and relevant. The population of children and adolescents living with HIV are often particularly difficult to engage in medical and psychosocial care, owing to high levels of stigma, economic concerns, and lack of nearby access to treatment. Thus, clinicians' approach to intervention implementation may vary by setting and patient. See Table 4.1 for an overview of a variety of empirically tested interventions.

Conclusion

In this chapter, we have reviewed the key considerations for children and adolescents growing up with HIV regarding their mental health, relationships, and transition to adult care. We recognized the specific issues facing this population in low-resource country settings and have stressed the importance of relying on strong evidence in developing interventions to support the mental and emotional well-being of children and adolescents engaged with clinical care. To conclude, we want to propose a number of key areas with the potential to add considerable value to what is already known about the psychosocial considerations of pediatric and adolescent HIV.

First, are young people generating their own understandings of and responses to the social stigma attached to HIV? Rather than imposing an adult understanding and concern about stigma and HIV onto children and young people, we must try and understand how these issues are understood and lived from their perspectives. Are they coming up with new ways to understand HIV itself, and new ways to configure the meanings it holds in relation to their sense of self and ways of relating to others? Second, how can psychosocial interventions be more genuinely engaged with the needs and perspectives of the population they are seeking to support? Third, in an era of HIV normalization, what opportunities can be afforded by the new ways of relating that children and adolescents growing up with HIV may well develop? This is a period in the history of HIV medicine which offers never-before-seen opportunities for inclusion and transformation in the social and sexual lives of people with HIV, and children and adolescents need to be appropriately included in the decision-making processes to ensure the promise of a post-AIDS world is available to all.

It is essential that we make no assumptions about what living with HIV will mean for children and adolescents in the coming years, and that attention continues to be paid to learning from the experts in this subject; that is, these young people themselves. In the face of considerable challenges, we may be surprised and encouraged by the resilience and capacities they display and can be assured that recognizing those strengths will offer meaningful insights that can help to keep our support systems dynamic in response to the changing needs of these young people.

Annotated Bibliography

Fair, C., & Albright, J. (2012). Don't tell him you have HIV unless he's 'the one': Romantic relationships among adolescents and young adults with perinatal HIV infection. *AIDS Patient Care & STDs*, *26*(12), 746–754. doi:10.1089/apc.2012.0290

Experiences with romantic relationships among youth with perinatally-acquired HIV are explored in this qualitative study. Relationship challenges included risk of rejection upon disclosure. However, participants also encouraged other youth living with HIV to have hope that they would find a supportive partner.

Kim, M., Mazenga, A., Yu, X., Devandra, A. Nguyn, C., & Sharp, C. (2015). Factors associated with depression among adolescents living with HIV in Malawi. *BMC Psychiatry*, *15*, 1–12. doi:10.1186/s12888-015-0649-9

This study examined contributory and protective factors associated with depression in adolescents with HIV in Malawi. Findings indicated that older age, less schooling, and experiences of bullying for taking medications were associated with increased risk for depression.

Persson, A., & Newman, C. (2012). When HIV-positive children grow up: A critical analysis of the transition literature in developed countries. *Qualitative Health Research*, *22*(5), 656–667. doi:10.1177/1049732311431445

This paper critically reviews the literature on transition to adult care, identifying a problematic framing of young people with perinatally acquired HIV as vulnerable and unprepared for adult life, without sufficient attention to understanding their potential strengths and capacities, nor documenting their own accounts of growing up with HIV/

References

Albright, J. N., & Fair, C. D. (2014). Providers caring for adolescents with perinatally-acquired HIV: Current practices and barriers to communication about sexual and reproductive health. *AIDS Patient Care and STDs*, *28*(11), 587–593. doi:10.1089/apc.2014.0162

Alonso, I., Molina, S., & Requejo, M. D. P. (2013). Multimodal digital storytelling: Integrating information, emotion and social cognition. *Review of Cognitive Linguistics*, *11*(2), 369–387. doi:10.1075/rcl.11.2.10alo

Azzopardi, C., Wade, M., Salter, R., Macdougall, G., Shouldice, M., Read, S., et al. (2014). Medical nonadherence in pediatric HIV: Psychosocial risks and intersection with the child protection system for medical neglect. *Child Abuse and Neglect*, *38*(11), 1766–1777. doi:10.1016/j.chiabu.2014.08.013

Battles, H. B., & Wiener, L. S. (2002). From adolescence through young adulthood: Psychosocial adjustment associated with long-term survival of HIV. *Journal of Adolescent Health, 30*(3), 161–168. doi:10.1016/S1054-139X(01)00341-X

Beegle, K., De Weerdt, J., & Dercon, S. (2006). Orphanhood and the long-run impact on children. *American Journal of Agricultural Economics, 88*(5), 1266–1272. doi:10.1111/j.1467-8276.2006.00943.x

Belzer, M. E., Kolmodin MacDonell, K., Clark, L. F., Huang , J., Olson, J., Kahana, S., et al. (2015). Acceptability and feasibility of a cell phone support intervention for youth living with HIV with nonadherence to antiretroviral therapy. *AIDS Patient Care STDS, 29*(6), 338–345. doi:10.1089/apc.2014.0282.

Bernays, S., Jarrett, P., Kranzer, K., & Ferrand, R. A. (2014). Children growing up with HIV infection: The responsibility of success. *The Lancet, 383*(9925), 1355–1357. doi:10.1016/S0140-6736(13)62328-4

Betancourt, T. S., Meyers-Ohki, S., Stulac, S. N., Barrera, A. E., Mushashi, C., & Beardslee, W. R. (2011). Nothing can defeat combined hands (Abashize hamwe ntakibananira): Protective processes and resilience in Rwandan children and families affected by HIV/AIDS. *Social Science and Medicine, 73*(5), 693–701. doi:10.1016/j.socscimed.2011.06.053

Betancourt, T. S., Meyers-Ohki, S. E., Charrow, A., & Hansen, N. (2013). Annual research review: Mental health and resilience in HIV/AIDS-affected children—A review of the literature and recommendations for future research. *Journal of Child Psychology and Psychiatry, 54*(4), 423–444. doi:10.1111/j.1469-7610.2012.02613.x

Brent, D. A., Melhem, N. M., Masten, A. S., Porta, G., & Payne, M. W. (2012). Longitudinal effects of parental bereavement on adolescent developmental competence. *Journal of Clinical Child and Adolescent Psychology, 41*(6), 778–791. doi:10.1080/15374416.2012.717871

Brown, L. K., Whiteley, L., Harper, G. W., Nichols, S., & Nieves, A. (2015). Psychological symptoms among 2032 youth living with HIV: A multisite study. *AIDS Patient Care and STDs, 29*(4), 212–219. doi:10.1089/apc.2014.0113

Chandwani, S., Abramowitz, S., Koenig, L., Barnes, W., & D'Angelo, L. (2011). A multimodal behavioral intervention to impact adherence and risk behavior among perinatally and behaviorally HIV-infected youth: Description, delivery, and receptivity of adolescent impact. *AIDS Education and Prevention, 23*(3), 222–235. doi:10.1521/aeap.2011.23.3.222.

Chen, X., Murphy, D. A., Naar-King, S., Parsons, J. T., & Adolescent Medicine Trials Network for HIV/AIDS Interventions. (2011). A clinic-based motivational intervention improves condom use among subgroups of youth living with HIV. *Journal of Adolescent Health, 49*(2), 193–198. doi:10.1016/j.jadohealth.2010.11.252.

Clark, C., Rodgers, B., Caldwell, T., Power, C., & Stansfeld, S. (2007). Childhood and adulthood psychological ill health as predictors of midlife affective and anxiety disorders: The 1958 British Birth Cohort. *Archives of General Psychiatry, 64*(6), 668–678. doi:10.1001/archpsyc.64.6.668

Cluver, L. D., Gardner, F., & Operario, D. (2008). Effects of stigma on the mental health of adolescents orphaned by AIDS. *Journal of Adolescent Health, 42*(4), 410–417. doi:10.1016/j.jadohealth.2007.09.022

Cluver, L. D., & Orkin, M. (2009). Cumulative risk and AIDS-orphanhood: Interactions of stigma, bullying and poverty on child mental health in South Africa. *Social Science and Medicine, 69*(8), 1186–1193. doi:10.1016/j.socscimed.2009.07.033

Collins, W. A. (2003). More than myth: The developmental significance of romantic relationships during adolescence. *Journal of Research on Adolescence, 13*(1), 1–24. doi:10.1111/1532-7795.1301001

Conner, L. C., Wiener, J., Lewis, J. V., Phill, R., Peralta, L., Chandwani, S., et al. (2013). Prevalence and predictors of drug use among adolescents with HIV infection acquired perinatally or later in life. *AIDS and Behavior, 17*(3), 976–986. doi:10.1007/s10461-011-9950-x

Dowshen, N., & D'Angelo, L. (2011). Health care transition for youth living with HIV/AIDS. *Pediatrics, 128*(4), 762–771. doi:10.1542/peds.2011-0068

Dowshen, N., Kuhns, L. M., Johnson, A., Holoyda, B. J., & Garofalo, R. (2012). Improving adherence to antiretroviral therapy for youth living with HIV/AIDS: A pilot study using personalized, interactive, daily text message reminders. *Journal of Medical Internet Research, 14*(2), e51. doi:10.2196/jmir.2015.

Elkington, K. S., Robbins, R. N., Bauermeister, J. A., Abrams, E. J., McKay, M., & Mellins, C. A. (2011). Mental health in youth infected with and affected by HIV: The role of caregiver HIV. *Journal of Pediatric Psychology, 36*(3), 360–373. doi:10.1093/jpepsy/jsq094

Ezeanolue, E. E., Wodi, A. P., Patel, R., Dieudonne, A., & Oleske, J. M. (2006). Sexual behaviors and procreational intentions of adolescents and young adults with perinatally acquired human immunodeficiency virus infection: Experience of an urban tertiary center. *Journal of Adolescent Health, 38*(6), 719–725. doi:10.1016/j.jadohealth.2005.06.015

Fair, C., & Albright, J. (2012). Don't tell him you have HIV unless he's 'the one': Romantic relationships among adolescents and young adults with perinatal HIV infection. *AIDS Patient Care & STDs, 26*(12), 746–754. doi:10.1089/apc.2012.0290

Fair, C., & Albright, J. (in press). I definitely want kids, but I think the risks are pretty high: Fertility desires and perinatal HIV transmission knowledge among adolescents and young adults with perinatally-acquired HIV. In P. Liamputtong (Ed.), *Children, young people and living with HIV/AIDS: A cross-cultural perspective*. Springer: Dordrecht, Netherlands.

Fair, C., Osherow, J., Albright, J., & McKeone, D. (2014). Medication adherence among youth with HIV: A case study of social work interventions. *Journal of Social Services and HIV/AIDS, 13*, 26–45.

Fair, C. D., Sullivan, K., Dizney, R., & Stackpole, A. (2012). It's like losing a part of my family: Transition expectations of adolescents living with perinatally acquired HIV and their guardians. *AIDS Patient Care and STDs, 26*(7), 423–429. doi:10.1089/apc.2012.0041

Fair, C. D., Sullivan, K., Dizney, R., & Stackpole, A. (2014). Knowledge of disease markers and quality of patient–provider interaction among adolescents with perinatally acquired HIV: Implications for transition to adult care. *Vulnerable Children and Youth Studies, 9*(2), 167–173. doi:10.1080/17450128.2013.861619

Fernet, M., et al. (2007). Issues of sexuality and prevention among adolescents living with HIV/AIDS since birth. *Canadian Journal of Human Sexuality, 16*(3/4), 101.

Foster, C., Judd, A., Tookey, P., Tudor-Williams, G., Dunn, D., Shingadia, D., … & Lyall, H. (2009). Young people in the United Kingdom and Ireland with perinatally acquired HIV: The pediatric legacy for adult services. *AIDS Patient Care & STDs, 23*(3), 159–166. doi:10.1089/apc.2008.0153

Foster, C., McDonald, S., Frize, G., Ayers, S., & Fidler, S. (2014). Payment by results–financial incentives and motivational interviewing, adherence interventions in young adults with perinatally acquired HIV-1 infection: A pilot program. *AIDS Patient Care STDS, 28*(1), 28–32. doi:10.1089/apc.2013.0262.

Funck-Brentano, I., Dalban, C., Veber, F., Quartier, P., Hefez, S., Costagliola, D., et al. (2005). Evaluation of a peer support group therapy for HIV-infected adolescents. *AIDS, 19*(14), 1501–1508.

Gilliam, P. P., Ellen, J. M., Leonard, L., Kinsman, S., Jevitt, C. M., & Straub, D. M. (2011). Transition of adolescents with HIV to adult care: Characteristics and current practices of the adolescent trials network for HIV/AIDS interventions. *Journal of the Association of Nurses in AIDS Care, 22*(4), 283–294. doi:10.1016/j.jana.2010.04.003

Hosek, S. G., Lemos, D., Harper, G. W., & Telander, K. (2011). Evaluating the acceptability and feasibility of Project ACCEPT: An intervention for youth newly diagnosed with HIV. *AIDS Education & Prevention, 23*(2), 128–144. doi:10.1521/aeap.2011.23.2.128.

Kaihin, R., Kasatpibal, N., Chitreechuer, J., & Grimes, R. M. (2015). Effect of an empowerment intervention on antiretroviral drug adherence in Thai youth. *Behavioral Medicine, 41*(4), 186–194. doi:10.1080/08964289.2014.911717.

Kumakech, E., Cantor-Graae, E., Maling, S., & Bajunirwe, F. (2009). Peer-group support intervention improves the psychosocial well-being of AIDS orphans: Cluster randomized trial. *Social Science and Medicine, 68*(6), 1038–1043. doi:10.1016/j.socscimed.2008.10.033

Lam, P. K., Naar-King, S., & Wright, K. (2007). Social support and disclosure as predictors of mental health in HIV-positive youth. *AIDS Patient Care and STDs, 21*(1), 20–29. doi:10.1089/apc.2006.005

Li, X., Naar-King, S., Barnett, D., Stanton, B., Fang, X., & Thurston, C. (2008). A developmental psychopathology framework of the psychosocial needs of children orphaned by HIV. *Journal of the Association of Nurses in AIDS Care, 19*(2), 147–157. doi:10.1016/j.jana.2007.08.004

Martinez, J., Harper, G., Carleton, R. A., Hosek, S., Bojan, K., Clum, G., … & The Adolescent Medicine Trials Network, J. (2012). The impact of stigma on medication adherence among HIV-positive adolescent and young adult females and the moderating effects of coping and satisfaction with health care. *AIDS Patient Care & STDs, 26*(2), 108–115. doi:10.1089/apc.2011.0178

Mellins, C. A., Smith, R., O'Driscoll, P., Magder, L., Brouwers, P., Chase, C., … & Matzen, E. (2003). High rates of behavioral problems in perinatally HIV-infected children are not linked to HIV disease. *Pediatrics, 111*(2), 384–393.

Miles, K., Edwards, S., & Clapson, M. (2004). Transition from paediatric to adult services: experiences of HIV-positive adolescents. *AIDS Care, 16*(3), 305–314. doi:10.1080/09540120410001665312

Murphy, M., Xinguang, C., Naar-King, S., Parsons, J., & Adolescent Trials Network (2010). Alcohol and marijuana use outcomes in the healthy choices motivational interviewing intervention for HIV-positive youth. *AIDS Patient Care & STDS, 26*(2), 95–100. doi:10.1089/apc.2011.0157.

Naar-King, S., Templin, T., Wright, K., Frey, M., Parsons, J. T., & Lam, P. (2006). Psychosocial factors and medication adherence in HIV-positive youth. *AIDS Patient Care and STDs, 20*(1), 44–47. doi:10.1089/apc.2006.20.44

Naar-King, S., Outlaw, A. Y., Sarr, M., Parsons, J. T., Belzer, M., Macdonell, K., et al. (2013). Motivational Enhancement System for Adherence (MESA): Pilot randomized trial of a brief computer-delivered prevention intervention for youth initiating antiretroviral treatment. *Journal of Pediatric Psychology, 38*(6), 638–648. doi:10.1093/jpepsy/jss132.

Naar-King, S., Parsons, J. T., Murphy, D., Kolmodin, K., Harris, D. R., & ATN 004 Protocol Team. (2010). A multisite randomized trial of a motivational intervention targeting multiple risks in youth living with HIV: Initial effects on motivation, self-efficacy, and depression. *Journal of Adolescent Health, 46*(5), 422–428. doi:10.1016/j.jadohealth.2009.11.198.

Newman, C. E., Persson, A., Miller, A., & Cama, E. (2014). Bridging worlds, breaking rules: Clinician perspectives on transitioning young people with perinatally acquired HIV into adult care in a low prevalence setting. *AIDS patient care and STDs, 28*(7), 381–393. doi:10.1089/apc.2013.0346

Newman, C. E., Persson, A., Miller, A., & Brown, R. J. (2015). Just take your medicine and everything will be fine: Responsibilisation narratives in accounts of transitioning young people with HIV into adult care services in Australia. *AIDS Care*, 1–6.

Orban, L. A., Stein, R., Koenig, L. J., Conner, L. C., Rexhouse, E. L., Lewis, J. V., et al. (2010). Coping strategies of adolescents living with HIV: Disease-specific stressors and responses. *AIDS Care, 22*(4), 420–430. doi:10.1080/09540120903193724

Parsons, G. N., Siberry, G. K., Parsons, J. K., Christensen, J. R., Joyner, M. L., Lee, S. L., et al. (2006). Multidisciplinary, inpatient directly observed therapy for HIV-1-infected children and adolescents failing HAART: A retrospective study. *AIDS Patient Care STDS, 20*(4), 275–284.

Patel, V., Flisher, A. J., Hetrick, S., & McGorry, P. (2007). Mental health of young people: A global public-health challenge. *The Lancet, 369*(9569), 1302–1313. doi:10.1016/S0140-6736(07)60368-7

Persson, A., & Newman, C. (2012). When HIV-positive children grow up: A critical analysis of the transition literature in developed countries. *Qualitative Health Research, 22*(5), 656–667. doi:10.1177/1049732311431445

Persson, A., Newman, C. E., & Miller, A. (2014). Caring for 'underground' kids: Qualitative interviews with clinicians about key issues for young people growing up with perinatally acquired HIV in Australia. *International Journal of Adolescence and Youth* (ahead-of-print), 1–15. doi:10.1080/02673843.2013.866149

Persson, A., Newman, C, E., & Miller, A. (in press). There's more to you than just this virus: Young people growing up with perinatally acquired HIV in Australia. In P. Liamputtong (Ed.), *Children, Young People and HIV/AIDS: A Cross-Cultural Perspective*. Dordrecht, The Netherlands: Springer.

Puccio, J. A., Belzer, M., Olson, J., Martinez, M., Salata, C., Tucker, D., et al. (2006). The use of cell phone reminder calls for assisting HIV-infected adolescents and young adults to adhere to highly active antiretroviral therapy: A pilot study. *AIDS Patient Care STDS, 20*(6), 438–444.

Rahill, G. J., Joshi, M., & Lescano, C. (2017). Cultural considerations for pediatric HIV research and practice. In T. Chenneville (Ed), *A Clinical Guide to Pediatric HIV*, 259–271. Dordrecht: Springer.

Raley, R. K., Crissey, S., & Muller, C. (2007). Of sex and romance: Late adolescent relationships and young adult union formation. *Journal of Marriage and Family, 69*(5), 1210–1226. doi:10.1111/j.1741-3737.2007.00442.x

Reisner, M. S. L., Mimiaga, M. J., Skeer, M. M., Perkovich, M. B., Johnson, M. C. V., & Safren, S. A. (2009). A review of HIV antiretroviral adherence and intervention studies among HIV-infected youth. *Topics in HIV Medicine, 17*(1), 14.

Ryscavage, P. A., Anderson, E. J., Sutton, S. H., Reddy, S., & Taiwo, B. (2011). Clinical outcomes of adolescents and young adults in adult HIV care. *JAIDS Journal of Acquired Immune Deficiency Syndromes, 58*(2), 193–197. doi:10.1097/QAI.0B013E31822D7564

Salama, C., Morris, M., Armistead, L., Koenig, L. J., Demas, P., Ferdon, C., et al. (2013). Depressive and conduct disorder symptoms in youth living with HIV: The independent and interactive roles of coping and neuropsychological functioning. *AIDS Care, 25*(2), 160–168. doi:10.1080/09540121.2012.687815

Sharma, N., Willen, E., Garcia, A., & Sharma, T. S. (2014). Attitudes toward transitioning in youth with perinatally acquired HIV and their family caregivers. *Journal of the Association of Nurses in AIDS Care, 25*(2), 168–175. doi:10.1016/j.jana.2013.01.007

Stangl, A. (2017). HIV-related stigma and children. In T. Chenneville (Ed), *A Clinical Guide to Pediatric HIV*, 297–315. Dordrecht: Springer.

Thurston, I. B., Decker, K., & Hardin, R. (2017). Antiretroviral medication adherence and disease management in pediatric populations. In T. Chenneville (Ed), *A Clinical Guide to Pediatric HIV*, 163–188. Dordrecht: Springer.

Travers, R., & Paoletti, D. (1999). Responding to the support needs of HIV positive lesbian, gay and bisexual youth. *Canadian Journal of Human Sexuality, 8*(4), 271–284.

UNAIDS. (2015). Leaders from around the world are All Into end the AIDS epidemic among adolescents [Press release]. Retrieved from http://www.unaids.org/en/resources/presscentre/pressreleaseandstatementarchive/2015/February/20150217_PR_all-in

Valenzuela, J. M., Buchanan, C. L., Radcliffe, J., Ambrose, C., Hawkins, L. A., Tanney, M., et al. (2011). Transition to adult services among behaviorally infected adolescents with HIV—A qualitative study. *Journal of Pediatric Psychology, 36*(2), 134–140. doi:10.1093/jpepsy/jsp051

Vijayan, T., Benin, A. L., Wagner, K., Romano, S., & Andiman, W. A. (2009). We never thought this would happen: Transitioning care of adolescents with perinatally acquired HIV infection from pediatrics to internal medicine. *AIDS Care, 21*(10), 1222–1229. doi:10.1080/09540120902730054

Wiener, L. S., Battles, H. B., & Wood, L. V. (2007). A longitudinal study of adolescents with perinatally or transfusion acquired HIV infection: Sexual knowledge, risk reduction self-efficacy and sexual behavior. *AIDS and Behavior, 11*(3), 471–478. doi:10.1007/s10461-006-9162-y

Wiener, L. S., Kohrt, B. A., Battles, H. B., & Pao, M. (2011). The HIV experience: Youth identified barriers for transitioning from pediatric to adult care. *Journal of Pediatric Psychology, 36*(2), 141–154. doi:10.1093/jpepsy/jsp129

Worden, J. W., & Silverman, P. R. (1996). Parental death and the adjustment of school-age children. *Omega: Journal Of Death & Dying, 33*(2), 91–102. doi:10.2190/p77l-f6f6-5w06-nhbx

Chapter 5
The Impact of Pediatric HIV on Families

Maryann Koussa Youssef, Danielle Harris and Mary Jane Rotheram-Borus

Introduction

Children become infected with the human immunodeficiency virus (HIV) via two major routes: perinatal infections and infections acquired by adolescents due to their sexual or drug-related behaviors. While these are two very different routes for infection, the predictable challenges for families when either a baby or an adolescent are infected are similar. The family has to support and cope on a daily basis with (Rotheram-Borus et al. 1998):

- Health issues: navigating a health system, encouraging adherence to antiretroviral (ARV) medications, coping with illnesses, and implementing healthy habits daily for eating, sleeping, and exercise, without alcohol and drug use.
- Mental health challenges around coping with a chronic illness; deciding who, when, and how to disclose to others; coping with depression or anxiety regarding a premature death; and recognizing and confronting stigma from others (Lamping et al. 1991; Leta et al. 2012; Rotheram-Borus et al. 1999a).
- Social relationships which are fundamentally reordered, especially sexual relationships which require protecting others from acquiring HIV, promoting testing among one's partners, and educating others about HIV.
- Post-death challenges regarding custody, creation of new family routines and life goals, and managing grief.

M.K. Youssef (✉) · D. Harris · M.J. Rotheram-Borus
University of California, Los Angeles, CA, USA
e-mail: MKoussa@mednet.ucla.edu

D. Harris
e-mail: DMHarris@mednet.ucla.edu

M.J. Rotheram-Borus
e-mail: mrotheram@mednet.ucla.edu

T. Chenneville (ed.), *A Clinical Guide to Pediatric HIV*,
DOI 10.1007/978-3-319-49704-4_5

The issues are different for the child who is infected perinatally and the adolescent who is infected behaviorally. Parents and siblings are the primary agents who must cope with caring for young children living with HIV—and, perhaps more important, the mother almost inevitably is herself coping with HIV. For an adolescent, serostatus can be hidden from family members, but in most cases, families know about their adolescent children's HIV infection (Rotheram-Borus et al. 1997). Adolescents manage their own disease daily, but parents react with a range of emotions: grief, rejecting their children, trying to micromanage their children's lives, and coping with HIV-related stressors.

This chapter will review the epidemiology of HIV among children infected by HIV, both in the US and globally; outline the intervention approaches for family, home-based, and clinic-based evidence-based interventions (EBI); and describe the types of structural and policy interventions which have been most influential in shifting the context and the rates of pediatric HIV. We will conclude with suggesting the path forward to address both perinatal and adolescent pediatric infections with regard to eliminating new infections and ensuring that youth currently infected by HIV are provided with the comprehensive services needed for a long, happy, and productive life.

Epidemiology of Pediatric HIV from 1981 to 2016

Perinatal infection is acquired during pregnancy and childbirth from a mother living with HIV (MLH) or during breastfeeding during the first few months of life. In the first 15 years of the epidemic, there were about 3 million perinatal infections. In the US, about 84% of these infections were among women who had a history of injection drug use or were immersed in a neighborhood with high rates of HIV due to high rates of drug dealing. Infections were focused in large urban centers along the Eastern seaboard, as the quality of heroin was far lower on the East coast compared to the West coast, and it took much longer to kill HIV if the injector was "heating their works" (AIDSVu 2013; Ciccarone and Bourgois 2003). Acquiring pediatric HIV early in the epidemic almost guaranteed that the child would die within five years, as physicians' abilities to cope with the opportunistic infections were limited. At that time, there was a 23% likelihood that a MLH would pass HIV to her baby (Newell et al. 1997).

Infants

Today, there are almost no perinatal infections in the US. The first major breakthrough in stopping and eliminating pediatric HIV occurred in 1996, with the demonstration that zidovudine (AZT)—an ARV administered during pregnancy—reduced transmission by 75% (Bryson 1996). Over the next few years, the rate of perinatal transmission from a MLH to her infant was further reduced to 0.2% with a combination of ARV therapies, caesarian section births, and administration of ARV to infants combined with a single feeding method for the first six months of life or through the cessation of breastfeeding (The Interagency Task Team 2015). In 2014, fewer than 100 infants were born with HIV in the US, almost all to mothers who had not received proper antenatal care or who were serious injection drug users (CDC 2016).

While the technologies to reduce infection were well known by about 2000, the broad diffusion and implementation of the procedures to eliminate perinatal transmission in high-income countries came from policy interventions. In the US, an Institute of Medicine Task Force in 1999 recommended and states promptly passed laws requiring opt-out HIV testing for pregnant women (CDC 2006). Even when these policies were demonstrated not to be cost-effective (Leibowitz et al. 2015), the mandate for opt-out maternal HIV testing became routine. The virtual elimination of perinatal HIV infection in high-income countries is the best example of a public health success to date of eliminating HIV transmission within a population at risk.

A similar pattern has not been found in low- and middle-income countries (LMIC). As more than 65% of the epidemic is in sub-Saharan Africa, perinatal transmission remains a major challenge today (UNAIDS 2014c). Currently, the rate of perinatal HIV testing is only 42% in Africa, 20 years after the efficacy of AZT was demonstrated, and far after the Global Fund and the President's Emergency Plan for AIDS Relief began committing $8 billion annually to stop HIV and provide ARV to LMIC. Annually, 9200 infants are born or acquire HIV during the first 18 months of life in South Africa alone (UNAIDS 2015a). This is a public health failure of major proportions.

Stopping perinatal HIV in LMIC, however, requires MLH to complete many tasks: getting tested for HIV; getting and adhering to ARV during pregnancy; disclosing to healthcare providers at the child's birth about her serostatus and then taking nevirapine; administering ARV to the infant for the first six weeks of life; and getting the infant tested with a polymerase chain reaction (PCR) laboratory test that requires two clinic visits about two weeks apart. Of the 3.4 million children under the age of 15 living with HIV worldwide, almost 90% live in sub-Saharan Africa (WHO 2012). In these areas, only 24% of children living with HIV obtain treatment. The remaining untreated children infected with HIV face 50% odds of dying before their second birthday (Newell et al. 2004). This is difficult for pregnant women who lack transportation (Finlayson and Downe 2013) and are insecure about how to get their family's next meal (38–49%) in the context of high rates of HIV stigma (McCoy et al. 2015; Tsai et al. 2012). Only about 25% of MLH complete all of these tasks to prevent mother-to-child transmission (PMTCT) in South Africa (le Roux et al. 2011). Thus, the rate of perinatal infection among women in sub-Saharan Africa women is believed to be about 4%, with a large, region-dependent range (Leach-Lemens 2011). Perinatal infection is claimed to be 2.7% in South Africa (Barron et al. 2012), but we observed a 4.5% rate in the Western Cape, the province with the best healthcare system in the country (le Roux et al. 2014; Rotheram-Borus et al. 2014a, 2016). The rates of HIV are often masked, however, by the high rates of infant mortality. In a trial which included all mothers in an urban township, 9% of the children died by three years of age. Some 30% of those children will be children living with HIV.

Daily life coping with HIV is the context in which families experience the most challenges. Mothers must have strategies to hide her HIV drugs, mask her frequent doctor's appointments, and deal with symptoms of disease that emerge. More than 18 million children have lost at least one parent to AIDS (UNAIDS 2015b). In families whose infants are at risk of becoming infected with HIV due to their mother's HIV, breastfeeding solely for six months is optimal. However, using a simple feeding method is frequently seen as counter to tribes' customs of providing alternative healing medicines, which are given routinely to all newborns by local faith healers. To refuse such ointments and drinks is offensive to the healer and, in conjunction with solely breastfeeding, may raise neighbors' suspicions about their children's HIV disease. Social isolation is one of the hallmarks of HIV infection. It is the mothers and older family members who most fear the social isolation of HIV.

Adolescents

Young children lack the capacity to understand their illness. Most parents do not disclose to children that they are HIV seropositive until the child becomes an adolescent (Sahay 2013). For many children, this is too late, as they have already become sexually active and could have transmitted HIV to their sexual partners. Historically, among HIV epicenters (e.g., San Francisco, Los Angeles, New York) in high-income countries, there are three prototypical scenarios in which adolescents (12–24 years old) become high risk or infected with HIV as described in the case examples below:

> Matthew is 16 years old, living in San Francisco and already knows he's different from other kids his age – he's gay. Matthew is afraid to tell his parents or experiment sexually with anyone from his high school for fear of being found out. Instead, he goes to the Castro District to meet men interested in sexual relationships. After a few visits, Matthew meets an older man who takes him to an upscale apartment and introduces him to a warm and intimate sexual relationship, as well as a range of drugs. The older man promises to take care of Matthew, provides him with drugs regularly, and invites him to move in. After a few months, the older man kicks Matthew out. Now alone and homeless, Matthew becomes addicted to methamphetamines. In time, Matthew finds his way back to his family home and discloses his sexual orientation to his parents but they are not accepting. After two years on his own, Matthew becomes HIV positive.

> Elena, a 14-year-old girl living in Los Angeles is depressed and uncomfortable with the changes in her body. She begins receiving attention from an older male neighbor next door and within weeks, the two begin a sexual relationship. The attention makes her feel desired so she begins to have romantic relationships with boys her own age as well. One of her partners introduces her to marijuana, which he claims enhances the sexual experience. Shortly thereafter, she begins to party in Hollywood, at first only on weekends, but then on a regular basis. The parties become more frequent and more intense, with heavy drinking and experimenting with harder substances. Older men proposition Elena often, and offer to

give her money in exchange for sex, which she uses to buy expensive clothes her family cannot afford. In time, she loses interest in school and her grades drop. Elena only wants to be around friends from her new lifestyle, who she considers her "real friends." She argues with her parents about changes in her behavior at home and school and eventually, decides to run away from home. A month later, she ends up in the Emergency Department with a bad infection; she is tested and has acquired HIV.

Michael is a young man living in the Bronx in New York who grew up without his biological father. His mother remarries but to a man who abuses her. Michael is protective of his mother so he has an extremely contentious relationship with his new stepfather. Without any allowance or means to make money, Michael turns to dealing drugs in hopes of providing him and his mother with the financial independence they need to leave his stepfather. When his stepfather realizes what Michael's up to, he kicks him out of the house. Living on the streets, Michael continues dealing drugs and eventually becomes addicted to heroin himself. Two years later, while detoxing, Michael finds out he is infected with HIV.

In each scenario, the adolescent is left vulnerable, is homeless, and has initiated drug use. They are all much more likely to barter sex as a means of survival in the form of shelter, money, or drugs to quell their habit. In the US, youth living with HIV (YLH) are about 74% male gay, bisexual, or transgender youth (GBTY), 5% heterosexual males, 71% African-American, 15% Latino, and 16% female. Nationally, the percentage of YLH aged 12–24 years has doubled since the year 2000 (CDC 2008, 2011). Among the 62,400 YLH aged 12–24 years, estimates are that only 10–40% know their serostatus (Zanoni and Mayer 2014). The relative risk is twice as high for African-American and Latino GBTY compared to white, non-Hispanic GBTY (CDC 2014). Having a sexual orientation as GBTY is highly stigmatizing (Kaufman and Adolescent Health Committee 2008; Swendeman et al. 2006), and youth are developmentally challenged about who, when, how, and what to disclose about their sexual orientation and HIV status (D'Angelo et al. 2001; Rotheram-Borus and Fernandez 1995).

Homelessness is also highly associated with HIV. Unfortunately, 42% of GBTY's parents eject their children when children disclose being gay, bisexual, or transgender (D'Augelli et al. 1998), resulting in 40% of homeless youth being GBTY (Durso and Gates 2012). Homeless youth (HY) are likely to have psychiatric disorders, have substance abuse problems (usually poly-substances, including alcohol), and have homes with high levels of conflict (sometimes because parents have substance abuse, or mental health problems themselves) (Lightfoot and Rotheram-Borus 2000; Rotheram-Borus et al. 2001a). Bartering sex is a means of survival among homeless youth (Greene et al. 1999; Rice et al. 2013). Oftentimes, ethnic minority youth are already stigmatized for being Black or Latino or poor. Adding the stigma of HIV is then overwhelming. The European Union (EU), African Union (AU), China, New Zealand, and India also reflect this pattern. Thus, risk of HIV comes both from youth's life circumstances, as well as a history of multiple behavioral risks.

Among YLH, only 36% are linked to health care and only 6% are virally suppressed (Zanoni and Mayer 2014). It is imperative that YLH achieve viral suppression in order to reduce the probability of infecting others, as well as increasing the length and quality of their own life. Yet, only 36–62% of YLH who know their serostatus are linked to medical care within 12 months of diagnosis (Hall et al. 2012; Zanoni and Mayer 2014). Young people are also more likely to drop out from care than adults 25 years of age older (Gardner et al. 2005; Hall et al. 2012). Existing studies suggest that few YLH remain in medical care more than a year, ensuring that ARV treatment adherence will also be low [approximately 50% (Fernandez et al. 2015)] (Belzer et al. 1999; Ferrand et al. 2015; Garofalo et al. 2015).

Again, the epidemiology of HIV is substantially different in high-income countries such as the US versus LMIC. In sub-Saharan Africa, about 70% of the epidemic is among women aged 15 or greater (UNICEF 2016). Young women aged 15–23 years old in South Africa have an HIV incidence of 9%, compared to about a 1.2% incidence in same-age male peers. Young women are also far more likely to be identified as YLH than their male peers because if they become pregnant, the girl is automatically tested for HIV, without a separate informed consent. Adolescent girls typically have partners about six years older than themselves and become pregnant with partners to whom they are not married.

The pattern is quite different among young men. Testing rates of adolescent males are typically below 15% in sub-Saharan Africa (Fox et al. 2013), and young men are far less likely to receive health care when ill (Leta et al. 2012). Substance use and abuse among young men is very high. In a recent study by our team in Cape Town, South Africa, most young men in 24 neighborhoods used alcohol in the last week (78%), with 29% of all young men self-reported going to bars on more than ten nights in the last month. Concurrently, 84% reported using marijuana in the last two weeks. These rates were confirmed with biomarkers of recent use (Rotheram-Borus and Tomlinson 2016). Similar to young people in high-income countries, YLH in LMIC face multiple stressors such as having their parents reject them for having acquired HIV, and feeling ashamed, as if the YLH has not lived up to the promise of his ethnic group. Going into an HIV clinic to seek care is also difficult. Typically, there are long lines and the young man will wait in the line outside where all of his friends and neighborhood can see him. However, unlike the youth in high-income countries, almost all youth in LMIC face the following challenges: lifelong unemployment rates of 30–50%, food insecurity, and dislocation from family tribal lands. These stressors emerge in a context in which the rates of interpersonal partner violence are about 25% and up to half of young men experience jail. While the rates of HIV are likely also high among GBTY men in Africa, being GBTY is more highly stigmatized and typically hidden with African men.

Thus, geography is destiny in HIV prevention and treatment. Those infected and affected by HIV are not found at equal rates in every community (AIDSVu 2013). Disparities in HIV are evident from access to ARV, linkage to care, and perinatal transmission, to disease stigma and rates of disclosure.

Intervention Approaches

Almost all EBI for HIV have focused on individuals (CDC 2015), reflecting a Western, largely American and European bias, for the organization of health services and interventions. These interventions emerge from a counseling literature whose roots are in an insight-oriented approach to improving the quality of one's life. This luxury is not useful in communities where 15–40% of the population is infected with HIV and HIV is confounded with large epidemics of tuberculosis (TB), malaria, schistosomiasis, alcoholism, and poverty. Each individual's disease radiates throughout their social networks, affecting families and communities. The solutions and EBI are needed for individuals, families, and communities—with structural interventions likely to have the largest impact on the most people (Blankenship et al. 2006; Rotheram-Borus 2000).

Beginning in 1994, our research group conducted eight randomized controlled trials with families and/or adolescents living with HIV. Table 5.1 summarizes the trials and the major findings from these trials with families living with HIV.

The structure of each of the interventions is similar. However, the trials were mounted in very different contexts and cultures, including the US, Thailand, China, South Africa, and Uganda. There are multiple modules in each of these interventions, with each module addressing a different HIV-related challenge. As noted in the introduction, the major issues are: health, mental health, social relationships, and post-death readjustment.

The specific solution to HIV-related health challenges has shifted dramatically over time. Early in the epidemic, parents living with HIV were primarily managing opportunistic infections in themselves and their children. This evolved to routinely monitoring one's CD4 count, viral load, and adoption of ARV in late-stage disease. In 2011, definitive evidence demonstrated that when ARV treatment reduces viral load to an undetectable level, HIV transmission is prevented (Cohen et al. 2011). Concurrently, another set of studies demonstrated that ARV treatment benefits individuals the most when initiated as soon as detection of HIV occurs (Baeten et al. 2012; Das et al. 2010; Thigpen et al. 2012). Finally, the possibility of a "functional cure" exists, especially if acute infection can be detected and aggressive ARV treatment is instituted during the phase of acute infection (Frange et al. 2015; Persaud and Luzuriaga 2014). Pediatric HIV creates the best opportunity for implementing and testing an HIV functional cure—infants are identified during the first three months of acute infection. Early initiation of treatment of infants with HIV is associated with control of viral reservoir burden and rapid and sustained decreases in viral reservoir burden over time—each is predictive of long-term HIV control (Nielsen-Saines et al. 2012; Persaud et al. 2014). Although demonstration of these functional cures is very rare, early and aggressive ARV treatment during acute infection has been associated with an extended period of complete viral quiescence, also known as HIV drug-free remission.

Some studies suggest HIV reservoirs from adolescents who were recently HIV infected may be more pliable and responsive to early combined ARV than that of

Table 5.1 Summary of studies on evidence-based interventions for families affected by HIV

Reference	Duration	Retention	Outcomes
• **TALC 1: Teens and Adults Learning to Communicate** Randomized controlled study: enhanced care (*n* = 153 parents, 205 adolescents) versus standard care (n = 154 parents, 207 adolescents) Data collected in New York City 1993–1995, followed until 2003, 48% Latino, 36% African-American Randomization worked well; 42% parents died Intervention was three modules: coping with illness; reducing risk; and planning a legacy			
#1	2 years	85% PLH 81.5% adolescents	Intervention adolescents reported significantly lower levels of emotional distress, multiple problem behaviors, conduct problems, and family-related stressors and higher levels of self-esteem than adolescents in the standard care condition. PLH in the intervention condition also reported significantly lower levels of emotional distress and multiple problem behaviors than control parents. Coping style, levels of disclosure regarding serostatus, and formation of legal custody plans were similar across PLH in both intervention conditions
#2	2 years	85% PLH 81.5% adolescents	Adolescents less emotionally distressed, fewer multiple problem behaviors, fewer conduct problems and family stressors than PLH less emotional distress, fewer multiple problem behaviors. No changes in coping, disclosure, custody plans; 13% PLH died
#3	4 years	87% PLH 79% adolescents	Fewer teenage parents, conduct problems tended to be lower than adolescents in the control. Fewer PLH were drug dependent and tended to less often relapse into substance use and use of passive coping lower than the control PLH. There was an erosion of earlier benefits in problem behaviors and emotional distress. 48% PLH died. Fewer adolescents became teenage parents, and conduct problems tended to be lower among intervention compared to control adolescents. Fewer parents were drug dependent and tended to relapse into substance use or use passive coping styles in the intervention compared to the control condition. The time–trend analysis showed that the significant reductions in problem behaviors and emotional distress previously observed over 15–24 months in the intervention condition, then eroded over time, and were nonsignificant at 48 months
#4	6 years	82% PLH 79% adolescents	Grandchildren of PLH reported significantly fewer internalizing and externalizing behavioral symptoms. When PLH/adolescent received an intervention compared to PLH/adolescents without an intervention. 51% PLH died

(continued)

Table 5.1 (continued)

Reference	Duration	Retention	Outcomes
#5	6 years	82% PLH 79% adolescents	Adolescents of PLH had high rates of any lifetime and recent anxiety disorders and post-traumatic stress disorder compared to control adolescents. Lifetime anxiety disorders were significantly associated with older age, baseline emotional distress and prior traumatic exposure, while lifetime depressive disorders were associated with female gender, parental bereavement, and prior traumatic exposure
#6	6 years	82% PLH 79% adolescents	Bereaved adolescents of PLH had significantly more emotional distress, negative life events, and contact with the criminal justice system than non-bereaved adolescents of PLH prior to parental death, though these behaviors did not remain significantly higher after parental death among bereaved compared to non-bereaved adolescents. Depressive symptoms and passive problem solving increased soon after parental death. One year subsequent to parental death, depression and passive problem solving were similar to the levels of non-bereaved peers. Only sexual risk behaviors increased following parental death among adolescents PLH compared to non-bereaved adolescents of PLH
#7	6 years	82% PLH 79% adolescents	Significantly more intervention adolescents were employed or in school, were less likely to receive public welfare payments, less likely to have psychosomatic symptoms, more likely to report better problem-solving and conflict resolution skills in their romantic relationships, expected to have a partner with a good job, and expected to be married when parenting compared to adolescents of PLH in the control condition. Intervention adolescents of PLH reported significantly less substance use three and six years later compared to adolescents of PLH in the control condition. Positive parental bonds reported at baseline reduced emotional distress at three years and increased positive future expectations at six years
• TALC 2: Teens and Adults Learning to Communicate Data collected in 2005–2006 in Los Angeles Randomized controlled trial; 173 MLH and their 289 adolescent children; 166 mothers without HIV; 62% Latino, 32% African-American Follow-up was conducted one time at 18 months			
#8	18 months	78%	Intervention MLH were more likely to monitor their own CD4 cell counts and their children were more likely to decrease alcohol and drug use compared to control condition
#9	18 months	78%	Adolescents in the intervention reported significantly more positive family bonds than control group. Greater participation by MLH predicted fewer family conflicts, and was indirectly associated with less adolescent sexual risk behavior at follow-up assessment
#10	18 months	78%	Less depression in the intervention compared to control

(continued)

Table 5.1 (continued)

Reference	Duration	Retention	Outcomes
• Philani 1: Cluster RCT of Home Visiting Intervention Data collected in 2006–2007 in Cape Town townships in South Africa 788 malnourished children ≤ 6 years old, receiving home visiting or not Intervention (n = 536 households) and control (n = 252 households) Randomization based on the Mentor Mother; Mentor Mothers assigned to neighborhoods are assigned households as interventions or control			
#11	12 months	90%	Children in the intervention condition were rehabilitated at a higher rate and sooner than children in the control condition, with sustained improvement over 12 months
• Philani 2: Cluster RCT of Home Visiting Intervention with randomization within the Mentor Mother's caseload Data collected in 2002–2004; 37 neighborhoods; 100% black households in South African townships 684 mothers with malnourished children; intervention (n = 500); control (n = 184)			
#12	12 months	94%	Malnourished children gained significantly more weight, faster when receiving home visits compared to a control condition, households with malnourished children without home visits
• Philani 3: Cluster RCT of Home Visiting Intervention Data collected in 2009–2010 in 24 neighborhoods; 100% black households in South African townships; 92% follow-up within 2 weeks post-birth Intervention (n = 644 households) and control (n = 594 households) in 12 neighborhoods 1238 pregnant women in 24 matched neighborhoods			
#13	6 months	87%	MLH in the intervention were 50% more likely to complete tasks to prevent vertical transmission, use one feeding method for 6 months, avoid birth-related medical complications, and have infants with healthy height-for-age measurements; were more likely to use condoms consistently, breastfeed exclusively for 6 months, and to have infants with healthier height-for-age measurements than MLH in the control condition
#14	6 months	87%	Improved infant growth among depressed intervention mothers compared to infants of antenatally depressed mothers in the control condition
#15	18 months	88%	Home visits enhance maternal/child health outcomes; including child growth and outcomes to prevent mother to child transmission
#16	18 months	89%	Significantly lower number of diarrhea episodes, increased rates and longer duration of breastfeeding; better infant growth patterns in the intervention compared to the control

(continued)

Table 5.1 (continued)

Reference	Duration	Retention	Outcomes
#17	36 months	87%	Mothers were less depressed, children less likely to be stunted, to have better vocabularies, less likely to be hospitalized compared to control mothers and children
#18	36 months	85%	Mothers less likely to have mental health symptoms in the intervention compared to control; alcohol and partner violence highly consistent over time and linked to depression
• **Masihambisane: Peer Mentor Interventions in Clinics** Data collected in 2008–2009; 100% black Africans in KwaZulu-Natal, South Africa 1200 black MLH attending 9 clinics; 5 intervention (n = 600 MLH) and 4 control clinics (n = 600 mothers)			
#19	6 months	89%	MLH were more likely to complete parent mother to child transmission tasks, use one feeding method for 6 months, avoid birth-related medical complications, and have infants with healthy height-for-age measurements. Mothers were more likely to use condoms consistently, breastfeed exclusively for 6 months, and have infants with healthy height-for-age measurements
#20	12 months	57%	MLH reported significantly fewer depressive symptoms of depression, fewer underweight infants, more likely to use one feeding method for six months and exclusively breastfeed their infants for at least 6 months in clinic-based intervention compared to a control condition
• **Family-2-Family: Intervention for Persons living with HIV and their Family Members** Data collected in 2007–2009 in Thailand in 4 district hospitals in Chang Rai and Korat (rural settings); Follow-up at 6, 12, 18, and 24 months 505 persons living with HIV and their families and 308 control adults and their families			
#21	24 months	88%	Intervention group reported significantly improved quality of life compared to the control condition
• **TEA 1** Intervention to decrease depressive symptoms and improve social support Data collection in 2009–2010 in Anhui Province, China 3-level intervention: gathering, time, and garden 79 families (88 PLH and 79 family members), intervention (n = 38) and control (n = 41)			
#22	6 months	94%	PLH and family members in intervention reported significant improvement in depressive symptoms, social support and family functioning compared to those in the control group

(continued)

Table 5.1 (continued)

Reference	Duration	Retention	Outcomes
• TEA 2 Intervention to access children's outcomes Data collection: 2009–2010 in Anhui Province, China 3-level intervention: gathering, time, and garden 79 families (88 PLH and 79 family members), intervention (n = 38) and control (n = 41)			
#23	3 and 6 months	100%	Some intervention effects related to children's psychological measures accompanied by the improvement in mental health of PLH and family members was observed
• TLC: Together Learning Choices Data collected in 1994–1999 at adolescent medical clinics- and community-based agencies in Los Angeles, New York City, San Francisco, Miami 37% Latino; 27% African-American Intervention (n = 208) and control (n = 102); adolescents age 13–29 years Three modules: reducing risk; promoting health; improving quality of life			
#24	15 months	70%	Significant reductions in abuse of multiple substances over time in the intervention compared to the control
#25	21 months	70%	Number of positive lifestyle changes and active coping styles increased. Social support coping also increased significantly. Fewer unprotected sexual acts, 45% fewer sexual partners, 50% fewer HIV-negative sexual partners, and 31% less substance use, on a weighted index, than those in the control condition
#26	21 months	70%	YLH in the Immediate Intervention Condition were significantly less emotionally distressed on multiple indices and decreased emotional distress even when controlling for HIV symptomatology than those in the control condition
• CLEAR: Choosing Life: Empowerment, Actions, Results, HIV Prevention and Health Promotion Intervention Data collection in 1999–2002 in Los Angeles, New York City, San Francisco; 42% Latino; 26% African-American; 23% white Telephone intervention (n = 59); individual intervention (n = 61); control delayed intervention (n = 55); Follow-up rates were at 3 months: 56, 78, and 86% 175 HIV + teens and YLH (age 13–29 years)			
#27	15 months	82%	Intervention YLH tended to have fewer sexual partners, used fewer drugs, reported less emotional distress and decrease in their use of antiretroviral therapies

(continued)

Table 5.1 (continued)

Reference	Duration	Retention	Outcomes
#28	15 months	82%	Percentage of protected sex was moderated by ethnicity, use of antiretroviral medications (ARV), healthcare utilization and mental health. Number of partners was moderated by anxiety and depression. When deciding if an intervention is appropriate and beneficial for an individual young person, consideration must be given to type of services the adolescents currently accesses and the adolescents mental health
#29	15 months	82%	Drug Abuse decreased significantly in the intervention compared to the control
#30	15 months	82%	Significant reductions in drug abuse of multiple substances over time in the intervention compared to the control
• **Efficacy of a Culturally Adapted HIV Intervention for YLH** Data collected in 2003–2004, 100% black Africans in Kampala, Uganda Intervention (n = 50) and control (n = 50) 18 session intervention in 3 modules: 6 sessions resilience, 6 sessions medical, and 6 sessions mental health			
#31	3 months	90%	Significantly more YLH used condoms consistently and decreased their number of sexual partners in the intervention compared to the control condition
• **Healthy Living Project, a multi-institutional collaborative research project** Data collected in 2000–2001, 1270 PLH in Los Angeles, Milwaukee, New York City, San Francisco; Follow-up rates: 86% at 5 months, 82% at 10 months, 81% at 15 months, 76% at 20 months Individual (n = 467); control (n = 489) 15 sessions: 5 risky behaviors, 5 medical adherence, and 5 mental health			
#32	25 months	77% 25 months	Intervention PLH reduced unprotected sexual intercourse with HIV-negative or unknown status partners, reduced substance use and depression and improved the quality of life compared to the control condition
#33	25 months	90%	Significantly greater reductions in unprotected risky sexual acts, the number of sexual partners of HIV-negative or unknown serostatus, alcohol or marijuana use, and hard drug use among the intervention group than among the control group. Intervention versus control of PLH homeless during the 25 months follow-up period
#34	25 months	77%	Reduced drug abuse risk acts among intervention compared to standard care

(continued)

Table 5.1 (continued)

Reference	Duration	Retention	Outcomes
• **Intervention to assist Health Care workers and Researchers working with PLH, MD for Life in Primary Health Care** Data collected in 2001–2003 in Los Angeles Motivational interviewing (n = 209), computerized delivery in waiting room (n = 325), motivational interviewing by physical control (n = 229) 529 healthcare workers and researchers			
#35	30 months	69%	PLH in the computerized delivery condition reported a significant decrease in the number of HIV–/unknown sexual partners and unprotected sex acts compared with the provider delivered motivational interviewing compared

MLH—mothers living with HIV; *PLH*—persons living with HIV; *YLH*—youth living with HIV

#1 **TALC 1** Family-Based Processes Associated with Adolescent Distress, Substance Use and Risky Sexual Behavior in Families Affected by Maternal HIV (Journal of Clinical Child & Adolescent Psychology), Lester, P., Stein, J. A., Bursch, B., Rice, E., Green, S., Penniman, T., & Rotheram-Borus, M. J. (2010)

#2 **TALC 1** An Intervention for Parents with AIDS and Their Adolescent Children (American Journal of Public Health), Rotheram-Borus, M. J., Lee, M. B., Gwadz, M., & Draimin, B. (2001)

#3 **TALC 1** Four-year behavioral outcomes of an intervention for parents living with HIV and their adolescent children (AIDS), Rotheram-Borus, M.J., Lee, M., Leonard, N., Lin, Y.Y., Franzke, L., Turner, E., Lightfoot, M. & Gwadz, M. (2003)

#4 **TALC 1** Intergenerational Benefits of Family-Based HIV Interventions (Journal of Consulting and Clinical Psychology Rotheram-Borus, M.J., Lester, P., Song, J., Lin, Y.Y., Leonard, N.R., Beckwith, L., Ward, M.J., Sigman, M. & Lord, L. (2006)

#5 **TALC 1** Adolescent Adjustment over Six Years in HIV-Affected Families (Journal of Adolescent Health), Rotheram-Borus, M. J., Stein, J. A., & Lester, P. (2006)

#6 **TALC 1** Adolescent Adjustment Before and After HIV-Related Parental Death (Journal of Consulting and Clinical Psychology), Rotheram-Borus, M. J., Weiss, R., Alber, S., & Lester, P. (2005)

#7 **TALC 1** Six-Year Intervention Outcomes for Adolescent Children of Parents with HIV (Archives of Pediatrics & Adolescent Medicine), Rotheram-Borus, M. J., Lee, M., Lin, Y. Y., & Lester, P. (2004)

#8 **TALC 2** Intervention outcomes among HIV-affected families over 18 months (AIDS and Behavior), Rotheram-Borus, M. J., Rice, E., Comulada, W. S., Best, K., Elia, C., Peters, K., Li, L., Green, S.and Valladares, E, E. (2012)

#9 **TALC 2** Intervening on conflict, parental bonds, and sexual risk acts among adolescent children of mothers living with HIV (MLH) (PLoS One), Rotheram-Borus, M. J., Stein, J. A., & Rice, E. (2014)

#10 **TALC 2** Rates and predictors of anxiety and depressive disorders in adolescents of parents with HIV (Vulnerable Children and Youth Services), Lester, P., Jane Rotheram-Borus, M., Lee, S. J., Comulada, S., Cantwell, S., Wu, N., & Ying Lin, Y. (2006)

#11 **Philani Intervention Program 1** Home visits by Mentor Mothers provide recovery from childhood malnutrition (Nutrition Journal) le Roux, I. M., le Roux, K., Comulada, W. S., Greco, E. M., Desmond, K. A., Mbewu, N., & Rotheram-Borus, M. J. (2010)

#12 **Philani Intervention Program 2** Home visits by neighborhood mentor mothers to improve children's nutrition in South Africa (Vulnerable Children), le Roux, I. M., le Roux, K., Mbeutu, K., Comulada, W. S., Desmond, K. A., & Rotheram-Borus, M. J. (2011)

#13 **Philani Intervention Program 3** Outcomes of home visits for pregnant mothers and their infants: a cluster randomized controlled trial (AIDS), le Roux, I. M., Tomlinson, M., Harwood, J.M., O'Connor, M.J., Worthman, C.M., Mbewu, N., Stewart, J., Hartley, M., Swendeman, D., Comulada, W.S. & Weiss, R.E. (2013)

#14 Community health workers improve child growth of antenatally-depressed mothers, 6. months (BMC Psychiatry), Tomlinson, M., Rotheram-Borus, M. J., Harwood, J., le Roux, I. M., O'Connor, M., & Worthman, C. (2015)

#15 A cluster randomized controlled effectiveness trial evaluating perinatal home visits (PLOS ONE), Rotheram-Borus, M.J., Tomlinson, M., Le Roux, I.M., Harwood, J.M., Comulada, S., O'Connor, M.J., Weiss, R.E. & Worthman, C.M. (2014)

#16 The impact of paraprofessional home visitors on infants' growth and health at 18 months (Vulnerable Children), e Roux, I. M., Rotheram-Borus, M. J., Stein, J., & Tomlinson, M. (2014)

#17 36 Month Outcomes of a Generalist Paraprofessional Perinatal Home Visiting Intervention in South Africa (Prevention Science), Tomlinson, M., Rotheram-Borus, M.J., Le Roux, I, Youssef, M., Nelson, S.H., Scheffler, A., Weiss, R.E., O'Connor, M., Worthman, C.M. (2016)

#18 Alcohol use partner violence and mental distress, 3 years post-birth (American Journal of Preventative Medicine), Rotheram-Borus, M. J., Tomlinson, M., Le Roux, I., & Stein, J. A. (2015)

#19 **MASI** A cluster randomized controlled trial evaluating the efficacy of peer mentors to support South African women living with HIV and their infants (PLOS ONE), Rotheram-Borus, M.J., Richter, L., van Heerden, A., van Rooyen, H., Tomlinson, M., Harwood, J.M., Comulada, W.S., & Stein, A. (2014)

#20 **MASI** Peer mentors to improve outcomes for pregnant mothers living with HIV (Trials), Rotheram-Borus, M.J., Richter, L., Van Rooyen, H., van Heerden, A., Tomlinson, M., Stein, A., Rochat, T., de Kadt, J., Mtungwa, N., Mkhize, L. & Ndlovu, L. (2011)

#21 **F2F** Efficacy of an Intervention for Families Living with HIV in Thailand: A Randomized Control Trial (AIDS & Behavior), Li, L., Liang, L. J., Lee, S. J., Iamsirithaworn, S., Wan, D., & Rotheram-Borus, M. J. (2012)

#22 **TEA** A multilevel intervention for HIV-affected families in China: Together for Empowerment Activities (Social Science & Medicine), Li, L., Ji, G., Liang, L. J., Ding, Y., Tian, J., & Xiao, Y. (2011)

#23 Effect of a Family Intervention on Psychological Outcomes of Children Affected by Parental HIV (AIDS & Behavior), Li, L., Liang, L. J., Ji, G., Wu, J., & Xiao, Y. (2014)

#24 **TLC** Reductions in Drug Use Among Young People Living with HIV (The American Journal of Drug and Alcohol Abuse), Scott Comulada, W., Weiss, R. E., Cumberland, W., & Rotheram-Borus, M. J. (2007)

#25 **TLC** Efficacy of a Preventive Intervention for Youths Living With HIV (American Journal of Public Health), Rotheram-Borus, M.J., Lee, M.B., Murphy, D.A., Futterman, D., Duan, N., Birnbaum, J.M., Lightfoot, M. & Teens Linked to Care Consortium (2001)

#26 **TLC** Improving the quality of life among young people living with HIV (Evaluation and Program Planning), Rotheram-Borus, M.J., Murphy, D.A., Wight, R.G., Lee, M.B., Lightfoot, M., Swendeman, D., Birnbaum, J.M. & Wright, W. (2001)

#27 **CLEAR** Prevention for Substance-Using HIV-Positive Young People Telephone and In-Person Delivery (JAIDS), Rotheram-Borus, M.J., Swendeman, D., Comulada, W.S., Weiss, R.E., Lee, M. & Lightfoot, M. (2004)

#28 **CLEAR:** Who Benefited from an Efficacious Intervention for Youth Living with HIV: A Moderator Analysis (AIDS & Behavior), Lightfoot, M., Tevendale, H., Comulada, W.S. & Rotheram-Borus, M.J. (2007)

#29 **CLEAR:** An HIV-Preventive Intervention for Youth Living With HIV (Behavior Modification), Lightfoot, M., Rotheram-Borus, M. J., & Tevendale, H. (2007)

#30 Reductions in drug use among young people living with HIV (American Journal of Drug and Alcohol Abuse), Scott Comulada, W., Weiss, R. E., Cumberland, W., & Rotheram-Borus, M. J. (2007)

#31 **SUIBI** Efficacy of a Culturally Adapted Intervention for Youth Living with HIV in Uganda (Prevention Science), Lightfoot, M. A., Kasirye, R., Comulada, W. S., & Rotheram-Borus, M. J. (2007)

#32 **Healthy Living** Randomized Controlled Trial of a Cognitive-Behavioral Intervention for HIV-Positive Persons: An Investigation of Treatment Effects on Psychosocial Adjustment (AIDS & Behavior), Carrico, A. W., Chesney, M. A., Johnson, M. O., Morin, S. F., Neilands, T. B., Remien, R. H., Rotheram-Borus, M. J., Wong, F. L. and NIMH Healthy Living Project Team (2009)

#33 **Healthy Living** Reducing Risky Sexual Behavior and Substance Use Among Currently and Formerly Homeless Adults Living With HIV (American Journal of public Health), Rotheram-Borus, M. J., Desmond, K., Comulada, W. S., Arnold, E. M., & Johnson, M. (2009)

#34 **Healthy Living** Effects of behavioral intervention on substance use among people living with HIV: the Healthy Living Project randomized controlled study (ADDICTION), Wong, F. L., Rotheram-Borus, M. J., Lightfoot, M., Pequegnat, W., Comulada, W. S., Cumberland, W., Weinhardt, L. S., Remien, R. H., Chesney, M. & Johnson, M. (2008)

#35 **MD for Life** Efficacy of Brief Interventions in Clinical Care Settings for Persons Living With HIV (JAIDS), Lightfoot, M., Rotheram-Borus, M. J., Comulada, W. S., Reddy, V. S., & Duan, N. (2010)

adults (Bryson 1996; Persaud and Luzuriaga 2014). This research team is mounting a trial to evaluate whether the viral reservoirs of adolescents can remain low, by identifying adolescents who are acutely infected (i.e., during the first three months of infection). The possibility of treating infants infected by HIV and adolescents during early infection, in particular, and the findings about long-term disease control, and quality and length of life when treatment is initiated means the health challenges are now focused on the HIV treatment continuum (HIV testing and early detection, linkage and retention in care, and consistent and lifelong adherence to ARV).

Again, the concept of an HIV treatment continuum focuses on individuals, not families. Neither infants nor adolescents will initiate or sustain health care and adherence to ARV without family support and community structures which will facilitate easily accessible, attractive, and consistent health regimens. Reports of pediatric adherence to ARV are based primarily on caretaker self-report and are highly variable (Vreeman et al. 2008). On average, studies from LMIC report greater than 75% adherence to pediatric ARV, while high-income countries report around 55% (Vreeman et al. 2008). LMIC perceive access to ARV as a real gift. In high-income countries, for example the US, it may be that patients are clear that missing one appointment only means rescheduling for a more convenient time for yourself, not a threat to have no more access to ARV.

In 2013, only 24% of children under the age of 14 living with HIV accessed ARV (UNAIDS 2014b). Pediatric treatment coverage is especially low in sub-Saharan Africa, extending to only 22% of children living with HIV (UNAIDS 2014b). Unfortunately, in the US, the mothers who become infected are often those who have the hardest time adhering to the optimal infant health regimens. Mothers who become infected are much more likely to be chronically homeless or to have unstable living situations with partners who are substance abusers or to have psychiatric disorders themselves.

Concurrently, many pediatric HIV cases in LMIC are AIDS orphans. Almost 18 million children have been orphaned by AIDS globally and, depending on the country, up to 12% of these AIDS orphans are themselves infected (UNAIDS 2015b). While the percentage of AIDS orphans is expected to decrease over time, currently there are many pediatrically infected children being taken care of by relatives or in orphanages. Especially in the LMIC with the highest prevalence of HIV, so many family members have died that there remain few or no family members to care for a child. In these settings, stigmatization of the child is much more prevalent, as their HIV status will be apparent to all caretakers and, likely, to their peers.

Among adolescents, the rates of ARV adherence are typically lower than among adults (Agwu et al. 2012; Kahana et al. 2015), and youth are 50% less likely to receive any care, for prevention or treatment of disease (Szilagyi 1998; Tsai et al. 2014). To be retained in care and to adhere on a regular basis to ARV medications lifelong is difficult. Innovations resulting in fewer pills being taken over longer periods of time will reduce patient burden: this is a high-priority HIV research agenda at the National Institutes of Health. Furthermore, these results increase the drive to identify HIV-seropositive persons early, to link and retain these persons in HIV care and to consistently have ARV medications delivered to the person in a timely manner (Grossman et al. 2013). Structural impediments to adherence are common, especially in LMIC. For example, in Africa, clinics and hospitals, especially in rural areas can go for periods of months without having sufficient ARV medications to serve the patients in need of treatment. This is particularly problematic for young children. The most affected countries (e.g., South Africa) prioritize maintaining drugs for infants and children over all other populations. Yet, the gap between intentions and action are substantial.

Another major challenge among adolescents is reducing the probability of transmitting to others, as most adolescents initiate sexual relationships during this developmental period (Finer and Philbin 2013). If adolescents achieve an undetectable viral load, protection by condoms or an additional protective strategy becomes unnecessary—transmission is rare with an undetectable viral load, while superinfection, the acquisition of multiple strains of HIV, was a worry early in the epidemic (Hemelaar 2012); there are only a very limited number of cases documenting superinfection, and controversy surrounds elevated consequences of having multiple viral strains (Smith et al. 2005). Thus, the best protection strategy for stopping transmission is now adherence to ARV.

The mental health challenges associated with HIV remain and are similar in both LMIC and high-income countries. Depression, alcohol, and drug abuse have consistently been found to be higher among YLH, as well as parents living with HIV (Parsons et al. 2008; Rotheram-Borus et al. 1999b). Rates of depression have repeatedly been documented of about 30% (le Roux et al. 2013; Rotheram-Borus et al. 2015a). Generally, MLH are far less likely to be effective parents, especially for children whose health is compromised by HIV (Murphy et al. 2010). Depressed MLH are even less likely to adhere to the tasks to prevent mother-to-child transmission (Tomlinson et al. 2015). Infant growth is slower (both height and weight), and children are more likely to be hospitalized when parents are living with HIV (Rotheram-Borus et al. 2016). Adolescents are also far less likely to remain adherent to ARV when depressed (Murphy et al. 2001) and when abusing drugs and alcohol frequently (Lightfoot and Rotheram-Borus 2000; Parsons et al. 2008). Thus, to reduce both perinatal and adolescent HIV transmission, treatment of mental health problems is a central need.

There have been multiple interventions with adults living with HIV that reduce depression among persons infected with HIV (Crepaz et al. 2014; Gonzalez et al. 2011; Sikkema et al. 2015). In our studies in South Africa with pregnant mothers living with HIV (Rotheram-Borus et al. 2011a; Rotheram-Borus et al. 2015b; Tomlinson et al. 2015) and among adolescent mothers living with HIV in rural South Africa (K. le Roux, in submission), there have been significant reductions in depression with visits from paraprofessional home visitors (Mentor Mothers) who are trained to support positive events and goal setting in the lives of pregnant women and new mothers, to encourage problem solving of daily hassles and relationships with partners and children, and to form a strong bond with the mothers in the community. The benefits accrue to seropositive mothers, as well as improving the parenting of depressed mothers.

In addition, substance abuse treatment improves adherence to ARV (Binford et al. 2012). When delivering interventions to families affected by HIV in the US historically, almost all had been heavily involved in drug abuse subcultures prior to learning that they were living with HIV. Learning that they might die, and in 1994 the time to death was expected to be 14.9 months (Rotheram-Borus et al. 2001a, b), these parents dramatically reduced their substance abuse. Becoming seropositive provided a wake-up call that led to living a higher quality of life. However, there is a small subset of mothers living with HIV in the US who continue to engage in poly-substance use throughout pregnancy and their children's early years. These women typically began sexual activity by the age of 12.5 years, are psychiatrically disturbed with major disorders, and have substantial challenges parenting young children. The two cases of seropositive infants who demonstrated prolonged control over HIV were born to two such mothers. These infants for whom a functional cure of HIV was hypothesized (Mississippi and Los Angeles) were observed only because their mothers had not adhered to their infant's or their own health (Morin 2014; National Institute of Allergy and Infectious Disease 2014). The mothers were only identified as seropositive at childbirth; the two infants had been treated aggressively with ARV for a few months; mothers became unstable and no longer sought or adhered to health care for several years; but the infants demonstrated excellent viral control and small viral reservoirs when re-identified at about two years of age.

In sub-Saharan Africa, living in a high prevalence neighborhood means that even one sexual partner has a relatively high probability of transmission. Women are far less likely to use alcohol or drugs than are men, especially in rural settings where access is typically limited to home brew. Among pregnant women, a one-session meeting is typically sufficient to significantly and substantially reduce alcohol use among pregnant women. We have found that it actually takes about five years post-birth for mothers to reinitiate alcohol use at the levels reported prior to pregnancy. Having home visits by a Mentor Mother can reduce use of alcohol for five years—an unexpected finding.

Among parents living with HIV, stigma, isolation, concerns about their children and a fear of premature death are major impediments to caretaking (Hackl et al. 1997). Children in families affected by HIV experience heightened stress, frequently demonstrate problem behaviors, and are less likely to successfully achieve their timely developmental milestones (Rotheram-Borus et al. 2012a). Both parent's and children's diagnoses are often kept secret from family and community members because of fear of discrimination. Fear of stigma prevents parents with HIV from reaching out to their friends and neighbors for assistance and encourages negative coping mechanisms, such as denial, hiding their health issues, and isolation (Hackl et al. 1997).

Stigma appears to be a much greater problem today in LMIC than in high-income countries (UNAIDS 2013). It is easier to hide one's healthcare treatment in the large urban settings in the US or EU. It is even easier now that HIV care is increasingly mainstreamed into primary healthcare settings.

In LMIC, HIV remains vertically integrated, that is, HIV testing sites and treatment centers are stand-alone clinics. This means anyone entering the clinic is going to be identified as seropositive. In one study, stigma, in particular, led 62% of 354 mothers living with HIV to take three years post-birth to reinitiate HIV treatment (Rotheram-Borus et al. 2015a). Mothers also hide their baby's illnesses from their families, often sending their children to grandparents, out of their partner's and neighbors' sight. Children who are placed with extended family members are those most likely to harmfully use mixed breastfeeding methods in order to maintain traditional feeding customs (Li et al. 2006; Rotheram-Borus et al. 2011b). Thus, stigma and discrimination grossly undermine effective prevention and intervention outcomes for families and leave children confused as to why they are mistreated by neighbors or peers (Ji et al. 2007). Any plans to improve outcomes require that community stigma be reduced to improve pediatric and family outcomes.

Another major set of challenges is in the area of social relationships. Sexual relationships among people infected with HIV are far more complex. Having an undetectable viral load offers the possibility of not needing to disclose one's serostatus while still protecting one's sexual partners from HIV. Today, in the US, at best 70% of parents living with HIV have undetectable viral loads. The percentage varies substantially by community. In Los Angeles, the rate appears to be about 40%, while San Francisco reports 75% viral suppression. In order to be virally suppressed, parents and adolescents with HIV must remain linked to care lifelong and take ARV consistently. In high-income countries, viral load testing can be easily obtained, but in a LMIC parents are only likely to get tested once a year (even when adhering to all medical regimens). Thus, knowing whether you are likely to transmit HIV is an unpredictable process in LMIC.

Those who do disclose their serostatus to partners have fewer mental health problems. In more than 63 countries, non-disclosure has been criminalized (UNAIDS 2012). Withholding the knowledge of being seropositive from a sexual partner can result in jail time. Yet, lifelong condom use is not attractive nor acceptable to either men or women, even if social acceptability leads persons to state they use condoms consistently. Serosorting is a strategy that has been advocated for GBTY since the early 1980s, but only among seropositive men (Smit et al. 2012). This means that two seropositive adults abandon condom use within their relationship. While this strategy has been seen as highly acceptable in high-income countries, this has not been a strategy ever stated in LMIC. All seropositive persons in LMIC are encouraged and told that lifelong condom use is the only protection strategy. The origins of this double standard are not clear. Because most adolescents in high-income countries and LMIC do not know their serostatus, serosorting is not a viable strategy for adolescents.

Delivery Sites

Throughout the discussion of interventions below, we have chosen to call paraprofessional community health workers, Mentor Mothers. Mentor Mothers have been used in clinics, for home visits, in recreational, school, and community sites throughout multiple interventions in South Africa and Los Angeles.

High-income countries have usually organized care delivery at health centers. Babies are treated in different clinics from their mothers, and adolescents are treated at adolescent medicine clinics, which will not serve other family members. The organization of care is for individuals, not families. In the US, almost all HIV is in urban centers, so that transportation and housing are sometimes available for families living with HIV. Most major HIV epicenters have residential group homes for YLH, as many are GBTY who have been ejected from their families or are chronically homeless. For example, in New York City, Housing Works serves 400 persons living with HIV, mostly young people. Larkin Street in San Francisco has also had a residential program for YLH since the late 1990s. One challenge with this type of care is the location of the services. Larkin Street is in the center of one of the neighborhoods with the highest HIV rates in San Francisco. The neighborhood also has the highest rate of substance abuse. When the Larkin Street residential program was new (Kennedy et al. 2000), we found that getting residential services was associated with substantial increases in serious drug use. The Tenderloin District has multiple medical marijuana dispensaries, and being seropositive qualified a YLH for medical marijuana. With unlimited marijuana, YLH could "trade up" for a consistent supply of more serious drugs. These are common challenges when health care is localized in high-risk neighborhoods.

Unfortunately, similar challenges occur in LMIC, especially in sub-Saharan Africa, the region most affected by HIV. Clinic-based services are likely to successfully engage from 30–50% of MLH (Rotheram-Borus et al. 2011c). Even when attempting to reorganize referral processes so that each seropositive pregnant mother is identified and linked to a supportive paraprofessional, linkage is not typically achieved. Peer support is an important strategy for improving health outcomes for HIV, malnutrition, and diabetes (Fisher et al. 2012; le Roux et al. 2011; Rotheram-Borus et al. 2011c). Peer support not only improves health outcomes, but has the advantage of allowing tasks to be shifted from healthcare professionals to paraprofessionals (WHO 2007). With the number of healthcare personnel available in LMIC unlikely to be sufficient to address HIV until the year 2050 (Samb et al. 2007), task-shifting to paraprofessionals may critically support MLH to cope with their HIV-related stressors.

Peer support programs have been broadly diffused throughout Africa. For example, the Mothers-2-Mothers Programme has linked MLH to newly diagnosed HIV-positive (+) Peer Mentors to prevent mother-to-child transmission throughout 717 sites across 11 countries (Futterman et al. 2010; Mothers2Mothers 2011; Teasdale and Besser 2008). We have examined the benefits of having clinic-based HIV + Peer Mentors on post-birth outcomes of MLH and their infants

(Richter et al. 2014; Rotheram-Borus et al. 2014a). To evaluate efficacy, we randomly assigned pregnant South African women by clinic to either a usual care or an enhanced care condition, in which peers who were living with HIV delivered a preventive intervention over eight meetings. MLH attended an average of four sessions; yet, even with aggressive outreach, 13% did not attend any sessions. MLH in the enhanced care reported significantly fewer depressive symptoms over time than MLH in the standard care condition. Compared to usual care, MLH in the enhanced care clinics were more likely to have infants who were longer and less likely to be malnourished (i.e., >2 SD below World Health Organization [WHO] guidelines for weight by age). MLH in the enhanced care were also more likely to use one feeding method for six months, requested their sexual partners to be tested for HIV more often, stopped using alcohol and drugs, and had larger social networks that they accessed more frequently over time compared to MLH in the usual care condition. However, there were no differences in healthcare adherence, acts to stop partner transmission, HIV disclosure, or self-reported stress.

While we were able to get uptake by 87% of mothers in the enhanced care condition at clinics, only half of MLH attended eight meetings. These MLH faced many barriers to attending interventions, especially in rural settings, which reflects more than 50% of sub-Saharan Africa. The clinics in LMIC are often large and require arriving by about 6 a.m. in order to enter a long que that will take all day to navigate. Each action needed on one day: getting physically evaluated, going through a program to prepare patients to consistently take medications, and actually receiving the medications—requires waiting in three separate lines.

Therefore, home visit by local women, who we called Mentor Mothers, was a second delivery strategy that we used in South Africa to improve MLH's consistent engagement in HIV care for their families. Demonstrating effective implementation strategies is particularly important for home visiting. Perinatal nurse home visiting is highly efficacious (Olds et al. 1988, 2002, 2014), even when mounted in LMIC within a randomized controlled trial (RCT) (Abbatt 2005; Aracena et al. 2009; Campbell and Scott 2011; Gardner et al. 2005; le Roux et al. 2013; Lewin et al. 2010; Nahar et al. 2012; Peacock et al. 2013; Rahman et al. 2009; Rotheram-Borus et al. 2014a; Sweet and Appelbaum 2004; Swider 2002; Tomlinson et al. 2015; Walker et al. 1991). Yet, when scaling these programs, efficacy disappears (Peacock et al. 2013). Why efficacy disappears is unknown. It could be insufficient management structures, a lack of control of resources, or a graft when large programs mount. The potential reasons for a failure to scale are many. When nurses visit pregnant and new mothers, there are benefits that have been demonstrated to persist for up to 20 years (Olds et al. 2014). Children do better in school, have fewer behavioral problems, are less likely to use drugs, or be arrested and detained in the criminal justice system in the US (Olds et al. 1998). The professional staff needed to implement perinatal HIV care globally will be insufficient until at least the year 2050 (Michalopoulos et al. 2015; National Scientific Council on the Developing Child 2007), let alone to also meet the demand for healthcare support with the emerging pandemic of non-communicable diseases (Singh and Sachs 2013; World Health Organization

African Region 2011). Therefore, task-shifting to paraprofessionals is needed (Patel et al. 2011).

The paraprofessional Mentor Mothers used in our interventions are typically local women who have never held previous jobs, have less than a high school education, and may or may not receive a stipend; supervision is often sparse or nonexistent. The paraprofessional Mentor Mother is typically trained to address one issue with information transfer only, not skill based. We implemented home visiting in Cape Town, South Africa, townships. Our implementation differed from usual practice by having multiple outcomes, selecting home visitors who were positive peer deviants (local role models), who were trained in cognitive behavior skills, rather than being taught to replicate a manual with fidelity, and who were monitored daily with mobile phone reports of their implementation (Rotheram-Borus et al. 2014b). Mentor Mothers were routinely accountable in our intervention to supervisors.

Our project, the Philani Intervention Model (le Roux et al. 2010), was another one of the successful programs in LMIC (Peacock et al. 2013). We conducted a cluster RCT of all pregnant women in 24 neighborhoods in the Cape Town townships, with random assignment based on neighborhood. We found benefits for mothers and children over 60 months. On average, Mentor Mothers visited households about 11 times through pregnancy and the first six months of life for about 31 min each visit. Compared to women not receiving home visits, women visited by Mentor Mothers used alcohol significantly less often in pregnancy, adhered to 50% more of the tasks to PMTCT, and had fewer infants with low birth weight. At six months, MLH were more likely to get their children tested for HIV and to administer an ARV, as well as to use condoms more often with their partner and to ask the partners to test for HIV. Mothers visited by Mentor Mothers were likely to breastfeed longer, with a higher percentage breastfeeding for six months. Infants in the intervention group had better growth. In particular, antenatally depressed mothers were significantly more likely to have babies that were similar in growth to non-depressed mothers, when visited by Mentor Mothers. These earlier benefits were sustained at 18 months with home visits associated with higher infant IQ on the Bayley Infant Scales and better growth measures (height, weight, weight/height, z-scores <2SD). At three years of age, mothers in the intervention were less depressed than mothers without home visits and their children had larger vocabularies, fewer child hospitalizations, less stunting, and more prosocial behaviors. Mothers in the intervention group were also far less likely to use alcohol five years past birth than mothers without home visits.

Another strategy is to have drop-in or scheduled small group or community meetings (typically not in the neighborhood in which the family with HIV lives). This is the strategy used in Project Teens & Adults Learning to Communicate (TALC) in New York City, Los Angeles, Korat and Chang Rai in Thailand, and in rural China. The initial Project TALC in New York City demonstrates the importance of designing scalable interventions from the conceptualization of an intervention. We designed a 24-session intervention that was not a scalable design. No parent with AIDS wanted to meet peers in their own neighborhood; therefore, we had to find a centralized delivery site and paid $55 for cab rides to this centralized site. Because of this cost, we delivered two intervention sessions back-to-back, with a meal in between. At a centralized site in Manhattan, mothers with AIDS and their children came on Saturdays from the Bronx, Staten Island, and Brooklyn. Most mothers were too ill and had too many small children to easily take the subway, so families were provided with a taxi ride and met for 7.5 h, with breakfast and lunch shared as unstructured sharing time. Two group meetings were held daily, sometimes only among parents, sometimes only among children, and sometimes in mixed age groups. The results were substantial over six years—as the problems were substantial and pervaded the lives of the families at the beginning of the trial. Both parents and their children got healthier. Parents gave up substance abuse, were less depressed and anxious, and became better parents. Adolescent children were less likely to initiate sex, had fewer sexual partners, had fewer babies, were less depressed, and were more likely to remain in school or to be employed. The grandchildren of the original parents with AIDS were found to be better adjusted six years following the intervention. These improvements were remarkable.

However, in Los Angeles, MLH were not drug abusers, did not have multiple partners, but were good mothers. They were undocumented and, therefore, kept out of many mainstream activities. However, the lives of MLH and their children were basically healthy. Among this group, the impact of the intervention among Latina MLH was far less dramatic. As the medications, clinical care, and access to ARV treatments have improved globally, the current model of preventive interventions has had their impact mainly on improving the quality of life, rather than on reducing the kinds of risks that result in new HIV infections and early death.

After the initial family interventions were delivered in the US, culturally tailored programs were designed for Asian and African countries. Tailoring and adaptation is both at the level of surface issues (change of language, scripts to be culturally sensitive; Domenech et al. 2011), as well as more structural and "deep." In this set of family-based interventions, the work in Thailand (Li et al. 2012) and China reflects the most major adaptations. In Thailand, Buddhism is by far the dominant spiritual belief. The Family-2-Family Program involved the framework of a "Strong Mind, Strong Body." While the concept of "mind" is not a basic tenet of work in the US, it is basic to the framing of a successful intervention in Thailand. In contrast, China does not have a strong spiritual belief currently and, since the Cultural Revolution, the leaders have discouraged organized religion. Therefore, the "Together for Empowerment Activities" (TEA) family intervention focused on community activities as a primary strategy for personal and family support. The intervention created activities within the family and among the community of families coping with HIV in order to achieve the targeted outcomes, as well as having individual components.

Variations on clinic, home visits, and community meetings have been documented globally and used across LMIC, as well as high-income countries. There are a number of variations on this theme by many different groups. There are advocacy groups formed to support persons living with HIV and families living with HIV in all countries—overcoming stigma to attend these groups is always a challenge. Most communities in the US currently offer "navigators" to persons living with HIV and their families, in order to enhance engagement and utilization of healthcare services and resources. Some countries are experimenting with having ARV drugs delivered automatically to a home with prescriptions renewed only every few years in order to reduce non-adherence due to lacking medications.

Perhaps the most promising are the mobile phone-based interventions aiming to achieve the same goals as the EBI previously mounted (uptake and adherence to physical and mental health regimens, optimizing social relationships, and coping with stigma) (Comulada 2014; Rotheram-Borus et al. 2012b; Tomlinson et al. 2013). Automated technological approaches, tailored for subgroups and individual youth's or parent's circumstances, will provide the designers of the next generation of HIV interventions robust strategies. As we identified when reviewing the HIV prevention manuals for adolescents, both mobile phone and interpersonal HIV EBI accomplish the following tasks (Ingram et al. 2008; Rotheram-Borus et al. 2009a, b; Swendeman et al. 2009):

- frame an issue (ARV are similar to a daily vitamin; live with HIV, not die);
- communicate knowledge regarding HIV (e.g., ARV adherence can stop HIV acquisition by sexual partners) which must be implemented successfully in a youth's life;
- remove barriers to reaching goals; and
- build social support to sustain the behavior.

Many different technologies can accomplish the same goals and function, especially for linking parents and YLH to a healthcare system (Lenhart et al. 2010). Recent research shows that 80% of youth own a personal media device, 98% go online daily, and, for 78% of youth, cell phones are their preferred mode of communication in high-income countries (Calear et al. 2013; Montero-Marin et al. 2015; Zullig et al. 2014). Most youth in the US own a cell phone, and the percentage increases with age (Calear et al. 2013). In the US, 89% of adolescents use text messages and the monthly average number of text messages sent and received is 2899 texts (Lenhart et al. 2010), and texts are a well-validated intervention strategy (Lester et al. 2010). The rates of texting are similar across income, ethnic, and racial backgrounds, reducing health disparities in intervention uptake (Lenhart et al. 2010). Reviews of text interventions have found that text messages increase ARV adherence (Belzer et al. 2015; Finitsis et al. 2014; Horvath et al. 2012; Lester et al. 2010; Pop-Eleches et al. 2011) as well as adherence to other chronic disease medical regimens (Mbuagbaw et al. 2015). Text messages are efficacious to change the health behaviors of YLH and to reduce sexual and drug use behaviors (Dowshen et al. 2012; Kachur et al. 2013; Levine et al. 2008; Ybarra et al. 2015). Features of text messaging are even clear: weekly is better than daily, follow-up phone calls are needed if there is no response to a weekly text, and direct step-by-step instructions are better than vague support (Ramanathan et al. 2012). Yet, while we prefer using text messaging, texting is a specific delivery modality.

The design and selection of a specific technology delivery format is flexible and can be adapted over time to reflect the tools used most often by youth.

Social media is used by 73% of American youth, with 24% of youth posting daily (Lenhart et al. 2010) and may present opportunities for additional engagement strategies. Patterns of use can shift rapidly over time, requiring constant monitoring to know the best platforms to reach young people. YLH can be engaged with mobile strategies (Rice and Barman-Adhikari 2014; Rice et al. 2011, 2007). It is not clear whether mobile technologies must be complemented and embedded in personal relationships.

Similar to text messaging, monitoring youth's behaviors and encouraging self-monitoring is also efficacious to increase adherence and to reduce risk behaviors (Berg et al. 2011; DiClemente et al. 2002; Guo et al. 2011; Mlunde et al. 2012). Self-management of daily routines between clinical visits is a basic skill necessary for every chronic health condition, including HIV. Self-monitoring, in particular, is a strategy that has been repeatedly found to improve self-management (Free et al. 2013; Ramanathan et al. 2012; Swendeman et al. 2015). Even if useful for self-management, mothers with infants infected with HIV will improve their children's health, if mothers' adherence improves. In a recent study by our team with seropositive adults, we found significant improvements in treatment adherence associated with self-monitoring (Swendeman et al. 2015). Self-monitoring includes active observation and recording of behaviors, emotional states, and their determinants and affect a core element of self-regulation (Baker and Kirschenbaum 1993; Snyder and Gangestad 1986; Swendeman et al. 2015).

Structural Interventions

Systematic changes in how health care is delivered are perhaps the easiest example available of a structural intervention. Most countries are moving to provide Option B+ to pregnant women. Option B+ means that pregnant MLH will be provided lifelong ARV. Malawi is one country in which this policy has been implemented. In three years, Malawi increased the coverage of pregnant women receiving ARV by more than 70%. In just one year, the implementation of Option B+ resulted in approximately 10,660 pregnant and breastfeeding women starting ARV—a 748% increase (CDC 2013). The drastic rise in ARV access and uptake in Malawi attributed to Option B+ has driven a substantial drop in perinatal transmission from 40% to less than 5% (WHO 2013). However, global diffusion of this option requires substantial reductions in drug pricing before it can be implemented. ARV price reductions and Option B+ are structural interventions.

A number of African countries are expected to comply with this recommendation (e.g., Botswana and South Africa in the year 2016). Recent data from Botsawana (Gaolathe et al. 2016) indicate that the global goals of 90-90-90 by 2020 may be achievable. In 30 communities in rural Botswana, more than 90% of persons living with HIV know their status, more than 90% are receiving ARV, and viral suppression is being achieved by 73% of all persons living with HIV. Botswana offers hope to the world that in mature epidemics, consistent application of innovations in the healthcare system and accessibility of ARV can result in population level change. These are the types of structural interventions which are going to be needed to eliminate HIV.

Families living with AIDS cannot effectively cope with children living with HIV alone. Their extended family and communities are critical to provide ongoing care and support (Rotheram-Borus et al. 2005). One of the main challenges for families is when HIV care is siloed. HIV clinics historically were easily identified because they only served people with HIV. As reviewed above, this organization of care invokes stigmatism from community members and avoidance by families affected by HIV. Structural interventions, such as anti-discrimination laws, were central to reducing stigma in high-income countries, but are almost nonexistent in LMIC. Ryan White was a young boy living in Indiana who was denied school because he was seropositive for HIV. His ejection from school led to initiation of significant and sustained funding for persons living with HIV, a funding stream that is central for survival and the quality of life for families living with HIV in the US. Ryan White funding provides access to ARV for persons infected with HIV, access to housing, access to wrap-around mental health services and ensures anti-discrimination laws for persons living with HIV. Passing the Ryan White legislation was a major structural intervention.

A second area for structural change is in the social determinants of HIV. Co-occurring with HIV is unemployment, intimate partner violence, being an AIDS orphan, and alcohol and drug abuse. In many LMIC, these social factors are endemic in the region (Rotheram-Borus et al. 2015a, b).

Similar challenges are found under conditions of war and civil unrest. There are few data on the rate of HIV in the eastern Congo or in Northern Uganda—each has experienced war for almost two generations. Missing young women captured by the Boko Haram are also highly likely to be at risk for multiple negative outcomes, among which is becoming seropositive and having an untreated and unidentified HIV-seropositive infant. These settings are not monitored by global donor agencies, even though it is well known that the outcomes are highly negative. Global intervention will be required before such conditions are rectified with major military initiatives likely to supersede public health interventions.

Given these data, economic interventions have been one of the structural interventions being evaluated most often to improve adherence to the HIV Treatment Continuum. In Brazil and Mexico, conditional cash transfers for maternal adherence to child health regimens have been highly successful at improving implementation of public health interventions (e.g., vaccinations, PMTCT) (Velez et al. 2014). Sub-Saharan African countries are now experimenting with similar strategies. In particular, behavioral economics and the use of "nudges" and incentives to optimize and make good health behaviors easy are now being studied in many communities and countries globally. These strategies are likely to replace many of our small group and labor-intensive counseling strategies, which have dominated the research literature on preventing pediatric HIV and its consequences since 1981.

Conclusion

The paradigm for stopping HIV has evolved quickly and dramatically over the last 40 years. Initially, HIV signified premature death. Now, families must cope with chronic disease management and multigenerational effects. Families living with HIV can expect normal life span. Cancer, TB, or malaria are far more likely to kill a person living with HIV (UNAIDS 2014a). Yet, having adequate treatment strategies and access to life-saving medications does not eliminate the burdens of HIV. Mothers, infants, children, adolescents, fathers and extended families must adjust daily and plan how to get the transportation, medication, sleep, food, and exercise that will promote health. The potential for stock-outs (i.e., periods in which ARV drugs are not available in a region or a set of hospitals and clinics), lack of insurance, mental health symptoms, drug abuse or the complexities of daily life to delay healthy daily routines is huge. As a field, we must move away from individualized counseling models toward structural interventions.

Acknowledgments This chapter was completed with support by grants from the National Institutes of Health MH58107, 5P30AI028697, and MH111391 and from the National Institute of Alcohol and Alcohol Abuse AA022919 and AA017104.

Annotated Bibliography

Bryson, Y. J. (1996). Perinatal HIV-1 transmission: Recent advances and therapeutic interventions. *AIDS, 10*(Suppl 3), S33–S42.

In HIV research, 1996 represents a significant year in breakthroughs in perinatal transmission of HIV during pregnancy and childbirth. Dr. Bryson also reviews the landmark AIDS Clinical Trials Group 076 which formally cited zidovudine as a viable form of prevention of perinatal transmission.

Cohen, M. S., Chen, Y. Q., McCauley, M., Gamble, T., Hosseinipour, M. C., Kumarasamy, N., … & HPTN 052 Study Team. (2011). Prevention of HIV-1 Infection with Early Antiretroviral Therapy. *New England Journal of Medicine, 365*(6), 493-505.

Dr. Cohen and his team definitively demonstrated that HIV transmission is preventable with early initiation of antiretroviral therapy among serodiscordant couples. This HIV Prevention Trials Network is a large scale randomized controlled trial conducted across nine of the most HIV-prevalent countries, ultimately regarded as evidencing proof-of-concept for HIV treatment as prevention.

Rotheram-Borus, M. J., le Roux, I. M., Tomlinson, M., Mbewu, N., Comulada, W. S., le Roux, K., et al. (2011). Philani Plus (+): A Mentor Mother community health worker home visiting program to improve maternal and infants' outcomes. *Prevention Science, 12*(4), 372.

The Philani Plus intervention in South Africa validates the World Health Organization recommendation of task shifting and the benefits of paraprofessionals in HIV prevention and care in low- and middle-income countries. This manuscript provides a comprehensive understanding of Dr. Rotheram's Mentor Mothers, and has since been adopted in several sites.

UNAIDS. (2014). *90-90-90: An ambitious treatment target to help end the AIDS epidemic*. Geneva, Switzerland: Joint United Nations Programme on HIV/AIDS UNAIDS. Retrieved from http://www.unaids.org/sites/default/files/media_asset/90-90-90_en_0.pdf

In 2014 the Joint United Nations Programme on HIV/AIDS (UNAIDS) published its targets for the future direction of HIV and goals to be achieved by 2020: 90% of people living with HIV aware of their status; 90% on treatment; 90% virally suppressed. This report guides current research and practice and set worldwide benchmarks.

References

Abbatt, F. (2005). *Scaling up health and education workers: Community health workers literature review*. London, UK: Department for International Development, Health Systems Resource Center.

AIDSVu. (2013). *Persons living with an HIV or AIDS diagnosis*. Retrieved from http://aidsvu.org/map/

Agwu, A. L., Fleishman, J. A., Korthuis, P. T., Siberry, G. K., Ellen, J. M., Gaur, A. H., … & the HIV Research Network. (2012). Disparities in anitretroviral treatment: A comparison of behaviorally-HIV-infected youth and adults in the HIV research Network. *Journal of Acquiried Immuno Deficiency Syndrome, 58*(1), 100–107.

Aracena, M., Krause, M., Pérez, C., Méndez, M. J., Salvatierra, L., Soto, M., et al. (2009). A cost-effectiveness evaluation of a home visit program for adolescent mothers. *Journal of Health Psychology, 14*(7), 878.

Baeten, J. M., Donnell, D., Ndase, P., Mugo, N. R., Campbell, J. D., Wangisi, J., … & Partners PrEP Study Team. (2012). Antiretroviral prophylaxis for HIV prevention in heterosexual men and women. *New England Journal of Medicine, 367*(5), 399–410.

Baker, R. C., & Kirschenbaum, D. S. (1993). Self-monitoring may be necessary for successful weight control. *Behavior Therapy, 24*(3), 377–394.

Barron, P., Pillay, Y., Doherty, T., Sherman, G., Jackson, D., Bhardwaj, S., et al. (2012). Eliminating mother-to-child HIV transmission in South Africa. *Bulletin of the World Health Organization, 2013*(91), 70–74.

Belzer, M. E., Fuchs, D. N., Luftman, G. S., & Tucker, D. J. (1999). Antiretroviral adherence issues among HIV-positive adolescents and young adults. *Journal of Adolescent Health, 25*(5), 316–319.

Belzer, M. E., Kolmodin MacDonell, K., Clark, L. F., Huang, J., Olson, J., Kahana, S. Y., … & Adolescent Medicine Trials Network for HIV AIDS Interventions. (2015). Acceptability and feasibility of a cell phone support intervention for youth living with HIV with nonadherence to antiretroviral therapy. *AIDS Patient Care STDS, 29*(6), 338–345.

Berg, C. A., King, P. S., Butler, J. M., Pham, P., Palmer, D., & Wiebe, D. J. (2011). Parental involvement and adolescents' diabetes management: the mediating role of self-efficacy and externalizing and internalizing behaviors. *Journal of Pediatric Psychology, 36*(3), 329–339.

Binford, M. C., Kahana, S. Y., & Altice, F. L. (2012). A systematic review of antiretroviral adherence interventions for HIV-infected people who use drugs. *Current HIV/AIDS Reports, 9*(4), 287–312.

Blankenship, K. M., Friedman, S. R., Dworkin, S., & Mantell, J. E. (2006). Structural interventions: Concepts, challenges and opportunities for research. *Journal of Urban Health, 83*(1), 59–72.

Bryson, Y. J. (1996). Perinatal HIV-1 transmission: Recent advances and therapeutic interventions. *AIDS, 10*(Suppl 3), S33–S42.

Calear, A. L., Christensen, H., Mackinnon, A., & Griffiths, K. M. (2013). Adherence to the MoodGYM program: Outcomes and predictors for an adolescent school-based population. *Journal of Affective Disorders, 147*(1–3), 338–344.

Campbell, C., & Scott, K. (2011). Retreat from Alma Ata? The WHO's report on Task Shifting to community health workers for AIDS care in poor countries. *Global Public Health, 6*(2), 125.

Centers for Disease Control. (2006). Achievements in public health. Reduction in perinatal transmission of HIV infection–United States, 1985–2005. *MMWR Morbidity and Mortality Weekly Report, 55*(21), 592–597.

Centers for Disease Control. (2008). *HIV/AIDS among youth: CDC HIV/AIDS fact sheet.* Retrieved from http://www.cdc.gov/hiv/resources/factsheets/pdf/youth.pdf

Centers for Disease Control. (2011). *HIV among youth: HIV/AIDS.* Retrieved from http://www.cdc.gov/hiv/group/age/youth/

Centers for Disease Control. (2013). Impact of an innovative approach to prvent mother-to-child transmission of HIV—Malawi, July 2011–September 2012. *MMWR (Morbidity and Mortality Weekly Report), 62*(8), 148–151.

Centers for Disease Control. (2014). *Risk by racial/ethnic groups: HIV/AIDS.* Retrieved from http://www.cdc.gov/hiv/group/racialethnic/

Centers for Disease Control. (2015). *Compendium of evidence-based interventions and best practices for HIV prevention.* Retrieved from http://www.cdc.gov/hiv/prevention/research/compendium/rr/complete.html

Centers for Disease Control. (2016). *HIV among pregnant women, infants, and children.* Retrieved from http://www.cdc.gov/hiv/group/gender/pregnantwomen/

Ciccarone, D., & Bourgois, P. (2003). Explaining the geographical variation of HIV among injection drug users in the United States. *Substance Use and Misuse, 38*(14), 2049–2063.

Cohen, M. S., Chen, Y. Q., McCauley, M., Gamble, T., Hosseinipour, M. C., Kumarasamy, N., et al. (2011). Prevention of HIV-1 infection with early antiretroviral therapy. *New England Journal of Medicine, 365*(6), 493–505.

Comulada, S. (2014). Mobile phone assessment in egocentric networks: A pilot study on gay men and their peers. *Conenctions, 31*(1), 43–51.

Crepaz, N., Tungol-Ashmon, M. V., Higa, D. H., Vosburgh, W., Mullins, M. M., Barham, T., et al. (2014). A systematic review of interventions for reducing HIV risk behaviors among people living with HIV in the United States, 1988-2012. *AIDS, 28*(5), 633–656.

D'Angelo, L. J., Abdalian, S. E., Sarr, M., Hoffman, N., & Belzer, M. (2001). Disclosure of serostatus by HIV infected youth: The experience of the REACH study. Reaching for Excellence in Adolescent Care and Health. *Journal of Adolescent Health, 29*(3 Suppl), 72–79.

D'Augelli, A. R., Hershberger, S. L., & Pilkington, N. W. (1998). Lesbian, gay, and bisexual youth and their families: Disclosure of sexual orientation and its consequences. *American Journal of Orthopsychiatry, 68*(3), 361–371.

Das, M., Chu, P. L., Santos, G. M., Scheer, S., Vittinghoff, E., McFarland, W., et al. (2010). Decreases in community viral load are accompanied by reductions in new HIV infections in San Francisco. *PLoS ONE, 5*(6), e11068.

DiClemente, R. J., Crosby, R. A., & Wingood, G. M. (2002). Enhancing STD/HIV prevention among adolescents: the importance of parenteral monitoring. *Minerva Pediatrica, 54*(3), 171–177.

Domenech Rodriguez, M. M., Baumann, A. A., & Schwartz, A. L. (2011). Cultural adaptation of an evidence based intervention: from theory to practice in a Latino/a community context. *American Journal of Community Psychology, 47*(1–2), 170–186.

Dowshen, N., Kuhns, L. M., Johnson, A., Holoyda, B. J., & Garofalo, R. (2012). Improving adherence to antiretroviral therapy for youth living with HIV/AIDS: A pilot study using personalized, interactive, daily text message reminders. *Journal of Medical Internet Research: JMIR, 14*(2), e51.

Durso, L. E., & Gates, G. J. (2012). *Serving our youth: Finding from a national survey of service providers working with lesbian, gay, bisexual and transgender youth who are homeless or at risk of becoming homeless.* Los Angeles: The Williams Institute with True Colors Fund and The Palette Fund.

Fernandez, M. I., Huszti, H. C., Wilson, P. A., Kahana, S., Nichols, S., Gonin, R., et al. (2015). Profiles of risk among HIV-Infected youth in clinic settings. *AIDS and Behavior, 19*(5), 918–930.

Ferrand, R., Ford, N., & Kranzer, K. (2015). Maximising the benefits of home-based HIV testing. *Lancet HIV, 2*(1), E4–E5.

Finer, L. B., & Philbin, J. M. (2013). Sexual initiation, contraceptive use, and pregnancy among young adolescents. *Pediatrics, 131*(5), 886–891.

Finitsis, D. J., Pellowski, J. A., & Johnson, B. T. (2014). Text message intervention designs to promote adherence to antiretroviral therapy (ART): A meta-analysis of randomized controlled trials. *PLoS ONE, 9*(2), e88166.

Finlayson, K., & Downe, S. (2013). Why do women not use antenatal services in low- and middle-income countries? A meta-synthesis of qualitative studies. *PloS Medicine, 10*(1), e1001373.

Fisher, E. B., Boothroyd, R. I., Coufal, M. M., Baumann, L. C., Mbanya, J. C., Rotheram-Borus, M. J., et al. (2012). Peer support for self-management of diabetes improved outcomes in international settings. *Health Affairs, 31*(1), 130–139.

Fox, K., Ferguson, J., Ajose, W., Singh, J., Marum, E., & Baggaley, R. (2013). Adolescent consent to HIV testing: A review of current policies and issues in sub-Saharan Africa. In *HIV and adolescents: Guidance for HIV testing and counselling and care for adolescents living wtih HIV.* Retrieved from http://apps.who.int/iris/bitstream/10665/95147/1/WHO_HIV_2013.141_eng.pdf

Frange, P., Faye, A., Avettand-Fenoel, V., Bellaton, E., Deschamps, D., Angin, M., … & ANRS Pediatric Cohort (2015). HIV-1 virological remission for more than 11 years after interruption of early initiated antiretroviral therapy in a perinatally infected child. *Journal of the International AIDS Society, 18*.

Free, C., Phillips, G., Galli, L., Watson, L., Felix, L., Edwards, P., … & Haines, A. (2013). The effectiveness of mobile-health technology-based health behaviour change or disease management interventions for health care consumers: A systematic review. *PLoS Medicine, 10*(1).

Futterman, D., Shea, J., Besser, M., Stafford, S., Desmond, K., Comulada, W. S., et al. (2010). Mamekhaya: A pilot study combining a cognitive-behavioral intervention and mentor mothers with PMTCT services in South Africa. *AIDS Care, 22*(9), 1093–1100.

Gaolathe, T., Wirth, K. E., Holme, M. P., Makhema, J., Moyo, S., Chakalisa, U., … & Botswana Combination Prevention Project study, T. (2016). Botswana's progress toward achieving the 2020 UNAIDS 90-90-90 antiretroviral therapy and virological suppression goals: a population-based survey. *Lancet HIV, 3*(5), e221–230.

Gardner, J. M., Powell, C. A., Baker-Henningham, H., Walker, S. P., Cole, T. J., & Grantham-McGregor, S. M. (2005). Zinc supplementation and psychosocial stimulation: Effects on the development of undernourished Jamaican children. *American Journal of Clinical Nutrition, 82*(2), 399–405.

Garofalo, R., Kuhns, L. M., Hotton, A., Johnson, A., Muldoon, A., & Rice, D. (2015). A randomized controlled trial of personalized text message reminders to promote medication adherence among HIV-positive adolescents and young adults. *AIDS and Behavior, 20*(5), 1049–1059.

Gonzalez, J. S., Batchelder, A. W., Psaros, C., & Safren, S. A. (2011). Depression and HIV/AIDS treatment nonadherence: A review and meta-analysis. *JAIDS (Journal of Acquired Immune Deficiency Syndromes), 58*(2), 181–187.

Greene, J. M., Ennett, S. T., & Ringwalt, C. L. (1999). Prevalence and correlates of survival sex among runaway and homeless youth. *American Journal of Public Health, 89*(9), 1406–1409.

Grossman, C. I., Purcell, D. W., Rotheram-Borus, M. J., & Veniegas, R. (2013). Opportunities for HIV combination prevention to reduce racial and ethnic health disparities. *American Psychologist, 68*(4), 237.

Guo, J., Whittemore, R., & He, G. P. (2011). The relationship between diabetes self-management and metabolic control in youth with type 1 diabetes: An integrative review. *Journal of Advanced Nursing, 67*(11), 2294–2310.

Hackl, K. L., Somlai, A. M., Kelly, J. A., & Kalichman, S. C. (1997). Women living with HIV/AIDS: The dual challenge of being a patient and caregiver. *Health and Social Work, 22*(1), 53–62.

Hall, H. I., Holtgrave, D. R., & Maulsby, C. (2012). HIV transmission rates from persons living with HIV who are aware and unaware of their infection. *AIDS, 26*(7), 893–896.
Hemelaar, J. (2012). The origin and diversity of the HIV-1 pandemic. *Trends in Molecular Medicine, 18*(3), 182–192.
Horvath, K. J., Nygaard, K., Danilenko, G. P., Goknur, S., Oakes, J. M., & Rosser, B. R. (2012). Strategies to retain participants in a long-term HIV prevention randomized controlled trial: Lessons from the MINTS-II study. *AIDS and Behavior, 16*(2), 469–479.
Ingram, B. L., Flannery, D., Elkavich, A., & Rotheram-Borus, M. J. (2008). Common processes in evidence-based adolescent HIV prevention programs. *AIDS and Behavior, 12*(3), 374–383.
Ji, G., Li, L., Lin, C., & Sun, S. (2007). The impact of HIV/AIDS on families and children—A study in China. *AIDS, 21*(Suppl 8), S157–S161.
Kachur, R., Mesnick, J., Liddon, N., Kapsimalis, C., Habel, M., David-Ferdon, C., … & Schindelar, J. (2013). *Adolescents, technology and reducing risk for HIV, STDs and pregnancy*. Retrieved from http://www.cdc.gov/std/life-stages-populations/adolescents-tech.htm
Kahana, S. Y., Fernandez, M. I., Wilson, P. A., Bauermeister, J. A., Lee, S., Wilson, C. M., et al. (2015). Rates and correlates of antiretroviral therapy use and virologic suppression among perinatally and behaviorally infected HIV+ youth linked to care in the United States. *Journal of Acquired Immuno Deficiency Syndrome, 68*(2), 169–177.
Kaufman, M., & Committee, Adolescent Health. (2008). Adolescent sexual orientation. *Paediatric Child Health, 13*(7), 619–630.
Kennedy, M., Springarn, R., Stanton, A., & Rotheram-Borus, M. J. (2000). A continuum of care model for adolescents living with HIV: Larkin Street Youth Center. *Drugs and Society, 16*, 87–105.
Lamping, D. L., Sewitch, M., Clark, E., Ryan, B., Gilmore, N., Grover, S. A., … & Di Meco, P. (1991). *HIV-related mental health distress in persons with HIV infection, caregivers, and family members/significant others: results of a cross-Canada survey*. Paper presented at the VII International Conference on AIDS: Science Challenging AIDS, Florence, Italy.
le Roux, I. M., le Roux, K., Comulada, W. S., Greco, E. M., Desmond, K. A., Mbewu, N., et al. (2010). Home visits by neighborhood Mentor Mothers provide timely recovery from childhood malnutrition in South Africa: Results from a randomized controlled trial. *Nutrition Journal, 9*, 56.
le Roux, I. M., le Roux, K., Mbeutu, K., Comulada, W. S., Desmond, K. A., & Rotheram-Borus, M. J. (2011). A randomized controlled trial of home visits by neighborhood mentor mothers to improve children's nutrition in South Africa. *Vulnerable Child Youth Studies, 6*(2), 91–102.
le Roux, I. M., Rotheram-Borus, M. J., Stein, J., & Tomlinson, M. (2014). The impact of paraprofessional home visitors on infants' growth and health at 18 months. *Vulnerable Child Youth Studies, 9*(4), 291–304.
le Roux, I. M., Tomlinson, M., Harwood, J. M., O'Connor, M., Worthman, C. M., Mbewu, N., et al. (2013). Outcomes of home visits for pregnant mothers and their infants: A cluster randomised controlled trial. *AIDS, 27*(9), 1461.
Leach-Lemens, C. (2011). South Africa's PMTCT programme reduces mother-to-child transmission to under 4%. In *Prevention of mother-to-child-transmission*. Retrieved from http://www.aidsmap.com/South-Africas-PMTCT-programme-reduces-mother-to-child-transmission-to-under-4/page/1880446/
Leibowitz, A. A., Garcia-Aguilar, A. T., & Farrell, K. (2015). Initial health assessments and HIV screening under the affordable care act. *PLoS ONE, 10*(9), e0139361.
Lenhart, A., Purcell, K., Smith, A., & Zickuhr, K. (2010). Social medica & mobile internet use among teens and young adults. In P. R. Center (Ed.), *Pew internet & American Life Project*, Washington, D.C.
Lester, R. T., Ritvo, P., Mills, E. J., Kariri, A., Karanja, S., Chung, M. H., et al. (2010). Effects of a mobile phone short message service on antiretroviral treatment adherence in Kenya (WelTel Kenya1): A randomised trial. *Lancet, 376*(9755), 1838–1845.
Leta, T. H., Sandoy, I. F., & Fylkesnes, K. (2012). Factors affecting voluntary HIV counselling and testing among men in Ethiopia: A cross-sectional survey. *BMC Public Health, 12*, 438.

Levine, D., McCright, J., Dobkin, L., Woodruff, A. J., & Klausner, J. D. (2008). SEXINFO: A sexual health text messaging service for San Francisco youth. *American Journal of Public Health, 98*(3), 393–395.

Lewin, S., Munabi-Babigumira, S., Glenton, C., Daniels, K., Bosch-Capblanch, X., van Wyk, B. E., … & Scheel, I. B. (2010). Lay health workers in primary and community health care for maternal and child health and the management of infectious diseases. *Cochrane Database Systematic Review, 3*, CD004015.

Li, L., Liang, L. J., Lee, S. J., Iamsirithaworn, S., Wan, D., & Rotheram-Borus, M. J. (2012). Efficacy of an intervention for families living with HIV in Thailand: A randomized controlled trial. *AIDS and Behavior, 16*(5), 1276–1285.

Li, L., Wu, S., Wu, Z., Sun, S., Cui, H., & Jia, M. (2006). Understanding family support for people living with HIV/AIDS in Yunnan, China. *AIDS & Behavior, 10*(5), 509–517.

Lightfoot, M., & Rotheram-Borus, M. J. (2000). Interventions for high-risk youth. In J. L. Peterson & R. J. DiClemente (Eds.), *Handbook of HIV prevention. AIDS prevention and mental health* (pp. 129–145). Dordrecht, Netherlands: Kluwer Academic Publishers.

Mbuagbaw, L., Mursleen, S., Lytvyn, L., Smieja, M., Dolovich, L., & Thabane, L. (2015). Mobile phone text messaging interventions for HIV and other chronic diseases: an overview of systematic reviews and framework for evidence transfer. *BMC Health Services Research, 15*.

McCoy, S. I., Buzdugan, R., Mushavi, A., Mahomva, A., Cowan, F. M., & Padian, N. S. (2015). Food insecurity is a barrier to prevention of mother-to-child HIV transmission services in Zimbabwe: A cross-sectional study. *BMC Public Health, 15*.

Michalopoulos, C., Lee, H., Duggan, A., Lundquist, E., Tso, A., Crowne, S. S., … & Knox, V. (2015). The mother and infant home visiting program evaluation: Early findings on the maternal, infant, and early childhood home visiting program. In *ACF Web Report*. Retrieved from http://www.acf.hhs.gov/sites/default/files/opre/mihope_report_to_congress_final_1.pdf

Mlunde, L. B., Poudel, K. C., Sunguya, B. F., Mbwambo, J. K. K., Yasuoka, J., Otsuka, K., … & Jimba, M. (2012). A call for parental monitoring to improve condom use among secondary school students in Dar es Salaam, Tanzania. *BMC Public Health, 12*.

Montero-Marin, J., Prado-Abril, J., Botella, C., Mayoral-Cleries, F., Banos, R., Herrera-Mercadal, P., … & Garcia-Campayo, J. (2015). Expectations among patients and health professionals regarding web-based interventions for depression in primary care: A qualitative study. *Journal of Medical Internet Research, 17*(3).

Morin, M. (2014). HIV disappears in 'Los Angeles baby,' doctors say. *Los Angeles Times*. Retrieved from http://articles.latimes.com/2014/mar/05/science/la-sci-sn-hivinfected-infant-deliver-in-long-beach-may-be-cured-20140305

Mothers2Mothers. (2011). *Moving forward and giving back*. Retrieved from http://www.m2m.org/files/pdf/2962_M2M_Annual_Report_2012_Online.pdf

Murphy, D. A., Marelich, W. D., Armistead, L., Herbeck, D. M., & Payne, D. L. (2010). Anxiety/stress among mothers living with HIV: Effects on parenting skills and child outcomes. *AIDS Care, 22*(12), 1449–1458.

Murphy, D. A., Wilson, C. M., Durako, S. J., Muenz, L. R., & Belzer, M. (2001). Antiretroviral medication adherence among the REACH HIV-infected adolescent cohort in the USA. *AIDS Care, 13*(1), 27–40.

Nahar, B., Hossain, M. I., Hamadani, J. D., Ahmed, T., Grantham-McGregor, S., & Persson, L. A. (2012). Effects of psychosocial stimulation on improving home environment and child-rearing practices: Results from a community-based trial among severely malnourished children in Bangladesh. *BMC Public Health, 12*(1), 622.

National Institute of Allergy and Infectious Disease. (2014). "Mississippi Baby" Now has detectable HIV, researchers find. *NIH News*. Rockville, MD: U.S. Department of Health and Human Services.

National Scientific Council on the Developing Child. (2007). *The science of early childhood development: Closing the gap between what we know and what we do*. Retrieved from http://developingchild.harvard.edu/resources/reports_and_working_papers/science_of_early_childhood_development/

Newell, M. L., Coovadia, H., Cortina-Borja, M., Rollins, N., Gaillard, P., Dabis, F., & Ias. (2004). Mortality of infected and uninfected infants born to HIV-infected mothers in Africa: A pooled analysis. *Lancet, 364*(9441), 1236-1243.

Newell, M. L., Gray, G., & Bryson, Y. J. (1997). Prevention of mother-to-child transmission of HIV-1 infection. *AIDS, 11*(Suppl A), S165–S172.

Nielsen-Saines, K., Watts, H., Veloso, V. G., Bryson, Y. J., Joao, E. C., Pilotto, J. H., … & NICHD HPTN 040/PACTG 1043 Protocol Team. (2012). Three postpartum antiretroviral regimens to prevent intrapartum HIV Infection. *New England Journal of Medicine, 366*(25), 2368–2379.

Olds, D., Henderson, C. R., Jr., Cole, R., Eckenrode, J., Kitzman, H., Luckey, D., et al. (1998). Long-term effects of nurse home visitation on children's criminal and antisocial behavior: 15-year follow-up of a randomized controlled trial. *JAMA, 280*(14), 1238–1244.

Olds, D. L., Henderson, C. R., Tatelbaum, R., & Chamberlin, R. (1988). Improving the life-course development of socially disadvantaged mothers: A randomized trial of nurse home visitation. *American Journal of Public Health, 78*(11), 1436.

Olds, D. L., Kitzman, H., Knudtson, M. D., Anson, E., Smith, J. A., & Cole, R. (2014). Effect of home visiting by nurses on maternal and child mortality: Results of a 2-decade follow-up of a randomized clinical trial. *JAMA Pediatrics, 168*(9), 800.

Olds, D. L., Robinson, J., O'Brien, R., Luckey, D. W., Pettitt, L. M., Henderson, C. R., Jr., et al. (2002). Home visiting by paraprofessionals and by nurses: A randomized, controlled trial. *Pediatrics, 110*(3), 486–496.

Parsons, J. T., Rosof, E., & Mustanski, B. (2008). The temporal relationship between alcohol consumption and HIV-medication adherence: A multilevel model of direct and moderating effects. *Health Psychology, 27*(5), 628–637.

Patel, V., Chowdhary, N., Rahman, A., & Verdeli, H. (2011). Improving access to psychological treatments: Lessons from developing countries. *Behaviour Research and Therapy, 49*(9), 523.

Peacock, S., Konrad, S., Watson, E., Nickel, D., & Muhajarine, N. (2013). Effectiveness of home visiting programs on child outcomes: A systematic review. *BMC Public Health, 13*(1), 17.

Persaud, D., & Luzuriaga, K. (2014). Absence of HIV-1 after treatment cessation in an infant reply. *New England Journal of Medicine, 370*(7), 678-678.

Persaud, D., Patel, K., Karalius, B., Rainwater-Lovett, K., Ziemniak, C., Ellis, A., … & Pediatric HIV/AIDS Cohort Study. (2014). Influence of age at virologic control on peripheral blood human immunodeficiency virus reservoir size and serostatus in perinatally infected adolescents. *JAMA Pediatrics, 168*(12), 1138–1146.

Pop-Eleches, C., Thirumurthy, H., Habyarimana, J. P., Zivin, J. G., Goldstein, M. P., de Walque, D., et al. (2011). Mobile phone technologies improve adherence to antiretroviral treatment in a resource-limited setting: A randomized controlled trial of text message reminders. *AIDS, 25*(6), 825–834.

Rahman, A., Iqbal, Z., Roberts, C., & Husain, N. (2009). Cluster randomized trial of a parent-based intervention to support early development of children in a low-income country. *Child: Care, Health and Development, 35*(1), 56.

Ramanathan, N., Swendeman, D., Comulada, W. S., Estrin, D., & Rotheram-Borus, M. J. (2012). Identifying preferences for mobile health applications for self-monitoring and self-management: Focus group findings from HIV-positive persons and young mothers. *International Journal of Medical Informatics, 82*(4), e38–e46.

Rice, E., & Barman-Adhikari, A. (2014). Internet and social media use as a resource among homeless youth. *Journal of Computer-Mediated Communication, 19*(2), 232–247.

Rice, E., Barman-Adhikari, A., Rhoades, H., Winetrobe, H., Fulginiti, A., Astor, R., et al. (2013). Homelessness experiences, sexual orientation, and sexual risk taking among high school students in Los Angeles. *Journal of Adolescent Health, 52*(6), 773–778.

Rice, E., Milburn, N. G., & Monro, W. (2011). Social networking technology, social network composition, and reductions in substance use among homeless adolescents. *Prevention Science, 12*(1), 80–88.

Rice, E., Milburn, N. G., & Rotheram-Borus, M. J. (2007). Pro-social and problematic social network influences on HIV/AIDS risk behaviours among newly homeless youth in Los Angeles. *AIDS Care, 19*(5), 697–704.

Richter, L., Rotheram-Borus, M. J., Van Heerden, A., Stein, A., Tomlinson, M., Harwood, J. M., et al. (2014). Pregnant women living with HIV (WLH) supported at clinics by Peer WLH: A cluster randomized controlled trial. *AIDS and Behavior, 18*(4), 706–715.

Rotheram-Borus, M. J., Ingram, B., Swendeman, D., & Flannery, D. (2009a). Common principles embedded in effective adolescent HIV prevention programs. *AIDS and Behavior, 13*(3), 387–398.

Rotheram-Borus, M., Swendeman, D., Lee, S.-J., Li, L., Amani, B., & Nartey, M. (2011a). Interventions for families affected by HIV. *Translational Behavioral Medicine, 2*, 1–14.

Rotheram-Borus, M. J. (2000). Expanding the range of interventions to reduce HIV among adolescents. *AIDS, 14*, S33–S40.

Rotheram-Borus, M. J., Draimin, B. H., Reid, H. M., & Murphy, D. A. (1997). The impact of illness disclosure and custody plans on adolescents whose parents live with AIDS. *AIDS, 11*(9), 1159–1164.

Rotheram-Borus, M. J., & Fernandez, I. (1995). Sexual orientation and development challenges experienced by gay and lesbian youths. *Suicide & Life-Threatening Behavior, 25*(Suppl), 26–34.

Rotheram-Borus, M. J., Flannery, D., Rice, E., & Lester, P. (2005). Families living with HIV. *AIDS Care, 17*(8), 978–987.

Rotheram-Borus, M. J., le Roux, I. M., Tomlinson, M., Mbewu, N., Comulada, W. S., le Roux, K., et al. (2011b). Philani Plus (+): A Mentor Mother community health worker home visiting program to improve maternal and infants' outcomes. *Prevention Science, 12*(4), 372.

Rotheram-Borus, M. J., Lightfoot, M., & Shen, H. (1999a). Levels of emotional distress among parents living with AIDS and their adolescent children. *AIDS and Behavior, 3*(4), 367–372.

Rotheram-Borus, M. J., Murphy, D. A., Kennedy, M., Stanton, A., & Kuklinski, M. (2001a). Health and risk behaviors over time among youth living with HIV. *Journal of Adolescence, 24* (6), 791–802.

Rotheram-Borus, M. J., Murphy, D. A., Swendeman, D., Chao, B., Chabon, B., Zhou, S., et al. (1999b). Substance use and its relationship to depression, anxiety, and isolation among youth living with HIV. *International Journal of Behavioral Medicine, 6*(4), 293–311.

Rotheram-Borus, M. J., Rice, E., Comulada, W. S., Best, K., Elia, C., Peters, K., et al. (2012a). Intervention outcomes among HIV-affected families over 18 months. *AIDS and Behavior, 16* (5), 1265–1275.

Rotheram-Borus, M. J., Richter, L., Van Rooyen, H., van Heerden, A., Tomlinson, M., Stein, A., et al. (2011c). Project Masihambisane: A cluster randomised controlled trial with peer mentors to improve outcomes for pregnant mothers living with HIV. *Trials, 12*, 2.

Rotheram-Borus, M. J., Richter, L. M., van Heerden, A., van Rooyen, H., Tomlinson, M., Harwood, J. M., et al. (2014a). A cluster randomized controlled trial evaluating the efficacy of peer mentors to support South African women living with HIV and their infants. *PLoS ONE, 9* (1), e84867.

Rotheram-Borus, M. J., Robin, L., Reid, H. M., & Draimin, B. H. (1998). Parent-adolescent conflict and stress when parents are living with AIDS. *Family Process, 37*(1), 83–94.

Rotheram-Borus, M. J., Stein, J. A., & Lin, Y. Y. (2001b). Impact of parent death and an intervention on the adjustment of adolescents whose parents have HIV/AIDS. *Journal of Consulting and Clinical Psychology, 69*(5), 763–773.

Rotheram-Borus, M. J., Swendeman, D., & Becker, K. D. (2014b). Adapting evidence-based interventions using a common theory, practices, and principles. *Journal of Clinical Child & Adolescent Psychology, 43*(2), 229.

Rotheram-Borus, M. J., Swendeman, D., Flannery, D., Rice, E., Adamson, D. M., & Ingram, B. (2009b). Common factors in effective HIV prevention programs. *AIDS and Behavior, 13*(3), 399.

Rotheram-Borus, M. J., & Tomlinson, M. (2016). *International AIDS Society conference*. South Africa: Durban.

Rotheram-Borus, M. J., Tomlinson, M., Gwegwe, M., Comulada, W. S., Kaufman, N., & Keim, M. (2012b). Diabetes buddies: Peer support through a mobile phone buddy system. *Diabetes Education, 38*(3), 357–365.

Rotheram-Borus, M. J., Tomlinson, M., Le Roux, I., & Stein, J. A. (2015a). Alcohol use, partner violence, and depression a cluster randomized controlled trial among Urban South African mothers over 3 years. *American Journal of Preventive Medicine, 49*(5), 715–725.

Rotheram-Borus, M. J., Tomlinson, M., Scheffler, A., Harris, D., & Nelson, S. (2016). Adjustment of a population cohort of South African children of mothers living with/and without HIV through three years post-birth. *AIDS and Behavior* (in press).

Rotheram-Borus, M. J., Tomlinson, M., Scheffler, A., & Le Roux, I. M. (2015b). Re-engagement in HIV care among mothers living with HIV in South Africa over 36 months postbirth. *AIDS, 17*, 2361–2362.

Sahay, S. (2013). Coming of age with HIV: A need for disclosure of HIV diagnosis among children/adolescents. *Journal of HIV/AIDS and Infectious Diseases, 1*, 1–7.

Samb, B., Celletti, F., Holloway, J., Van Damme, W., De Cock, K. M., & Dybul, M. (2007). Rapid expansion of the health workforce in response to the HIV epidemic. *New England Journal of Medicine, 357*(24), 2510–2514.

Sikkema, K. J., Dennis, A. C., Watt, M. H., Choi, K. W., Yemeke, T. T., & Joska, J. A. (2015). *Improving mental health among people living with HIV: A review of intervention trials in low- and middle-income countries*. Mental Health: Global. 2.

Singh, P., & Sachs, J. D. (2013). 1 million community health workers in sub-Saharan Africa by 2015. *Lancet, 382*(9889), 363.

Smit, P. J., Brady, M., Carter, M., Fernandes, R., Lamore, L., Meulbroek, M., et al. (2012). HIV-related stigma within communities of gay men: A literature review. *AIDS Care, 24*(4), 405–412.

Smith, D. M., Richman, D. D., & Little, S. J. (2005). HIV superinfection. *Journal of Infectious Diseases, 192*(3), 438–444.

Snyder, M., & Gangestad, S. (1986). On the nature of self-monitoring—Matters of assessment, matters of validity. *Journal of Personality and Social Psychology, 51*(1), 125–139.

Sweet, M. A., & Appelbaum, M. I. (2004). Is home visiting an effective strategy? A meta-analytic review of home visiting programs for families with young children. *Child Development, 75*(5), 1435–1456.

Swendeman, D., Ingram, B. L., & Rotheram-Borus, M. J. (2009). Common elements in self-management of HIV and other chronic illnesses: An integrative framework. *AIDS Care, 21* (10), 1321–1334.

Swendeman, D., Ramanathan, N., Baetscher, L., Medich, M., Scheffler, A., Comulada, W. S., et al. (2015). Smartphone self-monitoring to support self-management among people living with HIV: Perceived benefits and theory of change from a mixed-methods randomized pilot study. *Journal of Acquired Immune Deficiency Syndrome, 69*(Suppl 1), S80–S91.

Swendeman, D., Rotheram-Borus, M. J., Comulada, S., Weiss, R., & Ramos, M. E. (2006). Predictors of HIV-related stigma among young people living with HIV. *Health Psychology, 25* (4), 501–509.

Swider, S. M. (2002). Outcome effectiveness of community health workers: An integrative literature review. *Public Health Nursing, 19*(1), 11.

Szilagyi, P. G. (1998). Managed care for children: Effect on access to care and utilization of health services. *The Future of Children, 8*(2), 39–59.

Teasdale, C. A., & Besser, M. J. (2008). Enhancing PMTCT programmes through psychosocial support and empowerment of women: The mothers2mothers model of care. *Southern African Journal of HIV Medicine, 29*, 60.

The Interagency Task Team. (2015). *Monitoring & evaluation framework for antiretroviral treatment for pregnant and breastfeeding women living with HIV and their Infants: The Interagency Task Team IATT, WHO, UNICEF, CDC*. Retrieved from http://www.emtct-iatt.org/wp-content/uploads/2015/05/IATT-Framework-May-2015.pdf

Thigpen, M. C., Kebaabetswe, P. M., Paxton, L. A., Smith, D. K., Rose, C. E., Segolodi, T. M., ... & TDF2 Study Group. (2012). Antiretroviral preexposure prophylaxis for heterosexual HIV transmission in Botswana. *New England Journal of Medicine, 367*(5), 423–434.

Tomlinson, M., Rotheram-Borus, M. J., Doherty, T., Swendeman, D., Tsai, A. C., Ijumba, P., ... & Chopra, M. (2013). Value of a mobile information system to improve quality of care by community health workers. *South African Journal of Information Management, 15*(1).

Tomlinson, M., Rotheram-Borus, M. J., Harwood, J., le Roux, I. M., O'Connor, M., & Worthman, C. (2015). Community health workers can improve child growth of antenatally-depressed, South African mothers: A cluster randomized controlled trial. *BMC Psychiatry, 15*, 225.

Tsai, A. C., Bangsberg, D. R., Frongillo, E. A., Hunt, P. W., Muzoora, C., Martin, J. N., et al. (2012). Food insecurity, depression and the modifying role of social support among people living with HIV/AIDS in rural Uganda. *Social Science and Medicine, 74*(12), 2012–2019.

Tsai, Y., Zhou, F., Wortley, P., Shefer, A., & Stokley, S. (2014). Trends and characteristics of preventive care visits among commercially insured adoelscents, 2003–2010. *Journal of Pediatrics, 164*(3), 625–630.

UNAIDS. (2012). *Criminalisation of HIV non-disclosure, exposure and transmission: Background and current landscape*. Retrieved from http://www.unaids.org/sites/default/files/en/media/unaids/contentassets/documents/document/2012/BackgroundCurrentLandscapeCriminalisationHIV_Final.pdf

UNAIDS. (2013). *Global report: UNAIDS report on the global AIDS epidemic 2013*. Retrieved from http://www.unaids.org/sites/default/files/media_asset/UNAIDS_Global_Report_2013_en_1.pdf

UNAIDS. (2014a). *90-90-90: An ambitious treatment target to help end the AIDS epidemic*. Geneva, Switzerland: Joint United Nations Programme on HIV/AIDS UNAIDS. Retrieved from http://www.unaids.org/sites/default/files/media_asset/90-90-90_en_0.pdf

UNAIDS. (2014b). *Gap analysis on paediatric HIV treatment, care and support*. UNAIDS Programme Coordinating Board. Retrieved from http://www.unaids.org/sites/default/files/media_asset/20141117_Gap_Analysis_on_paediatric_ARVs.pdf

UNAIDS. (2014c). *The Gap report*. Geneva, Switzerland: Joint United Nations Program on HIV/AIDS (UNAIDS). Retrieved from http://www.unaids.org/sites/default/files/media_asset/UNAIDS_Gap_report_en.pdf

UNAIDS. (2015a). *2015 progress report on the global plan*. Retrieved from http://www.unaids.org/sites/default/files/media_asset/JC2774_2015ProgressReport_GlobalPlan_en.pdf

UNAIDS. (2015b). *AIDS by the numbers*. Retrieved from http://www.unaids.org/sites/default/files/media_asset/AIDS_by_the_numbers_2015_en.pdf

UNICEF. (2016). Great progress in reducing new HIV infections among children, but not fast enough. *UNICEF Data: Monitoring the situation of children and women*. Retrieved from http://data.unicef.org/hiv-aids/emtct.html

Velez, L. F., Sanitato, M., Barry, D., Alilio, M., Apfel, F., Coe, G., et al. (2014). The role of health systems and policy in producing behavior and social change to enhance child survival and development in low- and middle-income countries: an examination of the evidence. *Journal of Community Health, 19*(Suppl 1), 89–121.

Vreeman, R. C., Wiehe, S. E., Pearce, E. C., & Nyandiko, W. M. (2008). A systematic review of pediatric adherence to antiretroviral therapy in low- and middle-income countries. *Pediatric Infectious Disease Journal, 27*(8), 686–691.

Walker, S. P., Powell, C. A., Granthammcgregor, S. M., Himes, J. H., & Chang, S. M. (1991). Nutritional supplementation, psychosocial stimulation, and growth of stunted children—The Jamaican study. *American Journal of Clinical Nutrition, 54*(4), 642–648.

WHO. (2007). Task shifting to tackle health worker shortages. In *HIV/AIDS programme*. Retrieved from http://www.who.int/healthsystems/task_shifting_booklet.pdf

WHO. (2012). *Global HIV/AIDS response: Epidemic update and health sector progress towards universal access*. Retrieved from http://www.who.int/hiv/pub/progress_report2011/summary_en.pdf?ua=1

WHO. (2013). *Global update on HIV treatment 2013: Results, impact and opportunities Kuala Lumpur, Malaysia*. Retrieved from http://apps.who.int/iris/bitstream/10665/85326/1/9789241505734_eng.pdf?ua=1

World Health Organization African Region. (2011). *WHO Africal regional ministerial consultation on noncommunicable diseases*. Retrieved from http://www.who.int/nmh/events/2011/africa_ncds_background_paper.pdf

Ybarra, M. L., Prescott, T. L., Philips, G. L., 2nd, Bull, S. S., Parsons, J. T., & Mustanski, B. (2015). Iteratively developing an mHealth HIV prevention program for sexual minority adolescent men. *AIDS and Behavior, 20*(6), 1157–1172.

Zanoni, B. C., & Mayer, K. H. (2014). The adolescent and young adult HIV cascade of care in the United States: exaggerated health disparities. *AIDS Patient Care STDS, 28*(3), 128–135.

Zullig, L. L., Sanders, L. L., Shaw, R. J., McCant, F., Danus, S., & Bosworth, H. B. (2014). A randomised controlled trial of providing personalised cardiovascular risk information to modify health behaviour. *Journal of Telemedicine and Telecare, 20*(3), 147–152.

Chapter 6
HIV Prevention and Intervention in the School Setting

Audra St. John Walsh, Courtney Lynn, Katherine L. Wesley, Kimberly O'Leary and Tiffany Chenneville

Introduction

HIV is a domestic and international epidemic, and youth have been identified as a key population in need of broad support for both HIV prevention and treatment (US Department of Health and Human Services 2015). HIV disproportionately affects youth with more than 62,000 youth estimated to be living with HIV in the US in 2012 (Centers for Disease Control and Prevention [CDC] 2015d), many of whom attend public schools. Additionally, approximately 50% of Americans know someone with HIV. Although youth represent only 17% of the US population, they accounted for 26% of new HIV infections in 2010 (CDC 2015d), and it is estimated that the majority of people diagnosed with HIV before the age of 30 actually contracted the virus during adolescence. Furthermore, more than half of youth living with HIV in the US are unaware they are infected. HIV also disproportionately affects racial/ethnic and sexual minority youth and the poor. Consequently, youth at greatest risk of contracting HIV behaviorally already face social and economic disadvantages. With an 87% increase in HIV diagnoses from

A. St. John Walsh (✉) · C. Lynn · K.L. Wesley · K. O'Leary
University of South Florida, Tampa, FL, USA
e-mail: awalsh@health.usf.edu

C. Lynn
e-mail: clynn2@health.usf.edu

K.L. Wesley
e-mail: kwesley2@health.usf.edu

K. O'Leary
e-mail: kimberlyoleary@health.usf.edu

T. Chenneville
University of South Florida St. Petersburg, St. Petersburg, FL, USA
e-mail: chennevi@mail.usf.edu

T. Chenneville (ed.), *A Clinical Guide to Pediatric HIV*,
DOI 10.1007/978-3-319-49704-4_6

2005 through 2014, HIV infection was on a sharp rise among young black and Hispanic/Latino men who have sex with men (MSM). Although more recent data indicate that the increases in diagnoses among young ethnic/racial minority MSM have slowed, these youth remain a vulnerable population (CDC 2016).

Despite the continued HIV epidemic, recent medical advances have changed the outlook of HIV/AIDS for future generations. HIV is now considered a chronic, as opposed to a fatal, disease. Although no cure currently exists for HIV, most people living with HIV who are adherent to highly active antiretroviral therapy (HAART) are able to live long healthy lives, and the risk of HIV transmission, even from mothers with HIV to their children, can be dramatically decreased. However, prognosis relies on treatment adherence. When taken properly, HAART can make viral suppression possible, dramatically reducing levels of the virus in the body. Viral suppression typically results in optimal immune function for the individual and the ability to engage in healthy and productive life activities including work, leisure, intimate relationships, and bearing children, if desired. From a public health perspective, risk of HIV transmission is reduced dramatically with lower levels of the virus in the body. Thus, with little burden beyond taking daily medication and attending regular medical appointments, we can limit the number of new infections and continue to reduce the number of deaths due to AIDS. In fact, the Vision for the US National HIV/AIDS Strategy (US Department of Health and Human Services 2015) states:

> The United States will become a place where new HIV infections are rare and when they do occur, every person, regardless of age, gender, race/ethnicity, sexual orientation, gender identity or socio-economic circumstance, will have unfettered access to high quality, life-extending care, free from stigma and discrimination.

Although from a medical perspective, an AIDS-free generation is possible, there are a number of socioeconomic and psychosocial–developmental factors such as stigma, inadequate sexual education, increasing autonomy, risk behavior, victimization, and lack of social support, which may contribute to the rise of HIV cases among youth. In order to realize the vision described above, universal implementation of comprehensive HIV prevention and intervention efforts is essential.

Schools are uniquely poised to implement cost-effective efforts along the HIV prevention to intervention continuum and are critical for establishing health and wellness behaviors in youth (CDC 2015e; Lewallen et al. 2015). Almost fifty million youth attend US public schools (Davis and Bauman 2013). These youth are in school for at least six hours a day, approximately 180 days per year, totaling 14,040 h or 2340 days over the course of their educational careers. Second to being with their families, youth spend most of their lives in schools. Youth in schools are a captive audience during their most formative years. As such, schools play a critical role in promoting the academic, physical, social–emotional, and behavioral development of young people. Beyond academics, schools are responsible for ensuring student safety and for instilling healthy behaviors, many of which have the potential to endure long into adulthood (CDC 2015a). Schools are in a unique position to promote health behaviors including healthy eating habits, daily physical activity, and illness prevention. Schools can positively impact the lifelong attitudes and behavior that support overall health and well-being including those that reduce risk of HIV transmission and stigma (CDC 2015a). Therefore, the wide-reaching influence schools have on the health habits of millions of youth is critical when thinking about pediatric HIV along the prevention to intervention continuum.

Specifically, school-based universal and targeted HIV prevention as well as individualized interventions for youth living with HIV has the potential to reduce the pediatric HIV epidemic and improve the quality of life for youth infected with or affected by HIV. Intended for reference by educators, psychologists, social workers, counselors, parents, health professionals, and researchers interested in increasing their understanding of the issues surrounding pediatric HIV in the school setting, this chapter describes the impact of HIV and evidence-based interventions for youth infected with or affected by HIV and the importance of universal preventions and developmentally appropriate and comprehensive HIV education in the school setting within a three-tiered model of service delivery.

HIV and Youth: School-Related Considerations

As mentioned above, schools heavily influence the academic, physical, and social–emotional development of youth. This is true for all youth including those who have or are at risk of acquiring HIV. In the sections to follow, important considerations for thinking about the role of schools in HIV prevention and intervention efforts are described.

Developmental and Academic Considerations

Youth with HIV may face many unique developmental and academic challenges as a result of their chronic illness. In a systematic review of the literature, Sherr et al. (2014) identified several developmental challenges of youth with HIV. Executive functioning such as attention and visuospatial abilities as well as processing speed are cognitive categories presenting difficulties for these youth. For children born with HIV, the impact of the virus may be seen early in childhood with developmental delays, including cognitive, motor, or language delays (Whitehead et al. 2014). These delays may or may not last into school age. In a study comparing infants with HIV to those who were exposed to HIV but uninfected, researchers discovered infants with HIV scored significantly lower on motor and language development at baseline, three months, and six months compared to infants exposed but uninfected (Whitehead et al. 2014). However, by six months, the infants with HIV who had been taking HAART since birth were no longer considered delayed. This suggests that HAART may protect further decline in neurodevelopmental functioning. Thus, infants with HIV are in need of early screening and interventions to keep them from falling behind their same-age peers.

As youth born with HIV age into adolescence and young adulthood, they face challenges associated with living with the virus for a longer period of time. As the virus progresses, central nervous system dysfunction can lead to a decline in cognitive function and academic difficulties. Cognitive concerns may include memory and attention as well as a gradual progression into dementia (Donenberg and Pao 2005). As a result of these deficits, youth with HIV often experience low academic achievement and require additional educational support. In light of the neuropsychological symptoms associated with HIV, comprehensive assessment (e.g., developmental evaluation, neurocognitive assessment and monitoring, tests of attention/memory, norm-referenced achievement tests, and frequent monitoring with general outcome measures) is often warranted. Youth with advanced HIV infection may require intensive intervention and/or special education/exceptional student education (ESE) programming. See Nichols (2017) for more information on developmental considerations for children and youth with HIV.

Physical/Medical Considerations

Youth with well-managed or asymptomatic HIV may not present with physical needs that differ from their peers who do not have HIV (Reitz and Gallo 2015). However, those with symptomatic infection may experience a wide range of physical symptoms, which are affected by a variety of factors (e.g., different strains of HIV, length of time since infection, medication adherence, comorbid diseases; Martin et al. 2005). In fact, symptoms and treatment effects tend to be unique to each individual. Since HIV weakens the immune system, or decreases the number of CD4 cells (i.e., fighter cells) in the blood, symptoms associated with a compromised immune system may be present. For example, youth with symptomatic HIV may experience fatigue, weight loss, diarrhea, fever, and frequent opportunistic infections (e.g., thrush, cancer, pneumonia, herpes, tuberculosis; US Department of Health and Human Services 2015). Additionally, youth may experience mild to life-threatening side effects of HAART (e.g., headache, nausea, vomiting, diarrhea, dry mouth, anemia, kidney/liver dysfunction; Bindu and Anusha 2011). Youth receiving care for HIV attend frequent medical appointments and typically are prescribed a daily HAART medication regimen. See Rodriguez and Emmanuel (2017) for more information about medical considerations for children and youth with HIV.

Social–Emotional/Behavioral Considerations

Childhood and adolescence is characterized by many psychosocial and developmental changes. In addition to the typical personal and interpersonal challenges of adolescence, youth with HIV may experience increased stigma, challenges related to living with a chronic health condition, family stressors related to HIV, and difficult decisions about disclosure of their HIV status (Katz et al. 2013; Lee et al. 2015). As children transition into adolescence and young adulthood, they are presented with unique and often conflicting developmental influences. There is a growing need for autonomy/independence and an increase in risk-taking behavior that may conflict with their developing decisional capacity and cognitive/executive functioning (Panel on Antiretroviral Guidelines for Adults and Adolescents 2015).

For adolescents with health conditions, increasing autonomy means youth begin to take more ownership of their health and make independent health-related decisions (Buchanan et al. 2012). Developmental influences often result in adolescents and young adults managing their own health care less effectively than adults. Increased risk-taking behavior in adolescence may be the result of a low perception of risk when it comes to certain behaviors. Adolescents may engage in unsafe sexual behaviors and intravenous drug use both of which present a direct risk of contracting HIV. Non-injection drug and alcohol use also increases risk because these substances decrease inhibitions leading to risky sexual behavior. Most youth do not get tested for HIV for a variety of reasons to include a lack of information and/or misinformation about HIV and fear of HIV-related stigma. As a result, almost half of youth infected with HIV are unaware of their status (CDC 2015d) and, therefore, unknowingly may put sexual partners at risk. Moreover, condom use rates are low among youth, again due to a variety of factors to include a low perception of risk, which may result from the limited information provided to youth about sexual health. For some youth, such as young MSMs, sexual partners tend to be older and are more likely to have HIV (CDC 2015d). Youth affected by other socioeconomic issues such as homelessness, abandonment, and drug dependency are also at increased risk, particularly if they engage in sexual behavior in exchange for drugs, money, or shelter.

Along with the unique developmental influences of adolescence, young people living with HIV and families affected by HIV face additional challenges that make this time period one of particular vulnerability. In addition to the typical adolescent stressors, young people living with HIV have to deal with the negative stereotypes associated with HIV, which is linked with a very strong and negative stigma often serving as a barrier to HIV education, testing, treatment, and retention in care (Katz et al. 2013; Turan and Nyblade 2013). Stigma also is associated with poor medication adherence and an increase in risk-taking behavior (Mahajan et al. 2008). Many sexual and racial/ethnic minority youth with HIV fear or experience multiple stigmatizations and lack social support for engaging in important health behaviors (e.g., treatment adherence, safer sexual behavior). In a study of fifth-grade students, children were asked to draw an individual with a cold, a healthy person, a person with AIDS, and a person with cancer (Gonzalez-Rivera and Bauermeister 2007). Children depicted individuals with AIDS as being skinnier, having more accessories such as chains, tattoos, and piercings, and engaging in behaviors such as smoking or using drugs at a much higher rate than the individuals in other drawings. This suggests that stereotypes and stigma related to HIV can be seen as early as the age of 10.

One of the issues faced by children and adolescents living with HIV is that of medication management and adherence. Typically caregivers manage the medication of younger children living with HIV. Buchanan et al. (2012) identified a number of barriers to medication adherence reported by caregivers and their children to include youth forgetting to take their medication, avoiding it due to unpleasant taste, being unable to take medication because of being away from home, child refusal, and a lack of symptoms resulting in a denial of the health condition. Medication management and adherence are issues that need to be addressed with parents as well as youth throughout childhood and adolescence. As children grow into adolescents and young adults, the transition between parent management/adherence and self-management/adherence is important.

Youth living with HIV also face the unique challenge of disclosing their HIV status to family members, friends, and partners. Youth and young adults who reported more than one close friend and who had friends and family who continued to support them after disclosing their HIV-positive status perceived greater social support (Lee et al. 2015); despite this, many choose to keep their HIV status private, living in isolation from potential support from others. The topic of disclosure is an important issue and needs to be addressed when working with this population (e.g., when and how HIV status should be disclosed). For more information about disclosure, see Marhefka, Turner et al. (2017).

HIV also affects families of individuals living with HIV. The stigma associated with HIV isolates families; they often face economic hardships, and they tend to have poor quality of life as well as dissatisfaction with their own health status (Ji et al. 2007). Families are often responsible for providing emotional, social, and physical support to the individual living with HIV and can be intricately involved in their medical care. This involvement has the potential to lead to stress and resentment toward the individual with HIV. Additionally, parents may be uncomfortable discussing sexual behavior with their child or they may be reluctant to even disclose their child's status to him or her (Bor et al. n.d.) creating stress and tension among family members.

There is growing research on the emotional well-being of youth with HIV. In a sample of 34 youth with HIV aged 16–21 years, 85% met criteria for a DSM-IV Axis I diagnosis (Pao et al. 2000). Sixty-eight percent reported a diagnosis of a mood disorder at some point in their life, and 44% met criteria for a current mood disorder. In addition, 59% had a lifetime history of substance use or dependence and 29% met criteria for conduct disorder. For the majority of these youth, their HIV diagnosis followed a psychiatric diagnosis. A study comparing children with HIV to children who were perinatally exposed but uninfected found no differences in behavioral outcomes. However, 52% of the overall sample had elevated scores on at least one subscale of the Conners' Parent Rating Scale (i.e., conduct, learning, psychosomatic, impulsivity–hyperactivity, or anxiety). This suggests that other environmental effects (e.g., drug exposure) may be at play and contributing to some of the mental health problems of these youth. Findings from both of these studies suggest young people with HIV are at risk of experiencing mental or behavioral health issues often requiring intervention in the school setting. For more information about the psychosocial issues facing children and adolescents with HIV, see Albright, Fair, and Newman (2017).

Legal Considerations

The US Department of Education ensures all youth, with and without disabilities, have the right to a free and appropriate public education in a safe environment free from harassment—this includes youth living with HIV. These rights are protected by laws such as Section 504 of the Rehabilitation Act of 1973, the Americans with Disabilities Act, Public Law 94–142 (also known as the Individuals with Disabilities Education Act [IDEA]), the Family Education Rights and Privacy Act (FERPA) of 1974 (1974, amended in 1994), and additional case law. Despite the intent of these laws to protect youth, it is left up to individual school districts and schools to interpret and set school policy. School personnel, students, families, and communities tend to have strong and varying reactions when social and health policies enter the educational domain (Chenneville 2008a, 2014). Stinnett et al. (2004) found that many educators were misinformed and unaware of their beliefs about youth with HIV. As such, they tended to unfairly scrutinize, blame, and express unwarranted fear of contracting HIV through casual contact. Thus, even with protections in place, due to the strong negative social stigma and misinformation, students with HIV continue to face discrimination in schools. Well-known cases of school-based discrimination and violence against youth with HIV include the cases of Ryan White, an adolescent with HIV who was denied free and appropriate education on the basis of his HIV status, and the Rays brothers who lived with HIV and whose home was burned down after advocating for unfettered admission to school. As recent as 2011, the US Department of Justice found that the Milton Hershey School in Pennsylvania violated the Americans with Disabilities Act by refusing to enroll a student on the basis of his HIV-positive status (AIDS Law Project of Pennsylvania 2014).

In light of this enduring negative stigma and ongoing discrimination, confidentiality is of critical importance. FERPA is a federal law protecting the confidentiality of student records. All schools receiving federal funding must comply with this law which states release of student records necessitates written permission from the parent or student (over the age of 18) and must be provided only to those with a legitimate "need to know" (Policy Studies Associates 1997). However, the "need to know" is not explicitly defined in FERPA, and as such, there is considerable variability among schools and districts in terms of determining who has a "need to know." This means that schools are responsible for safeguarding student records and, for students who have disclosed HIV status to school personnel, determining who needs to know this information. Chenneville (2008b) found decisions about disclosure of confidential medical information based on FERPA's "need to know" policy varied among elementary school principals based on diagnosis and the presence of symptomatology.

HIV-Specific Educational Policies

Comprehensive Policy on HIV in Schools

Considering the discretion allowed in the interpretation of federal law and policy, it is important for schools and districts to outline their school-/district-specific policy for HIV in the schools (Simmonds and Chanock 1993). The National Association of State Boards of Education (NASBE) collaborated with the US Centers for Disease Control and Prevention's (CDC) Division of Adolescent and School Health to publish guidelines for developing educational policies concerning HIV in the school setting (NASBE 2001). These guidelines identify important areas to address when creating policy to include school attendance, employment, confidentiality/disclosure, infection control, athletics, prevention, and staff development. Moreover, these guidelines reiterate the need for a school-specific policy that expressly states (1) all students with HIV have the right to attend school in a safe and respectful atmosphere without discrimination or harassment, (2) employees with HIV are not to be discriminated against, (3) confidentiality of an individual's HIV status needs to be emphasized in a way that expresses its importance, (4) universal infection control guidelines should be followed at all times, (5) participation in physical education and other athletic activities is not contingent on the student's HIV status, (6) related services such as counseling should be offered for youth affected by HIV, (7) staff development regarding HIV should be provided, and (8) prevention education should be provided with the goal being to "promote healthful living and discourage the behaviors that put people at risk of acquiring HIV" (NASBE 2001, p. 4). However, a review by Chenneville (1999) revealed that many schools did not have a comprehensive policy specific for HIV but simply referred to federal/state law. As discussed previously, this can lead to subjective interpretation by school personnel with risk of being swayed by misguided influences. The extent to which schools and districts currently adopt their own specific HIV policy tailored for their school and population of youth is unknown.

HIV and Sex Education

Until very recently, the federal government only funded abstinence-only programs in schools, which taught only about abstinence until marriage. Currently, fewer than half of the states in the US require both sex education and HIV education in public schools (Guttmacher Institute 2016). Among these, there is great variability in the required content and divisive debate remains over the merits of abstinence-only versus comprehensive sexuality education. This is problematic because while abstinence is the only 100% effective method of HIV prevention, it is not realistic for everyone. As discussed previously, youth are engaging in sexual activity, and abstinence-only education is inadequate for providing youth with the information and skills required to make safer choices for their sexual health.

HIV Prevention and Intervention in the School Setting: A Multi-Tiered Approach

A multi-tiered model of service delivery can be used to address HIV in the school setting along the prevention to intervention continuum (Chenneville 2008a, 2014). Several professional fields use a tiered framework for the delivery of services. For example, in the public health field, the Public Health Prevention Model organizes prevention/intervention service delivery along a continuum of support based on population needs (Kazak 2006). In the field of education, response to intervention (RTI) utilizes three tiers to deliver services along the continuum of prevention to intervention. Chenneville (2008a) was the first to introduce a best practice approach for addressing HIV in the school setting using the three-tiered model, which recently was updated (Chenneville 2014). Similarly, Walsh and Chenneville (2013) adapted the four-level World Health Organization (WHO) model (Wyn et al. 2000) to describe a school change model to address HIV in the school setting. In this chapter, we retain the three-tiered model Chenneville (2008a, 2014) proposed, but incorporate aspects of Walsh and Chenneville's (2013) modified WHO model for school change related to HIV (Fig. 6.1).

Level or Tier 1: Primary Prevention Efforts

Level or Tier 1 represents primary prevention, which involves universal intervention efforts aimed at all students and school staff. Such efforts are designed to prevent the spread of HIV by increasing awareness, decreasing HIV-related stigma, and promoting safer sexual practices and other behaviors to minimize the risk of HIV transmission.

Universal Precautions Training

It is imperative that school personnel, students, and all members of the school community receive training on universal precautions regardless of the known presence of a student or employee with HIV (National Association of School Psychologists [NASP] 2012). Universal precautions refer to behaviors and practices for responding to situations involving exposure to blood and other bodily fluids. Some examples include wearing latex gloves when handling blood or bodily fluids, using special containers for disposing of contaminated sharp objects, and cleaning hard surfaces with a disinfectant. In the US, the Occupational Safety and Health Administration also mandates schools have a blood-borne pathogen exposure plan. More information about universal precautions is available from the CDC (2007), the American Academy of Pediatrics (AAP 2007), and the WHO (2007).

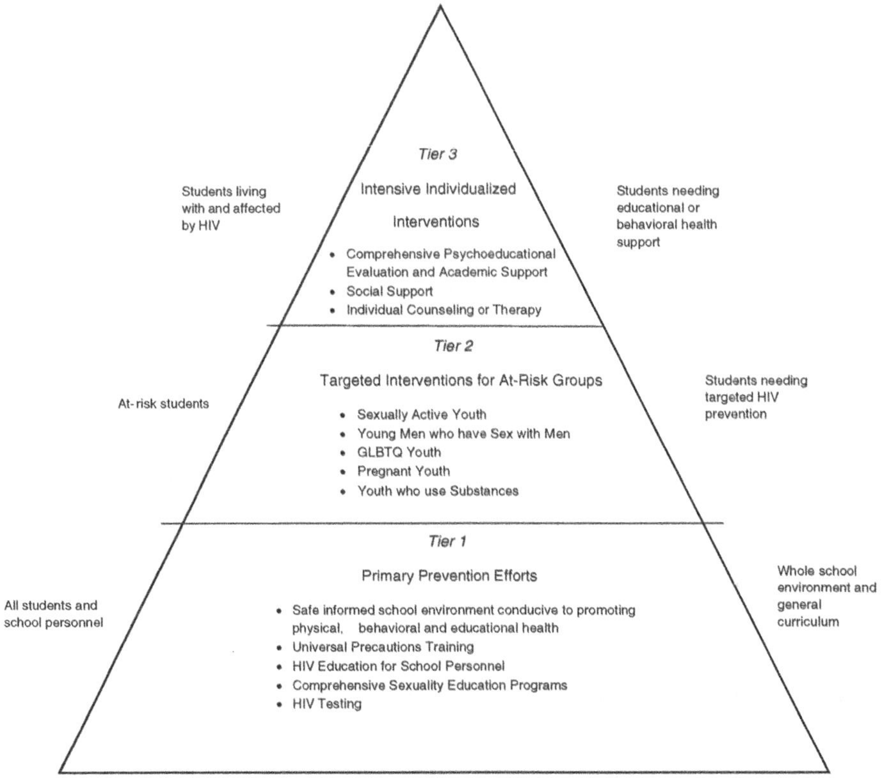

Fig. 6.1 A multi-tiered approach to HIV prevention and intervention in the school setting. Source: Modified from models proposed by Chenneville (2008a, 2014) and Walsh and Chenneville (2013)

HIV Education for School Personnel

In order to prevent the spread of HIV and eliminate its associated stigma, educators need to be trained in medically accurate and factual information about HIV. One of the primary reasons for educator training is so teachers and staff are able to effectively deliver HIV-related information as part of comprehensive sexuality education programs (Walsh and Chenneville 2013). Anderman et al. (2009) compared the efficacy of permanent classroom teachers to temporary health educators when teaching pregnancy and HIV prevention. Students valued the information more, perceived more motivational classroom atmospheres, and saw the teacher as more credible when the information was delivered from a regular classroom teacher. Additionally, adolescents who were sexually active at the time of the program engaged in more classroom discussion on HIV and pregnancy prevention with the regular classroom teachers than did their non-sexually active counterparts. These findings highlight the importance of permanent classroom teachers being trained with accurate information about HIV as students may feel more comfortable conversing about HIV and sexuality with familiar adults in the school setting.

School personnel who are not responsible for providing sexuality education also should receive HIV education so they are able to combat myths and misperceptions as they arise. This may help reduce HIV-related stigma (Walsh and Chenneville 2013). Adults who are accurately informed about HIV are better equipped to educate youth and model behavior/attitudes that will reduce stigma (NASP 2012). As described previously, HIV-related stigma is negatively associated with protective behaviors, HIV testing, and medication adherence, all of which contribute to HIV transmission. Thus, stigma-reduction efforts are an important aspect of HIV prevention initiatives.

Comprehensive Sexuality Education Programs

The American Academy of Pediatrics' Committee of Psychosocial Aspects of Child and Family Health and Committee on Adolescence (AAP 2001), the American Psychological Association (APA 2005), the National Association of School Nurses (NASN 2012), the Centers for Disease Control and Prevention (CDC 2010), and the National Association of School Psychologists (NASP 2012) recommend comprehensive sexuality education. Comprehensive sexuality education programs aim to promote health protective behaviors (e.g., condom use) and reduce sexual risk behaviors (e.g., number of sex partners) both of which can prevent the spread of HIV (Chin et al. 2012).

Those who oppose comprehensive sexuality education claim that comprehensive sexuality education results in increased sexual behavior. Research does not support this claim. For example, Lindberg and Maddow-Zimet (2012) analyzed data from the 2006–2008 National Survey of Family Growth and conducted face-to-face interviews with participants about the type of reproductive health education they received. They found participants who received educational programs that combined information about "how to say no" (i.e., abstinence) with information about protective behaviors (e.g., birth control to include condom use) were more likely to delay sexual intercourse, have higher levels of condom/contraception use, and have sexual partners of a similar age. In comparison, participants who received educational programs that taught only "how to say no" (i.e., abstinence-only) were more likely to have delayed onset of sexual intercourse, but were less likely to display any of the other protective health behaviors. Similarly, in their meta-analysis of sexuality education programs, Chin et al. (2012) included 82 studies that employed comprehensive risk reduction, 50 of which were randomized controlled trials (RCTs) and 32 which were non-randomized controlled trials (non-RCTs). Twenty-three studies of abstinence education were included, 10 of which were RCTs and 13 of which were non-RCTs. Results indicated that comprehensive risk-reduction programs (i.e., comprehensive sexuality education) decreased sexual activity and sexual risk behaviors (i.e., number of sex partners, unprotected sexual activity, and biologic outcomes) and increased protective behaviors (e.g., condom use). Abstinence-only education programs only decreased sexual activity with results differing by study design. When non-RCTs were compared to RCTs, significantly larger effects were found for non-RCTs. Chin et al. (2012) concluded that comprehensive risk-reduction programs had a positive impact on public health by both decreasing sexual activity and increasing protective sexual behaviors, but urged readers to interpret the effects of abstinence education programs with caution as many of the studies reviewed were poorly designed. Furthermore, Chin et al. (2012) reviewed program costs and found that among the eight studies that used individually packaged interventions, the program with the lowest cost per person was the program that was administered in the schools. Overall, research supports the utility of comprehensive sexuality programs for reducing sexual risk behaviors and increasing protective behaviors, thus adding support for including such programs into school curricula.

Based on a comprehensive review of the literature, Walcott et al. (2008) identified characteristics of effective HIV school-based prevention programs. According to their review, effective programs are theoretically driven (e.g., social learning theory, theory of planned behavior). Programs grounded in theory tend to be better developed and have a larger evidence base. In addition, effective programs include adequate training of program facilitators who are responsible for delivering the program. Comprehensive sexuality education programs that include information about and provide access to contraceptives are more effective than programs that focus exclusively on abstinence. Effective programs teach students specific skills for reducing sexual risk behaviors as well as how to address social pressures (i.e., negotiation, peer pressure, refusal) using a wide array of teaching methods (e.g., storytelling, real-life situations, and games) designed to keep students engaged. Programs involving shorter sessions over a longer period of time are more effective than longer sessions that cover more material. Finally, effective programs are those that are developmentally appropriate, culturally sensitive, and gender specific and address behaviors associated with different sexual orientations. See Table 6.1 for a review of evidence-based programs that possess these characteristics.

One school-based intervention, the School HIV/AIDS Education Program (SHEP), delivered in Zambian schools addressed HIV prevention, stigma, and sexual risk behavior and showed promise for increasing student knowledge of HIV prevention and decreasing stigma and sexual risk behaviors (Denison et al. 2012). SHEP is delivered by trained volunteer peer educators, typically between 18 and 25 years old, during weekly 40-min lessons. In addition to the lessons, SHEP also provides coordinated extracurricular activities for students, a library and counseling for students, community education, and workshops for teachers. Students participating in the SHEP program were 1.6 times more likely to correctly answer questions about HIV transmission and prevention. Additionally, students in the SHEP program were nearly two times more likely to positively answer questions

Table 6.1 Description of evidence-based school-based HIV prevention programs

Program	Description	Targeted population	Behavioral findings
Reducing the risk: building skills to prevent pregnancy, HIV and STD (Fourth Edition; Barth 2003)	• Comprehensive pregnancy and STI/HIV prevention curriculum • Covers abstinence and safer sex • Student workbook available in English and Spanish	High school, grades 9–12	Delayed onset of sex and increased condom/other contraceptive use when implemented as part of a comprehensive health education class
AIDS prevention for adolescents in school (Walter and Vaughan 1993)	• Six-session program delivered by regular classroom teachers (1-day in-service training recommended for teachers) • Covers HIV/AIDS information, how to appraise risk behaviors, myths about peers' sexual behaviors, values clarification, negotiation skills, and discussions of purchasing and using condoms	High school, grades 9–12 (recommended for urban high school students)	Reduced number of sexual partners and increased condom use
Draw the line/respect the line: middle school intervention to reduce sexual risk behavior (Marín et al. 2003)	• Latino-sensitive approach • Features English or Spanish worksheets • Covers abstinence and safer sex • Discusses social pressures, challenges to personal limits, and refusal skills	Middle school, grades 6–8	Delayed sexual initiation among boys only (no behavioral effects for middle school girls)
Youth AIDS prevention project (Levy et al. 1993)	• Designed for high-risk, African-American youth • Covers STI/HIV and substance abuse prevention • Ten classroom sessions for 7th grade and five "booster sessions" for 8th grade	Middle school, grades 7 and 8	Increased condom use and intentions to use condoms in the future
Safer choices (ETR Associates 1998)	• 2-Year prevention program • Covers abstinence and safer sex • Five primary components: school organization, staff development, peer resources/school environment, parent education, and school/community linkages	High school, grades 9–12	Reduced number of sexual partners and increased condom use
Get real about AIDS (Main et al. 1994)	• Comprehensive pregnancy and STI/HIV prevention curriculum • Covers abstinence and safer sex • Three components: information, skills, and vulnerability/personal impact	Three curriculum levels: Grades 4–6 Grades 6–9 Grades 9–12	Reduced number of sexual partners and increased condom use

Source Modified from table depicted in Walcott et al. (2008)

about attitudes toward individuals with HIV. While there is a growing body of research focused on HIV-related stigma, research that focuses on interventions that can be delivered in school settings is needed. For more information about HIV-related stigma, please see Stangl and Sievwright (2017).

HIV Testing

HIV testing is considered an important aspect of prevention as people who know they have HIV can receive treatment, including HAART that reduces the viral load of HIV in the blood, subsequently reducing the spread of HIV to others (CDC 2015e). The CDC recommends universal and routine HIV testing for all youth above the age of 12, and the AAP (2011) recommends youth between 16 and 18 years of age be tested at least once. While HIV prevalence among adolescents is increasing, HIV testing among this population remains low. In fact, the CDC's National Youth Risk Behavior Survey (YRBS) on student health risk behaviors found only 13% of high school students had been tested for HIV (CDC 2014). The CDC (2014) and NASP (2012) recommend schools use YRBS data to identify trends in their local area regarding HIV testing, promote communication between parents and adolescents, and educate students about HIV and other sexually transmitted infections (STIs), as well as the types of tests available, testing locations, hours of operation, and costs. Referrals to school-based or school-linked clinics where HIV testing is performed also are recommended.

Research suggests HIV testing is more common among students who receive school-based HIV education (13%) compared to those who do not (10%; CDC 2007). Without exhausting resources, schools can play a critical role in facilitating access to HIV testing. For example, school-based referral programs have been widely successful for connecting students to youth-friendly community healthcare providers (Dittus et al. 2014; Lezin et al. 2010). Establishing ties with health centers and other organizations within the community is critical for providing adequate referral information. Additionally, although more expensive, schools may offer on-site testing in association with the school-based clinic. Despite the benefits of this approach, school districts may not allow on-site testing for a number of reasons. First, school-based testing requires that school personnel, parents, and community leaders acknowledge that youth engage in risk behavior such as sexual activity and drug use—topics that are often easier to ignore or deny. Furthermore, positive results require follow-up action, which may present barriers in the school setting. For example, despite the fact that all states allow minors to consent to STI testing without parental consent, schools may feel obligated to inform parents of HIV testing and results (Guttmacher Institute 2016). Since a positive test result must also be confirmed with another test, it would be necessary for schools to develop a plan for linking students with agencies to conduct follow-up confirmatory testing. Likewise, obtaining a positive result in a school may also make schools feel responsible for linking youth with appropriate health care, a service that is beyond the scope of services provided by most schools.

Indeed, a number of schools across the US have demonstrated their commitment to HIV education, testing, and referral for services. A School Health Policies and Programs study found that among high schools in the US, 85% teach how HIV is transmitted, 77% teach how HIV is diagnosed and subsequently treated, and 76% teach how to find reliable information and services regarding HIV to include information about HIV counseling and testing (Kann et al. 2007). School-based health centers, such as those in Seattle Public Schools, provide a model for the provision of free on-site clinical services for students (e.g., HIV counseling and testing). Another example is Philadelphia Public School District where education, screening, and treatment are provided for some STIs through the City of Philadelphia Public Health Department (Coffee et al. 2015). These programs are laudable and can serve as models for other school districts.

Level or Tier 2: Targeted Interventions for at-Risk Groups

Level or Tier 2 represents secondary prevention and involves more intensive intervention efforts targeted to at-risk groups, which are layered on top of Tier 1 initiatives. Certain risk behaviors (e.g., unprotected sexual activity, substance use) put students at higher risk of contracting HIV, and the CDC (2016) supports the use of empirically sound and cost-effective interventions for at-risk populations. At-risk youth can be identified in a variety of ways to include school-wide screening for risky behavior and/or teacher/staff referrals. Once at-risk groups are identified, prevention/intervention efforts specifically designed to target risky behavior can be implemented. Directing efforts toward the specific behaviors that put an individual at risk of contracting or transmitting HIV can be effective for intervention. For example, youth who are known or suspected to engage in risky sexual behavior and/or substance use may benefit from targeted interventions designed to reduce unsafe behavior and increase adaptive behavior. Key at-risk populations and evidence-based interventions are discussed below.

Sexually Active Youth

Students who are sexually active have an increased risk of contracting HIV (CDC 2015e). Despite barrier protection (e.g., condoms) that helps reduce the risk of transmission, many students do not use barrier protection (CDC 2010). According to the CDC (2010), 46% of adolescents reported having had sexual intercourse at least once and 39% reported they did not use a condom the last time they had sexual intercourse.

A number of community-based interventions (generally at the group level) designed to decrease risky sexual behavior can be used in schools. The CDC (2015c) identifies high impact prevention programs designed to reduce HIV infections that are evidence based, cost-effective, and scalable; many have multifaceted foci, ranging from decreasing risk of HIV and other sexual risk to increasing social skills and decision-making. For example, Project AIM is a 12-session intervention, which encourages youth and adolescents (11–14 years of age) to explore a number of health activities such as personal interests, social surroundings, and planning and decision-making for the future (Clark et al. 2005). This type of future-oriented program has demonstrated effectiveness for decreasing sexual risk-taking behaviors among African-American students. Another example is the Collaborative HIV Prevention and Adolescent Mental Health Project (CHAMP; McKay et al. 2004). This evidence-based family intervention seeks to address and prevent health and mental health problems in African-American and Latino youth affected by poverty. This project targets families specifically, but may be adapted for schools and focuses on many interpersonal issues in order to decrease risk of HIV. Community-based programs that focus on social skills training have effectively enhanced consistent condom use in the past (e.g., DiClemente and Wingood 1995). Programs focusing on self-advocacy and social skills can also affect sexual outcomes. These programs can emphasize sexual self-control, assertiveness, pride, communication skills, proper condom use, and developing communication about consistent condom use.

Young Men Who Have Sex with Men

MSM have been the group most severely affected by HIV (CDC 2016). It is estimated that in 2014, 80% of HIV diagnoses in youth were among men who identify as gay or bisexual (CDC 2016). However, young MSM may or may not identify as gay or bisexual. Therefore, when targeting at-risk youth, it is important to avoid making assumptions based on sexual identity. Rather, identification of risk should be based on behavior, not labels. Particular interventions of note for MSM include: interventions that focus on knowledge of HIV, sexual interpersonal dynamics, and factors that impact HIV risk behavior. One such intervention, *Many Men, Many Voices*, is aimed at African-American MSM and shows promise for reducing risky HIV-related behaviors (Kelly et al. 1989).

Lesbian, Gay, Bisexual, Transgender, and Questioning Youth

Youth who identify as lesbian, gay, bisexual, transgender, or questioning (LGBTQ) comprise a large number of people diagnosed with HIV (CDC 2016). Although it is important to focus on behaviors rather than labels in order to avoid stigmatization, many established interventions have focused on individuals identifying as LGBTQ. Therefore, this section is included in order to provide the necessary foundation of evidence-based treatment, with an established focus on this targeted group.

Safe spaces for youth who identify as LGBTQ are important within the school setting and can foster HIV awareness and bolster HIV prevention efforts. Gay-Straight Alliances (GSAs), for example, are an established strategic intervention designed to interrupt homophobic school environments. Various qualitative analyses have examined different school practices including the provision of physical and emotional safe spaces through organizations such as GSAs which can aid in disrupting homophobic school environments though the creation of supportive accepting communities and a sense of safety and empowerment among members (e.g., Mayberry et al. 2011). Further, research has identified different strategies at various levels (e.g., organizational, systemic) toward creating safe spaces for youth who identify as LGBTQ and their allies (Currie et al. 2012). Although outside the domain of school-monitored activities, online support groups and discussion boards also have proven useful for reducing HIV risk among people who identify as LGBTQ (Ybarra et al. 2014). When referring students for outside counseling, it is important to consider factors that may contribute to discrimination and only make referrals to agencies known to be LGBTQ-friendly.

Youth Who Are Pregnant

Fortunately, recent years have seen a sizable decrease in the rate of mother-to-child transmission of HIV, at least in the US (CDC 2006a). Pregnant women who are treated with medication can dramatically reduce the risk of transmission to their unborn child. With medication, the rate of mother-to-child transmission can be less than 2% (CDC 2006a). Without adequate medical intervention, transmission rates from mother to child can be upwards of 15–45%. Unfortunately, many women in general are not aware of their HIV status (Hall et al. 2015). For students who are pregnant, it is essential to provide opportunities for prenatal care, HIV testing, and, if positive, HIV treatment.

For pregnant women, there are two different approaches to HIV testing: opt-in or opt-out. Opt-in testing requires pregnant women to agree to an HIV test, usually in writing; opt-out testing, on the other hand, involves including an HIV test in a standard battery of prenatal tests conducted on pregnant women. In the opt-out approach, pregnant women may decline the HIV test. Across the US, the opt-in approach results in variable testing rates from 25 to 69%, while the opt-out approach has resulted in testing rates of 85% and higher (Branson et al. 2008). CDC surveillance report statistics over the last decade support the use of the opt-out approach, and the CDC officially recommends universal opt-out HIV testing for pregnant women early in every pregnancy (CDC 2006b).

Youth Who Use Substances

Drug and alcohol use put adolescents at greater risk of contracting HIV and other STIs (CDC 2011). While needle sharing can directly increase HIV risk for youth who engage in intravenous drug use, substance use in general can lead to risky sexual behaviors given the decrease in inhibitions associated with alcohol and drug use. Although treatment for substance abuse is generally beyond the scope of services provided in schools, school-based interventions and referrals can be utilized. Education about substance abuse and treatment can be incorporated into the curriculum, as can education related to social skills training and resisting peer pressure. Outside referrals for more intensive treatment can also be made. For example, students can be referred for social skills training, stress management training, peer mentoring, cognitive behavioral therapy (CBT), or substance rehabilitation programs. While outside referrals contain certain barriers (e.g., financial limitations, transportation difficulties), some programs and clinics may be willing to work with schools or families. Establishing school-community partnerships is therefore recommended.

Level or Tier 3: Individualized Interventions for Students Infected with or Affected by HIV

Level or Tier 3 represents tertiary prevention and involves the most intensive and individualized interventions aimed at alleviating existing school/health problems. Tier 3 provides individualized interventions for students who are infected with or affected by HIV. Specifically, interventions at Tier 3 are focused on preventing reinfection or transmission to others and diminishing the psychosocial and psychoeducational impacts of HIV (Chenneville 2008a, 2014). Often students with HIV may not disclose their status to the school so school personnel may not be aware of the impact of HIV on a student. As a result, there is a paucity of research on interventions for youth with HIV delivered in the school setting. Despite this lack of research, students with HIV may need a range of interventions and services in academic, social–emotional, and behavioral domains. As discussed previously, state and federal laws protect the privacy of students with HIV. For students who do disclose their HIV status to school officials, FERPA guidelines dictate that further disclosure (e.g., to other teachers or staff) be made only on a "need to know" basis. Perceptions of who "needs" to know vary and may depend on other factors such as disease status and symptomatology (Chenneville 2008b). Nonetheless, in cases where a student's HIV status is known, the interventions below may be useful.

Comprehensive Psychoeducational Evaluation and Academic Support

Tier 3 services may include a comprehensive psychoeducational evaluation of a student with HIV. Best practice recommendations include using ecological assessment methods to determine functioning across the domains of intelligence, achievement, adaptive skills, attention and concentration, memory, and psychosocial functioning (Chenneville 2008a, 2014; NASP 2012). Additionally, assessing and/or monitoring language skills among young children may be important for determining the impact of HIV on development (Pumariega et al. 2006). Gathering baseline data is important, especially for students recently diagnosed, to allow for monitoring over time. The use of standardized, norm-referenced assessments and tests as well as curriculum-based measurement and functional behavioral assessment may provide information relevant for the development and implementation of academic interventions. Evaluation also may be needed to determine eligibility for special education/ESE services under IDEA (2004) or for accommodations under Section 504 of the Rehabilitation Act of 1973 (1973).

Social Support

Students with HIV may experience increased psychological symptoms including social stress and preoccupation with their illness (Lam et al. 2007). Students may experience fear related to disclosure of their HIV status or social isolation. They may need support engaging with peers, participating in social activities, and making decisions about disclosing their status to peers. Students with HIV may also need support around loss and trauma experienced due to HIV (e.g., death, loss of social relationships). These issues may also arise in students who are affected by a family member or loved one with HIV. Additionally, these youth may need support to help them cope with the impact of HIV on their family. Research suggests that one strategy to promote resilience in students affected by HIV is connecting them with extracurricular activities and supports (e.g., teachers, competent adults, structured extracurricular activities) at school. For example, Zhao et al. (2014) found a positive correlation between interest in extracurricular activities and self-esteem among children affected by parental HIV in China (Zhao et al. 2014). Similarly, these researchers found that youth affected by parental HIV with medium to high interest in extracurricular activities to include reading, sports, science, music, painting, and playing chess indicated lower levels of depression and loneliness. Schools provide many opportunities for youth to engage in extracurricular activities, and school personnel can help encourage engagement in these activities to support students infected with and affected by HIV.

Individual Counseling or Psychotherapy

Students with HIV may need individual counseling or psychotherapy to address issues related to their diagnosis, living with a chronic illness, disclosure, grief and bereavement, suicidal thoughts, depression, or anxiety among other issues. When providing counseling to students with HIV, the focus should be on the issues the student brings to the table and not only the HIV diagnosis (Chenneville 2008a, 2014). After all, youth with HIV are more similar to than different from their peers and, therefore, are facing similar issues as other children and adolescents. Nonetheless, there is some evidence to suggest that youth with HIV may experience guilt, low self-esteem, and worries about death (Pumariega et al. 2006). Students affected by the loss of a loved one due to AIDS or students who have a family member or loved one with HIV also may need help working through the mourning process (Fielden et al. 2006). Cognitive behavioral therapy (CBT) and connection with an adult who cares (e.g., counselor) can lead to short-term symptom reduction for students experiencing a loss (Mullen and Storie 2012). Counseling for grief and bereavement should explore the student's feelings and reactions to the loss as well as identify and create support systems (Sandoval et al. 2009). Timing is important as therapy surrounding grief and loss is most effective when it focuses on normalizing grief and is provided closer to the time of the loss (Currier et al. 2007).

Youth with HIV are at high risk of depression (Arseniou et al. 2014; Pao et al. 2000). Health and Wellness CBT (H&W CBT; Kennard et al. 2014) focuses on reducing depression, increasing adherence, and promoting mental health in youth 16–24 years of age diagnosed with HIV and depression. H&W CBT is delivered in 14 sessions over six months and is a manualized intervention that can be fitted to individual needs. Stage 1 of treatment incorporates psychoeducation on depression, HIV, and CBT, treatment options, and goal setting. Stage 2 focuses on reducing symptoms and teaching skills to manage mood, increase behavioral activation, and restructure cognitions. Stage 3 teaches wellness strategies and modifications to lifestyle to promote and attain wellness. A preliminary study showed reduction in depression symptoms and better medication adherence across participants. The nature of H&W CBT as a manualized intervention, and favorable initial outcomes, shows promise for use in schools with students with HIV and co-occurring depression to foster wellness.

Motivational interviewing (MI) is a client-centered approach to increasing intrinsic motivation to change through four processes: engaging, focusing, evoking, and planning (Miller and Rollnick 2013). MI is an effective strategy for students who are ambivalent to change and can be used in school settings to address a range of academic and behavior problems (Herman et al. 2014). MI is able to target a range of behaviors for students with HIV including increasing medication adherence, improving engagement in academics, and decreasing substance use. MI has been used with youth with HIV in clinic settings to target risk behaviors (e.g., medication adherence, substance use, risky sexual behavior). A brief four-session MI intervention, Healthy Choices, delivered to youth (16–24 years of age) with HIV showed reductions in depression and growth in willingness to change targeted risk behaviors over three months (Naar-King et al. 2010). Results were seen in youth who participated in at least two MI sessions. Healthy Choices also looked at condom use and alcohol use among youth with HIV. The intervention was effective in reducing the number of times youth engaged in unprotected sex (Chen et al. 2011) and also was effective in reducing alcohol use among youth with HIV (Murphy et al. 2012). While the intervention was delivered in adolescent medicine clinics, applications are recommended for community settings to increase engagement and accessibility and could be implemented in the schools.

Choosing Life: Empowerment! Action! Results! (CLEAR) is a modularized intervention targeting youth with HIV who use substances (Rotheram-Borus et al. 2004). The intervention consists of three modules with six individual sessions in each module. Module 1 targets physical health including medication adherence, Module 2 targets risky sexual and substance behavior including condom use, and Module 3 targets feelings and emotions impacting quality of life. The intervention design involves one-on-one sessions that can be implemented in a variety of settings. The intervention teaches participants relaxation and meditation strategies, self-instruction techniques, self-efficacy skills, and how to use routines to stay healthy (CDC 2015b). Youth receiving the intervention significantly increased their condom use with HIV-positive and HIV-negative partners compared to individuals in the waitlist control group (CDC 2015b; Rotheram-Borus et al. 2004).

Considerations for Researchers

Because students and families are hesitant to disclose HIV status to schools due to fear of stigma and discrimination, there is little research available on the experience of youth infected with or affected by HIV in school settings. This speaks to the need for school-based HIV stigma-reduction research, but also highlights that barriers exist to conducting school-based research in the area of pediatric HIV. For example, issues related to consent and assent present as barriers. Specifically, well-intended IRBs, designed to protect human participants, often present roadblocks to conducting research with minors who are considered a vulnerable population. Research in the area of HIV often involves minors who identify with sexual and gender minority groups, which further complicates IRB decisions related to protecting vulnerable youth. As Chenneville et al. (2010a) advocate, it is important to find a balance between protection and autonomy when working with youth with HIV given that over-protection may unnecessarily diminish autonomy. Mustanski and Fisher (2016) highlighted the health inequities that result when IRBs, in their desire to protect vulnerable populations, deny communities the potential benefits associated with participating in research. Fisher et al. (2016) examined attitudes toward guardian permission to participate in an HIV-related study and also preparedness to provide informed, voluntary, and rational self-consent among youth who identified as sexual or gender minorities. Findings revealed these youth were capable of consenting to research procedures that are age and population appropriate, providing further evidence of the importance of IRB decisions that promote the autonomy of youth. Chenneville et al. (2010a) introduced a model for balancing protection and autonomy that includes an assessment of decisional capacity. The importance of decisional capacity as a construct for consideration when working with youth with HIV is highlighted elsewhere in the literature (Chenneville et al. 2010b, 2014, 2015).

Community-based participatory research (CBPR) is worthy of consideration when conducting school-based research in the area of pediatric HIV. CBPR is a multi-disciplinary approach, wherein questions and goals materialize in conversation with the population of interest who, in this case, are students infected with or affected by HIV. In traditional research, populations of interest are *studied* but are not part of the overall research process. The traditional model frames the researcher as expert and is lacking because it does not incorporate the wisdom and ideas generated from people with lived experience around the topic of interest. In CBPR, individuals who are the focus of the research are actively engaged in every stage of the research process from conception to implementation to the dissemination of findings. Partnering with youth can generate useful knowledge while fostering youth development, empowerment, and engagement. This approach can benefit students in school settings by facilitating intergenerational partnerships resulting in interventions, systemic changes, and community mobilization. Youth gain immediate impact through their involvement in CBPR projects as opposed to only when research results are published, which can take many years. As Viswanathan et al. (2004) explain, the sharing of knowledge and experiences that is inherent in CBPR helps bridge the gap between researchers and communities by building trust and culturally appropriate methods and practices. This, of course, assumes CBPR is implemented correctly, which requires that power be distributed equally among members of the research team (Muhammad et al. 2015). The National Institutes of Health (2015) supports CBPR as evidenced by the number of CBPR projects funded annually.

Beyond research addressing the needs of students living with or directly affected by HIV, there continues to be a need for HIV prevention research in school settings. It is important for scientists to maintain awareness of political factors that can affect school-based research. Nonetheless, research on developmentally appropriate, cost-effective, and time-efficient evidence-based universal and targeted interventions is needed. HIV prevention can be incorporated into larger programs of research aimed at sexual health and health disparities among youth.

Conclusion

The severity of the pediatric HIV epidemic demands wide-reaching prevention and interventions for youth. Schools are uniquely positioned to implement cost-effective efforts along the HIV prevention to intervention continuum and, thus, alter the course of the epidemic by influencing the attitudes and behavior of millions of youth. A multi-tiered approach incorporating primary, secondary, and tertiary prevention strategies can be effective for reducing HIV transmission and improving outcomes for youth who are infected or affected by HIV.

Annotated Bibliography

CDC. (2015). *Schools play a key role in HIV/STD and teen pregnancy prevention*. Retrieved from: http://www.cdc.gov/features/hivstdprevention/

This website provides background information on the importance of schools in preventing HIV/STD and teen pregnancy. Suggestions on how schools can support HIV and STD prevention and testing are described. The article concludes by giving a brief overview of the funding and assistance offered by the CDC.

Chenneville, T. (2014). Best practices in responding to HIV in the school setting. In A. Thomas & P. Harrison (Eds.), *Best practices in school psychology (6th edition)*. Bethesda, MD: National Association of School Psychologists.

This chapter begins with an overview of HIV including prevalence and incidence, transmission, symptoms, and treatment. Basic considerations regarding legal issues and professional standards are described. Lastly, the chapter outlines best practices for responding to HIV in the school setting using a multi-tiered services model.

National Association of School Psychologists. (2012). *Supporting students with HIV/AIDS* [Position statement]. Bethesda, MD: Author.

This position statement contains examples of prevention and intervention efforts that schools should take including safety precautions as well as HIV/AIDS education for students, school personnel, and parents. Interventions need to consider confidentiality/legal issues and focus on psychoeducation and psychosocial factors. Disclosure, bereavement, and research/training issues are also discussed.

U.S. Department of Health and Human Services. (2015). National HIV/AIDS strategy: Overview. Retrieved from: https://www.aids.gov/federal-resources/national-hiv-aids-strategy/overview/

This website offers an overview of the *National HIV/AIDS Strategy for the United States: Updated to 2020*. The vision is for the United States to become a place where HIV rarely occurs and when it does occur there is adequate care. The goals and indicators of progress toward goals are described.

Walcott, C. M., Meyers, A. B., & Landau, S. (2008). Adolescent sexual risk behaviors and school-based sexually transmitted infection/HIV prevention. *Psychology in the Schools, 45*, 39–51. doi:10.1002/pits

This article describes risk and protective factors for adolescent sexual risk behaviors including demographic, social-contextual, and intrapersonal factors. Characteristics of effective STI/HIV prevention programs are described and evidence-based prevention and intervention programs are presented. For each program, the theory, description, targeted population, and behavioral findings are summarized.

References

AIDS Law Project of Pennsylvania. (2014). *Background on the Milton Hershey School case*. Retrieved from http://www.aidslawpa.org/background-on-the-milton-hershey-school-case/

Albright, J. N., Fair, C. D., & Newman, C. (2017). Psychosocial Considerations for Children and Adolescents with HIV. In T. Chenneville (Ed), *A Clinical Guide to Pediatric HIV*, 73–94. Dordrecht: Springer.

American Academy of Pediatrics. (2001). Sexuality education for children and adolescents. *Pediatrics, 108*(2), 498–502.

American Academy of Pediatrics. (2007). Infection prevention and control in pediatric ambulatory settings. *Pediatrics, 105*(6), 650–665. doi:10.1542/peds.2007-1734

American Academy of Pediatrics. (2011). Adolescents and HIV infection: The pediatrician's role in promoting routine testing. *Pediatrics, 128*(5), 1023–1029. doi:10.1542/peds.2011-1761

American Psychological Association. (2005). *Based on the research, comprehensive sex education is more effective at stopping the spread of HIV infection, says APA committee.* Retrieved from http://www.apa.org/news/press/releases/2005/02/sex-education.aspx

Anderman, E. M., Lane, D. R., Zimmerman, R., Cupp, P. K., Phebus, V. (2009). Comparing the efficacy of permanent classroom teachers to temporary health educators for pregnancy and HIV prevention instruction. *Health Promotion Practice, 10*(4), 597–505. doi:10.1177/1524839907309375

Arseniou, S., Arvaniti, A., Samakouri, M. (2014). HIV infection and depression. *Psychiatry and Clinical Neuroscience, 68*(2), 96–109. doi:10.1111/pcn.12097

Barth, R. (2003). *Reducing the risk: Building skills to prevent pregnancy, HIV, and STD* (4th ed.). Scotts Valley, CA: ETR Associates.

Bindu, H. A., & Anusha, N. (2011). Adverse effects of highly active anti-retroviral therapy (HAART). *Journal of Antivirals & Antiretrovirals, 3*, 60–64. doi:10.4172/jaa.1000037

Bor, R., Evans, A., Levitt, D. (n.d.). *Families living with HIV.* Retrieved from https://www.aamft.org

Branson, B. M., Handsfield, H. H., Lampe, M. A., Janssen, R. S., Taylor, A. W., Lyss, S. B., et al. (2008). Revised recommendations for HIV testing of adults, adolescents, and pregnant women in health-care settings. *Journal of the National Medical Association, 100*(1), 131–147.

Buchanan, A., Montepiedra, G., Sirois, P., Kammerer, B., Garvie, P., Storm, D., et al. (2012). Barriers to medication adherence in HIV-infected children and youth based on self- and caregiver report. *Pediatrics, 129*(5), 1244–1251. doi:10.1542/peds.2011-1740.

Centers for Disease Control and Prevention. (2006a). Achievements in public health. Reduction in perinatal transmission of HIV infection–United States, 1985–2005. *Morbidity and Mortality Weekly Report, 55*(21), 592.

Centers for Disease Control and Prevention. (2006b). Revised recommendations for HIV testing of adults, adolescents, and pregnant women in health-care settings. *Morbidity and Mortality Weekly Report, 55*, 14.

Centers for Disease Control and Prevention. (2007). HIV testing among high school students—United States, 2007. *Morbidity and Mortality Weekly Report, 58*, 665–668.

Centers for Disease Control and Prevention. (2010). Youth risk behavior surveillance-United States, 2009. *Morbidity and Mortality Weekly Report, 59.*

Centers for Disease Control and Prevention. (2011). *High-impact HIV prevention: CDC's approach to reducing HIV infections in the United States.* Retrieved from http://www.cdc.gov/hiv/policies/hip/hip.html

Centers for Disease Control and Prevention. (2014). Youth risk behavior surveillance—United States, 2013. *Morbidity and Mortality Weekly Report, 63.*

Centers for Disease Control and Prevention. (2015a). *Adolescent and school health.* Retrieved from http://www.cdc.gov/healthyyouth/index.htm

Centers for Disease Control and Prevention. (2015b). *Compendium of evidence-based interventions and best practices for HIV prevention; choosing life: Empowerment, actions, results (CLEAR).* Retrieved from https://www.cdc.gov/hiv/pdf/research/interventionresearch/compendium/rr/cdc-hiv-clear_best_rr.pdf

Centers for Disease Control and Prevention. (2015c). *High-impact HIV prevention: CDC's approach to reducing HIV infections in the United States.* Retrieved from http://www.cdc.gov/hiv/policies/hip/hip.html

Centers for Disease Control and Prevention. (2015d). *HIV among youth fact sheet.* Retrieved from http://www.cdc.gov/hiv/group/age/youth/

Centers for Disease Control and Prevention. (2015e). *Schools play a key role in HIV/STD and teen pregnancy prevention.* Retrieved from http://www.cdc.gov/features/hivstdprevention/, http://www.cdc.gov/hiv/prevention/research/compendium/rr/clear.html

Centers for Disease Control and Prevention. (2016). *HIV among youth.* Retrieved from http://www.cdc.gov/hiv/group/age/youth/index.html

Chen, X., Murphy, D. A., Naar-King, S., & Parsons, J. T. (2011). A clinic-based motivational intervention improves condom use among subgroups of youth living with HIV. *Journal of Adolescent Health, 49*, 193–198. doi:10.1016/j/jadohealth.2012.11.252

Chenneville, T. (1999). *An analysis of HIV/AIDS policies in Florida's schools* (Thesis). University of South Florida.

Chenneville, T. (2008a). Best practices responding to pediatric HIV/AIDS in the school setting. In A. Thomas & J. Grimes (Eds.), *Best practices in school psychology V* (pp. 177–194). Bethesda, MD: The National Association of School Psychologists.

Chenneville, T. (2008b). Results from an empirical study of school principals' decisions about disclosure of HIV status. *Journal of HIV/AIDS Prevention & Education for Adolescents & Children, 8*(2), 9–30. doi:10.1300/J499v08n02_02.

Chenneville, T. (2014). Best practices in responding to HIV. In P. L. Harrison & A. Thomas (Eds.), *Best practices in school psychology: Systems-level services* (pp. 423–436). Bethesda, MD: National Association of School Psychologists.

Chenneville, T., Clutter, M., Hintz, S., Walsh, A., Emmanuel, P., Lujan-Zilberman, J., et al. (2015). Decisional capacity and medication adherence among youth with HIV. *AIDS Care, 27* (3), 338–341. doi:10.1080/09540121.2014.993582

Chenneville, T., Machacek, M., Tan, R., Lujan-Zilberman, J., Emmanuel, P., & Rodriguez, C. (2014). Decisional capacity among youth with HIV: Results from the MacArthur competence tool for treatment. *AIDS Patient Care and STDs, 28*(8), 1–8. doi:10.1089/apc.2013.0374

Chenneville, T., Sibille, K., & Bendell-Estroff, D. (2010a). Decisional capacity among minors with HIV: A model for balancing autonomy rights with the need for protection. *Ethics and Behavior, 20*(2), 83–94. doi:10.1080/10508421003595901

Chenneville, T., Sibille, K., Lujan-Zilberman, J., Rodriguez, C., Brown, M., & Emmanuel, P. (2010b). Medical decisional capacity among children with HIV: Results from a pilot study. *AIDS Care, 22*(11), 1359–1366. doi:10.1080/09540121003758499

Chin, H. B., Sipe, T. A., Elder, R., Mercer, S. L., Chattopadhyay, S. K., Jacob, V., & Santelli, J. (2012). Guide to community preventive services: The effectiveness of group-based comprehensive risk-reduction and abstinence education interventions to prevent or reduce the risk of adolescent pregnancy, human immunodeficiency virus, and sexually transmitted infections. Two systematic reviews for the guide to community preventive services. *American Journal of Preventive Medicine*, 42272–42294. doi:10.1016/j.amepre.2011.11.006

Clark, L., Miller, K., Nagy, S., Avery, J., Roth, D., Liddon, N., et al. (2005). Adult identity mentoring: Reducing sexual risk for African-American seventh grade students. *Journal of Adolescent Health, 37*, 337. doi:10.1016/j.jadohealth.2004.09.024

Coffee, G., Fenning, P., & Wells, T. L. (2015). *Promoting youth sexual health: Home, school, and community collaboration*. New York, NY: Routledge.

Currie, S., Mayberry, M., & Chenneville, T. (2012). Destabilizing anti-gay environments through gay-straight alliances: Possibilities and limitations through shifting discourses. *The Clearing House: A Journal of Educational Strategies, Issues, and Ideas, 85*(2), 56–60.

Currier, J. M., Holland, J. M., & Neimeyer, R. A. (2007). The effectiveness of bereavement interventions with children: A meta-analytic review of controlled outcome research. *Journal of Clinical Child and Adolescent Psychology, 36*(2), 253–259. doi:10.1080/15374410701279669

Davis, J., & Bauman, K. (2013). *School Enrollment in the United States: 2011. U.S. Department of Commerce, Economics and Statistics Administration, U.S. Census Bureau.* Retrieved December 15, 2015 from www.census.gov

Denison, J. A., Tsui, S., Bratt, J., Torpey, K., Weaver, M. A., & Kabaso, M. (2012). Do peer educators make a difference? An evaluation of a youth-led HIV prevention model in Zambian schools. *Health Education Research, 27*(2), 237–247. doi:10.1093/her/cry093

DiClemente, R. J., & Wingood, G. M. (1995). A randomized controlled trial of an HIV sexual risk —Reduction intervention for young African-American women. *JAMA, 274*, 1271–1276. doi:10.1001/jama.1995.03530160023028

Dittus, P. J., De Rosa, C. J., Jeffries, R. A., Afifi, A. A., Cumberland, W. G., Chung, E. Q., … Ethier, K. A. (2014). The project connect health systems intervention: Linking sexually experienced youth to sexual and reproductive health care. *Journal of Adolescent Health, 55*(4), 528–534. doi: 10.1016/j.jadohealth.2014.04.005

Donenberg, G. R., & Pao, M. (2005). Youths and HIV/AIDS: psychiatry's role in changing epidemic. *Journal of the American Academy of Child and Adolescent Psychiatry, 44*(8), 728–747. doi:10.1097/01.chi.0000166381.68392.02

ETR Associates. (1998). *Safer choices*. Scotts Valley, CA.

Family Educational Rights and Privacy Act of 1974, 20 U.S.C. § 1232 g (1974).

Fielden, S. J., Sheckter, L., Chapman, G. E., Alimenti, A., Forbes, J. C., Sheps, S., … Frankish, J. C. (2006). Growing up: Perspectives of children, families, and service providers regarding the needs of older children with perinatally-acquired HIV. *AIDS Care, 18*, 1050–1053. doi:10.1080/09540120600581460

Fisher, C. B., Arbeit, M. R., Dumont, M. S., Macapagal, K., & Mustanski, B. (2016). Self-consent for HIV prevention research involving sexual and gender minority youth reducing barriers through evidence-based ethics. *Journal of Empirical Research on Human Research Ethics, 11* (1), 3–14. doi:10.1177/1556264616633963

Gonzalez-Rivera, M., & Bauermeister, J. A. (2007). Children's attitudes toward people with AIDS in Puerto Rico: exploring stigma through drawings and stories. *Qualitative Health Research, 17*(2), 250–263. doi:10.1177/1049732306297758

Guttmacher Institute. (2016). State policies in brief: Sex and education. Washington, DC: Author.

Hall, H. I., An, Q., Tang, T., Song, R., Chen, M., Green, T., et al. (2015). Prevalence of diagnosed and undiagnosed HIV infection—United States, 2008–2012. *MMWR Morbidity and Mortality Weekly Report, 64*(24), 657–662.

Herman, K. C., Reinke, W. M., Frey, A. J., & Shepard, S. A. (2014). *Motivational interviewing in schools: Strategies for engaging parents, teachers, and students*. New York: Springer Publishing Company.

Individuals with Disabilities Education Act of 2004, 20 U. S. C. § 1400. (2004).

Ji, G., Li, L., Lin, C., & Sun, S. (2007). The impact of HIV/AIDS on families and children: A study in China. *AIDS, 21*, S157–S161. doi:10.1097/01.aids.0000304712.87164.42

Kann, L., Tellijohann, S. K., & Wooley, S. F. (2007). Health education: Results from the school health Policies and programs study 2006. *Journal of School Health, 77*, 408–434. doi:10.1111/j.1746-1561.2007.00228.x

Katz, I., Ryu, A., Onuegbu, A., Rsaros, C., Weiser, S., Bangsberg, D., et al. (2013). Impact of HIV-related stigma on treatment adherence: Systemic review and meta-synthesis. *Journal of the international AIDS Society, 16*, 1–25. doi:10.7448/ias.16.3.18640

Kazak, A. E. (2006). Pediatric psycholosical preventative health model (PPPHM): Research, practice, and collaboration in pediatric family systems medicine. *Families, Systems, and Health, 24*(4), 381–395.

Kelly, J. A., St. Lawrence, J. S., Hood, H. V., & Brasfield, T. L. (1989). Behavioral intervention to reduce AIDS risk activities. *Journal of Consulting and Clinical Psychology, 57*, 60–67. doi:10.1037/0022-006X.57.1.60

Kennard, B. D., Brown, L. T., Hawkins, L., Risi, A., Radcliffe, J., Emslie, G. J., … Adolescent Trials Network for HIV/AIDS Interventions. (2014). Development and implementation of health and wellness CBT for individuals with depression and HIV. *Cognitive and Behavioral Practice, 21*, 237–246

Lam, P. K., Naar-King, S., & Wright, K. (2007). Social support and disclosure as predictors of mental health in HIV-positive youth. *AIDS Patient Care, 21*, 20–29. doi:10.1089/apc.2006.005
.

Lee, S., Yamazaki, M., Harris, R., Harper, G. W., & Ellen, J. (2015). Social support and human immunodeficiency virus-status disclosure to friends and family: Implications for human immunodeficiency virus-positive youth. *Journal of Adolescent Health, 57*, 73–80. doi:10.1016/j.jadohealth.2015.03.002

Levy, S., Flay, B., & Handler, A. (1993). *Youth AIDS prevention project*. Los Altos, CA: Sociometrics Corporation.

Lewallen, T., Hunt, H., Potts-Datema, W., Zaza, S., & Giles, W. (2015). The whole school, whole community, whole child model: A new approach for improving educational attainment and healthy development for students. *Journal of School Health, 85*(11), 729–739.

Lezin, N., Witt, S., Taylor, J., & Bliesner, J. (2010). *PATHS: Providing access to HIV testing through schools: a resource guide for schools*. Scotts Valley, CA: ETR Associates.

Lindberg, L. D., & Maddow-Zimet, I. (2012). Consequences of sex education on teen and young adult sexual behaviors and outcomes. *Journal of Adolescent Health, 51*, 332–338. doi:10.1016/j.jadohealth.2011.12.028

Mahajan, A. P., Sayles, J. N., Patel, V. A., Remien, R. H., Ortiz, D., ... Coates, T. J. (2008). Stigma in the HIV/AIDS epidemic: a review of the literature and recommendations for the way forward. *AIDS (London, England), 22*(Suppl. 2), S67.

Main, D. S., Iverson, D. C., McGloin, J., Banspach, S. W., Collins, J. L., Rugg, D. L., & Kolbe, L. J. (1994). *Get real about AIDS*. Evanston, IL: AGC Educational Media.

Marhefka, S. L., Turner, D. E., & Chenneville, T. (2017). HIV Disclosure in Pediatric Populations: Who, What, When to Tell, and then What?. In T. Chenneville (Ed), *A Clinical Guide to Pediatric HIV*, 189–227. Dordrecht: Springer.

Marín, B., Coyle, K., Gómez, C., & Kirby, D. (2003). *Draw the line/Respect the line*. Scotts Valley, CA: ETR Associates.

Martin, L. R., Williams, S. L., Haskard, K. B., & DiMatteo, M. R. (2005). The challenge of patient adherence. *Therapeutics and Clinical Risk Management, 1*(3), 189–199.

Mayberry, M., Chenneville, T., & Currie, S. (2011). Challenging the sounds of silence: A qualitative study of gay-straight student alliances and school reform efforts. *Education and Urban Society, 45*(3), 307–339. doi:0013124511409400

McKay, M. M., Chasse, K. T., Paikoff, R., McKinney, L. D., Baptiste, D., Coleman, D., ... Bell, C. C. (2004). Family-level impact of the CHAMP Family Program: A community collaborative effort to support urban families and reduce youth HIV risk exposure. *Family process, 43*, 79–93. doi:10.1111/j.1545-5300.2004.04301007.x

Miller, W. R., & Rollnick, S. (2013). *Motivational interviewing: Helping people change (Applications of motivational interviewing)* (3rd ed.). New York: Guilford.

Muhammad, M., Wallerstein, N., Sussman, A. L., Avila, M., Belone, L., & Duran, B. (2015). Reflections on researcher identity and power: The impact of positionality on community based participatory research (CBPR) processes and outcomes. *Critical Sociology, 41*(7–8), 1045–1063. doi:10.1177/0896920513516025

Mullen, J. A., & Storie, M. S. (2012). Treating complicated grief. In S. E. Brock & S. R. Jimerson (Eds.), *Best practices in school crisis prevention and intervention* (2nd ed., pp. 671–679). Bethesda, MD: National Association of School Psychologists.

Murphy, D. A., Chen, X., Naar-King, S., & Parsons, J. T. (2012). Alcohol and marijuana use outcomes in the healthy choices motivational interviewing intervention for HIV-positive youth. *AIDS Patient Care and STDs, 26*(2), 95–100. doi:10.1089/apc.2011.0157

Mustanski, B., & Fisher, C. B. (2016). HIV rates are increasing in gay/bisexual teens: IRB barriers to research must be resolved to bend the curve. *American Journal of Preventive Medicine,*. doi:10.1016/j.amepre.2016.02.026

Naar-King, S., Parsons, J. T., Murphy, D., Kolmodin, K., & Harris, D. R. (2010). A multisite randomized trial of a motivational intervention targeting multiple risks in youth living with HIV: Initial effects on motivation, self-efficacy, and depression. *Journal of Adolescent Health, 46*, 422–428. doi:10.1016/j.jadohealth.2009.11.198

National Association of School Nurses. (2012). *School health education about human sexuality*. Retrieved from: http://www.nasn.org/PolicyAdvocacy/PositionPapersandReports/NASNPositionStatementsFullView/tabid/462/ArticleId/43/School-Health-Education-about-Human-Sexuality-Revised-2012

National Association of School Psychologists. (2012). *Supporting students with HIV/AIDS [Position Statement]*. Bethesda, MD: Author.

National Association of State Boards of Education. (2001). *Someone at school has AIDS: A complete guide to education policies concerning HIV infection* (2nd ed.). Alexandria, VA: National Association of State Boards of Education.

National Institutes of Health. (2015). Community-based participatory research. Retrieved from https://obssr-archive.od.nih.gov/scientific_areas/methodology/community_based_participatory_research/index.aspx

Nichols, S. (2017). Developmental considerations for children and youth with HIV. In T. Chenneville (Ed), *A Clinical Guide to Pediatric HIV*, 43–72. Dordrecht: Springer.

Panel on Antiretroviral Guidelines for Adults and Adolescents. (2015). *Guidelines for the use of antiretroviral agents in HIV-1-infected adults and adolescents.* Retrieved from http://aidsinfo.nih.gov/contentfiles/lvguidelines/AdultandAdolescentGL.pdf

Pao, M., Lyon, M., D'Angelo, L., Schuman, W., Tipnis, T., & Mrazak, D. (2000). Psychiatric diagnoses in adolescents seropositive for the human immunodeficiency virus. *Archives of Pediatric and Adolescent Medicine, 15*(3), 240–244. doi:10.1001/archpedi.154.3.240

Policy Studies Associates. (1997). Protecting the privacy of student education records. *Journal of School Health, 67*(4), 139–140. doi:10.1111/j.1746-1561.1997.tb03433.x

Pumariega, A. J., Shugart, M. A., & Pumariega, J. B. (2006). HIV/AIDS among children and adolescents. In F. Fernandez & P. Ruiz (Eds.), *Psychiatric aspects of HIV/AIDS* (pp. 259–266). Philadelphia, PA: Lippincott Williams & Wilkins.

Rehabilitation Act of 1973, 34 C. F. R. Part 104 § 504. (1973).

Reitz, M. S., & Gallo, R. C. (2015). Human immunodeficiency viruses. In: J. E. Bennett, R. Dolin, & M. J. Blaser (Eds.), *Mandell, Douglas, and Bennett's principles and practice of infectious diseases* (8th ed., Ch. 171). Philadelphia, PA: Elsevier Saunders.

Rodriguez, C., & Emmanuel, P. (2017). Medical implications of HIV for children and adolescents. In T. Chenneville (Ed), *A Clinical Guide to Pediatric HIV*, 15–42. Dordrecht: Springer.

Rotheram-Borus, M. J., Swendeman, D., Comulada, S., Weiss, R. E., Lee, M., & Lightfoot, M. (2004). Prevention for substance-using HIV-positive young people; telephone and in-person delivery. *Journal of Acquired Immune Deficiency Syndromes, 37*(2), S68–S77. doi:10.1097/01.qai.0000140604.57478.67

Sandoval, J., Scott, A. N., & Padilla, I. (2009). Crisis counseling: An overview. *Psychology in the Schools, 46*, 246–256. doi:10.1002/pits.20370

Sherr, L., Croome, N., Castaneda, K. P., Bradshaw, K., & Romero, R. H. (2014). Developmental challenges in HIV infected children: An updated systematic review. *Children and Youth Services Review, 45*, 74–89. doi:10.1016/j.childyouth.2014.03.040

Simmonds, R. J., & Chanock, S. (1993). Perspectives on human immunodeficiency virus infections. *Pediatric Infectious Disease Journal, 12*, 845–52.

Stangl, A., & Sievwright, K. (2017). HIV-Related Stigma and Children. In T. Chenneville (Ed), *A Clinical Guide to Pediatric HIV*, 297–315. Dordrecht: Springer.

Stinnett, T. A., Cruce, M. K., & Choate, K. T. (2004). Influences on teacher education student attitudes toward youth who are HIV+. *Psychology in the Schools, 41*(2), 211–219. doi:10.1002/pits.10123

Turan, J., & Nyblade, L. (2013). HIV-related stigma as a barrier to achievement of global PMTCT and maternal health goals: A review of the evidence. *AIDS Behavior, 17*, 2528–2539. doi:10.1007/s10461-013-0446-8

U.S. Department of Health and Human Services. (2015). *Symptoms of HIV.* Retrieved from https://www.aids.gov/hiv-aids-basics/hiv-aids-101/signs-and-symptoms/

Viswanathan, M., Ammerman, A., Eng, E., Gartlehner, G., Lohr, K. N., Griffith, D., … Whitener, L. (2004). Community-based participatory research: Assessing the evidence: Summary. In AHRQ Evidence Report Summaries. Rockville (MD): Agency for Healthcare Research and Quality (US); 1998–2005. 99. Available from: http://www.ncbi.nlm.nih.gov/books/NBK11852/

Walcott, C. M., Meyers, A. B., & Landau, S. (2008). Adolescent sexual risk behaviors and school-based sexually transmitted infection/HIV prevention. *Psychology in the Schools, 45*(1), 39–51. doi:10.1002/pits

Walsh, A., & Chenneville, T. (2013). Addressing HIV in the school setting: Application of a school change model. *Advances in School Mental Health Promotion, 00*, 1–14. doi:10.1080/1754730X.2012.760918

Walter, H. J., & Vaughan, R. D. (1993). *AIDS prevention for adolescents in school*. Los Altos, CA: Sociometrics Corporation.

Whitehead, N., Potterton, J., & Coovadia, A. (2014). The neurodevelopment of HIV-infected infants on HAART compared to HIV-exposed but uninfected infants. *AIDS Care, 26*(4), 497–504. doi:10.1080/09540121.2013.841828

World Health Organization. (2007). *Standard precautions in health care*. Retrieved from http://www.who.int/csr/resources/publications/EPR_AM2_E7.pdf

Wyn, J., Cahill, H., Holdsworth, R., Rowling, L., & Carson, S. (2000). MindMatters, a whole-school approach promoting mental health and wellbeing. *Australian and New Zealand Journal of Psychiatry, 34*, 594–601.

Ybarra, M. L., DuBois, L. Z., Parsons, J. T., Prescott, T. L., & Mustanski, B. (2014). Online focus groups as an HIV prevention program for gay, bisexual, and queer adolescent males. *AIDS Education and Prevention: Official Publication of the International Society for AIDS Education, 26*(6), 554.

Zhao, J., Peilian, C., Li, X., Tam, C. C., & Zhao, G. (2014). Extracurricular interest as a resilience building block for children affected by parental HIV/AIDS. *AIDS Care, 26*(6), 758–762.

Chapter 7
Antiretroviral Medication Adherence and Disease Management in Pediatric Populations

Idia B. Thurston, Kristina Decker and Robin Hardin

Overview of HIV Adherence in Youth

Rates of HIV and Medication Adherence in Pediatric Populations

The HIV epidemic impacts many children and adolescents in the US as well as globally. By the end of 2013, approximately 3.2 million children were living with HIV around the world with 91% of these children living in sub-Saharan Africa (World Health Organization 2013). Perinatal HIV infection has been relatively well-managed in the US, with current estimates suggesting that fewer than 200 infants with HIV are born each year (AIDSInfo 2015). However, rates of perinatal infection continue to be high in developing countries, and transmission rates are as high as 45% in some regions (World Health Organization 2013). In 2010, it was estimated that only 2900 children under the age of 12 in the US were HIV positive (ChildHealth 2011; Woolston 2015). However, rates among youth aged 13–24 are large and growing. In fact, youth accounted for approximately 26% of all new HIV infections in 2010 (CDC 2012). Notably, there are significant gender differences in the HIV epidemic among youth, with close to 80% of all new HIV infections occurring in male youth. Specifically, young men who have sex with men (YMSM) are most at risk for contracting HIV with infection rates of 19% (CDC 2015b). Racial and ethnic disparities in HIV infection are also evident. Specifically, Black

I.B. Thurston (✉) · K. Decker · R. Hardin
University of Memphis, Memphis, TN, USA
e-mail: bthrston@memphis.edu

K. Decker
e-mail: kdecker@memphis.edu

R. Hardin
e-mail: rnhardin@memphis.edu

T. Chenneville (ed.), *A Clinical Guide to Pediatric HIV*,
DOI 10.1007/978-3-319-49704-4_7

youth are disproportionately infected with HIV at rates of 57% compared to Latino (20%) and White (20%) youth (CDC 2015b). The differential impact of the HIV epidemic on certain groups of youth and the role that intersecting identities have in contributing to even greater risk (e.g., among Black YMSM) highlight the need to understand unique factors that affect disease management and HIV medication adherence overall but even more so among these vulnerable populations who are most impacted by HIV/AIDS.

HIV-related morbidity and mortality rates have significantly decreased over the past several years owing to advances in antiretroviral therapy (ART). Updated guidelines from the Word Health Organization recommend treating HIV with ART as soon as possible rather than waiting until a certain CD4 count level given the impact of HIV on cognitive functioning and the protective role of starting medications early (IAPAC 2015). However, the success of HIV therapies is completely dependent on having high levels of HIV medication in the body, and therefore, adherence to ART is critical (Bartlett 2002; Chesney 2003; Paterson et al. 2000). Successful long-term treatment of HIV requires that individuals take at least 90–95% of their antiretroviral medications in order to receive maximum benefit (Chesney 2003; Reisner et al. 2009). However, even when the treatment regimen is simple (i.e., taking one pill once a day), maintaining adherence at such rates can be difficult for adults living with HIV, a challenge that is even more pronounced among youth. Specifically, research suggests adherence rates among youth to range between 28–69% (Chesney 2003; Murphy et al. 2005; Reisner et al. 2009), a rate that is much lower than in adults (Becker et al. 2002). While concerning, this low rate is not entirely surprising given that medication adherence poses unique challenges for children and adolescents due to various developmental concerns (such as reliance on caregivers, identity formation, risk taking, and behavioral experimentation associated with adolescence) and still developing cognitive function (Reisner et al. 2009). Considering the detrimental consequences of untreated HIV (AIDSInfo 2014), increasing medication adherence among youth is a top priority.

Disparities in HIV Medication Adherence

Although young people are at risk for low adherence, there are notable disparities in adherence rates across various sociodemographic groups. Specifically, racial and ethnic minorities not only carry a higher burden of the HIV epidemic compared to Whites but also have lower rates of medication adherence than Whites, a gap that has been maintained since the beginning of ART treatment (Cunningham et al. 2000; Gebo et al. 2005). Caregivers' level of education has also been shown to affect their children's adherence with higher levels of caregiver education being associated with higher rates of adherence (Reisner et al. 2009; Williams et al. 2006). Among adolescents and young adults (AYAs), those who drop out of high school are less likely to adhere to their medication regimens (Murphy et al. 2005). Similarly, youth from low socioeconomic (SES) backgrounds are less adherent to their HIV medications than youth from higher SES backgrounds (Rudy et al. 2009). This finding is likely driven by the myriad of risks associated with living in poverty. Specifically, families living in poverty are at greater risk for a number of stressful life events (e.g., increased exposure to violence, higher rates of substance abuse, and limited resources) that have been associated with higher levels of non-adherence (Crespo-Fierro 1997; Malee et al. 2011; Mellins et al. 2004). Consistent with many other chronic illnesses, as youth age their rates of non-adherence increase (Williams et al. 2006). This association may be related to the transition of medication-taking responsibility from parent-driven among younger children to adolescent-led as youth age. Notably, this transition of responsibility of care from parent to adolescent is rarely orchestrated in an organized manner, and factors that may interfere with an adolescents' ability to take medication autonomously, such as their developmental level, emotional functioning, psychological needs, or cognitive abilities, are rarely considered before making the transition (Naar-King et al. 2006b). Disparities in medication adherence by gender are also prominent. Research has also shown that male youth are more likely to adhere to ARTs than female youth (Williams et al. 2006). Given significant disparities in adherence rates by race/ethnicity, socioeconomic status, age, and gender, interventions aimed at increasing HIV adherence should not only target these youth but also develop innovative and customized strategies to address these concerns in order to be successful.

Adherence Among Youth with Behaviorally (BaHIV) and Perinatally (PaHIV) Acquired HIV

While most children under age 12 contracted HIV via perinatal transmission (i.e., from mother to child during pregnancy, labor and delivery, or breastfeeding), since the 1990s, there has been a significant decline (ovcr 90%) in the US with respect to the number of children with PaHIV due to numerous efforts aimed at prenatal HIV testing and interventions for mothers (CDC 2012). Unfortunately, rates of perinatal infection remain high in developing countries with rates up to 45% in certain regions (World Health Organization 2013). Notably, there are disparate medication adherence patterns between children and adolescents who were infected with HIV perinatally versus behaviorally (i.e., via unprotected vaginal or anal sex, injection drug use, or blood transfusion). Research has shown that youth with PaHIV tend to be more adherent to HIV medication regimens compared to youth with BaHIV (Chandwani et al. 2012). This may be related to the unique adherence challenges and barriers that are faced by youth with BaHIV and PaHIV.

Youth with PaHIV possess different treatment needs compared to youth with BaHIV. It is not uncommon for youth with PaHIV to have extensive treatment histories, drug resistance from years of being on antiretroviral therapy, and inconsistent treatment adherence over time (Hazra et al. 2010; Koenig et al. 2011).

Youth with PaHIV are also more likely to be in advanced stages of HIV disease and have more complicated antiretroviral regimens than youth with BaHIV who have not been infected with HIV for long. The consequences of non-adherence are also different, such that missing a dose for youth with PaHIV may be more detrimental to medication efficacy since they are prescribed less potent medication regimens because of commonly acquired medication resistance related to simply being on medication regimens for extended periods of time (Hazra et al. 2010). Although rates of adherence are higher overall, youth with PaHIV tend to report more barriers to medication adherence than youth with BaHIV (MacDonell et al. 2013).

On the other hand, youth with BaHIV tend to have a greater preoccupation with HIV-related stigma and privacy concerns, especially with respect to the possibility of their HIV status being revealed without their consent, which may have a negative impact on medication adherence (MacDonell et al. 2013). Further, adjusting to life living with a chronic illness, especially one highly associated with negative stigma, as well as managing issues of disclosure can pose specific challenges to medication adherence, such as sticking to a strict medication routine/schedule and managing experiences of stigma (Valenzuela et al. 2011). Stigma may be especially worse for youth with BaHIV compared to youth with PaHIV related to their mode of HIV infection (e.g., unprotected anal sex in same sex relationships) (Radcliffe et al. 2010). Youth with BaHIV who use substances are at even greater risk for medication non-adherence as they report more barriers to taking HIV medications as prescribed (MacDonell et al. 2013). Given these differences in adherence by mode of HIV infection, interventions should consider differential targets when addressing the unique needs of youth with PaHIV and BaHIV.

Barriers and Facilitators to Antiretroviral Therapy Adherence

Among youth with HIV/AIDS, factors that influence adherence to antiretroviral therapy (ART) are complex and multifaceted. While some barriers and facilitators to ART adherence apply broadly to many children and adolescents, nuances across youth developmental levels necessitate a discussion of barriers and facilitators that utilizes a developmentally responsive approach. Additionally, irrespective of developmental functioning, youth tend to become less adherent to medication regimens with increasing age (Kahana et al. 2013); thus, it is critical to emphasize the unique contextual influences on adherence as youth age. Despite biological, psychological, and social differences in various developmental groups (e.g., toddlerhood, early childhood, middle childhood, and adolescence), a limited number of studies consider developmental differences in adherence. Specifically, research on many pediatric chronic conditions such as asthma, diabetes, and gastrointestinal disorders has typically examined adherence across a broad age range without necessarily distinguishing among specific developmental groups (Rapoff 2010).

Studies on ART adherence tend to distinguish between childhood/early adolescence and adolescence/young adulthood or simply to examine a broad age range (e.g., 0–18 year olds). This trend in the pediatric HIV literature may be related to stark decreases in maternal-to-child HIV transmission rates in the US, which has resulted in a shrinking population of children under age 12 living with HIV in the US (CDC 2015a), a significant stride in the fight against the HIV epidemic. It should be noted that global transmission rates have decreased 58% with most countries outside of the sub-Saharan African region achieving very low rates of mother-to-child HIV transmission (WHO 2015). Therefore, while we acknowledge the existence of incremental developmental differences across various age groups, given limitations in the literature, we will frame our discussion of barriers and facilitators to adherence in the developmental context of childhood (ages 0–12) and adolescence/young adulthood (ages 13–25).

Barriers to ART Adherence in Childhood

Psychosocial Factors

Among younger children, adherence to ART is typically reliant on the caregiver (Buchanan et al. 2012). Therefore, considering the association between caregiver characteristics and adherence is critical. In a study of children aged between 3 and 13 years, worse parent–child communication, higher caregiver stress, lower caregiver quality of life, and lower caregiver cognitive functioning were associated with decreased child adherence to ART (Mellins et al. 2004). Additionally, higher caregiver psychological distress (Marhefka et al. 2006) and substance use (Naar-King et al. 2006a) have also been associated with decreased ART adherence. Furthermore, caregivers of youth in childhood and early adolescence reported difficulty adhering to their child's regime due to forgetfulness (Merzel et al. 2008; Vreeman et al. 2015) and decreased schedule structure during summer months (Merzel et al. 2008).

As children transition to school-age, unique barriers to adherence associated with school attendance become important. Specifically, caregivers may struggle with ART regimens that require taking a dose at school as this typically requires disclosing the child's HIV status to school staff and potentially stigmatizing the child further as well as put the child at risk for unintentional disclose of their HIV status (Merzel et al. 2008). In general, disclosure of seropositive status may act as a barrier to adherence because caregivers may not want to give their child medications in front of others and risk seropositive status disclosure (Vreeman et al. 2015; Wrubel et al. 2005). Additionally, caregiver concern over morning medication doses that could elicit potentially impairing side effects (e.g., diarrhea) has been associated with decreased adherence (Wrubel et al. 2005). This effect might be more pronounced for young children who are just starting school, given that parents may be reluctant to create an added burden of medication management to the already stressful school adjustment period.

Caregiver reports of child behavioral concerns, such as impulsivity, hyperactivity, and learning difficulties, have been associated with decreased adherence (Malee et al. 2011). Malee et al. (2011) suggest that behavioral difficulties may impede parent attempts to promote youth adherence and child willingness or ability to follow regimen directions. It should be noted that these behavioral difficulties are also associated with increasing age and thus are relevant to adolescents as well (Malee et al. 2011).

Treatment Regimen

Difficulty with pill swallowing may present a barrier for younger children. However, as children develop, taking ART that is not in pill form (i.e., syrup) is actually associated with decreased adherence (Nichols et al. 2012). Nichols and colleagues suggest that as children approach school-age, having a non-pill-based medication may be a barrier to adherence due to poor taste of the medication and the requirement to measure volume of medication—adding an extra step to the medication routine. Caregivers report increased concern for their child's level of distress when they experience various side effects of ART, such as nausea, diarrhea, and fatigue (Koenig and Bachanas 2006). Increased caregiver concern about ART side effects has been associated with decreased adherence (Wrubel et al. 2005). Additionally, child vomiting following medication administration created caregiver indecision about whether or not medications should be readministered, thus impacting regimen adherence (Wrubel et al. 2005). Just as youth experience regimen fatigue, caregivers also report experiencing regimen fatigue. This fatigue has been associated with increased likelihood of skipping ART doses when children are resistant to take medications (Wrubel et al. 2005).

Facilitators to ART Adherence in Childhood

While research findings highlight an array of barriers to adherence among children, few studies utilize a more strength-based approach by exploring developmentally specific facilitators of adherence. Among middle childhood youth with PaHIV who demonstrate confusion or fatigue over having to take medications, adherence is facilitated when caregivers disclose their seropositive status to them (Merzel et al. 2008). Status disclosure and education about one's HIV diagnosis may provide children with a clear rationale and strong motivation to continue taking medications as prescribed. This also alludes to the positive effect of open parent–child communication in facilitating adherence in childhood.

Treatment Regimen

Children demonstrated higher medication adherence when caregivers other than the biological parent(s) administered medications (Malee et al. 2011). Malee et al. (2011) hypothesized that biological caregivers diagnosed with HIV may acknowledge and sympathize with adherence difficulties more so than other caretakers, thus allowing room for more instances of non-adherence. Regarding pill-swallowing barriers, caregivers reported that inventive strategies such as mixing medication with food or dissolving medications in water facilitated adherence (Merzel et al. 2008; Wrubel et al. 2005). Adherence partnerships between caregivers and youth have also been associated with increased adherence (Merzel et al. 2008). These partnerships included activities such as sorting all pills for the upcoming week together or taking daily medications at the same time. Additionally, arranging with medical care providers to take medication two times per day, rather than three (i.e., reducing the medication regimen burden), allowed families to withhold diagnosis from the youth's school and was associated with increased adherence (Merzel et al. 2008).

Barriers to ART Adherence in Adolescence/Young Adulthood

Psychosocial Factors

During adolescence and young adulthood, primary responsibility for monitoring ART regimens tends to shift from the caregiver to the adolescent or young adult (Buchanan et al. 2012; Merzel et al. 2008). However, it should be noted that the nature of this transition is often informal, disorganized, and inconsistent, leaving room for multiple adherence difficulties. Further, with greater independence and choice regarding when to take medications, many developmentally specific factors especially prominent in adolescence and young adulthood may arise and influence adherence. For example, a developmentally congruent desire for independence and autonomy may be expressed as non-adherence (Fields et al. 2012). Furthermore, adolescents may rebel against instructions to follow a certain medication regimen, if the messaging comes from the caregiver or another person perceived to be an "authority figure" due to the developmentally congruent experience of reactance (i.e., the tendency of young people to act in opposing ways when they perceive that their choices are being limited or taken away) (Fields et al. 2012; Simoni et al. 2007). Typical developmental beliefs of invincibility and decreased consideration of the link between behaviors and consequences may also negatively impact adherence among AYA. Study findings highlight that AYAs tend to prioritize present emotions or desires above taking their medications, which underscores an inattention to long-term health consequences (Casey et al. 2008; Fields et al. 2012).

High rates of emotional concerns and substance use among adolescents living with HIV are also implicated in non-adherence (Koenig and Bachanas 2006).

Mental health concerns, such as increased depressive symptoms, are associated with decreased medication adherence (Hosek et al. 2005; Mellins et al. 2011; Murphy et al. 2001). Research findings indicate that youth experiencing depressive symptoms may report lower motivation to take medications and/or may experience a sense of hopelessness associated with living HIV and taking medications regularly (Fields et al. 2012). Furthermore, engagement in substance use has been associated with decreased adherence (Hosek et al. 2005; Mellins et al. 2011; Fields et al. 2012). AYAs have reported delaying or skipping doses to avoid a feared interaction between the substances and their ART (Fields et al. 2012).

During adolescence and young adulthood, as peer relationships become an important aspect of development, fear of peer rejection and discrimination based on HIV serostatus may become especially relevant. Among teenagers and young adults, dose skipping or complete non-adherence may function to avoid social and peer rejection (Koenig and Bachanas 2006; Reisner et al. 2009). Generally, experience with HIV-related stigma and discrimination has been associated with decreased adherence (Reisner et al. 2009). Among youth with BaHIV, infection typically occurs during adolescence or young adulthood, and thus, the youth may engage in self-blame or experience internalized stigma and delay onset of taking HIV medications (Fields et al. 2012). Regarding seropositive status disclosure, AYA may struggle with disclosing their HIV status to friends and family. Concern about or fear of disclosure of HIV status to friends or family may motivate youth to skip medication to prevent others from seeing the medications or witnessing them taking medications (Rao et al. 2007). As AYAs begin spending more time with peer groups and even moving away from home, disclosure of status may become an even more salient barrier as youth have to make decisions about who, when, and how to disclose their status.

Structural Factors

As AYAs become independent and take responsibility for their health care, structural barriers may play an increasingly important role in ART adherence. Specifically, youth who experienced problems with medical insurance were less likely to be adherent to medication regimens (Rudy et al. 2010). Additional structural concerns, such as problems with school or work, difficulty managing family or childcare, and experiencing a greater number of structural barriers, have been associated with decreased adherence (Rudy et al. 2010). Unstructured lifestyle and trying to balance a number of domains such as school, work, college lifestyle, and social outings are also associated with decreased adherence (Fields et al. 2012; Koenig and Bachanas 2006). Particularly relevant to AYA with BaHIV is the potential for familial or caregiver alienation or abandonment upon status disclosure. This estrangement from family has been associated with inconsistent housing and instability, which in turn is related to decreased ART adherence (Koenig and Bachanas 2006).

Treatment regimen

As previously discussed among younger children, factors associated with the medications themselves have been associated with non-adherence. Consistent with younger children's experiences, the desire to avoid medication side effects has been associated with AYA non-adherence (Fields et al. 2012). Additionally, as youth age, increased pill burden and increased dosing times due to potential resistance that develops over time (Fields et al. 2012), as well as avoiding reminders of their HIV infection (MacDonell et al. 2013), may function as barriers to adherence. AYA also frequently reported decreased adherence because they simply forgot to take a dose of medication or intentionally did not take the medication to avoid side effects, such as nausea or diarrhea (MacDonell et al. 2013).

Facilitators to ART Adherence in Adolescence/Young Adulthood

Similar to research on young children, studies exploring strength-based factors that promote adherence among AYA are limited. Regarding psychosocial factors, higher levels of life satisfaction, lower levels of psychological distress, and the belief that medication would improve quality of life are related to ART adherence (Reisner et al. 2009). Additionally, Chenneville et al. (2015) found that AYA with increased understanding of HIV demonstrated greater medication adherence within the preceding seven days. As adolescents develop, increased understanding of HIV and the risks of medication non-adherence paired with psychosocial factors (distress, quality of life) may reflect critical components for adherence given that adolescent behaviors are heavily influenced by their emotions (Casey et al. 2008).

Best Practices in Adherence Measurement

Because adherence to ART is critical to prevent infection and suppress viral load among youth with HIV, valid and reliable measures of adherence are essential (Martin et al. 2009). Research on the prevalence of adherence among youth yields considerably variable rates, which some researchers attribute to inconsistent measures of medication adherence (Martin et al. 2009). While adherence to ART can be estimated directly via markers in bodily fluids, many researchers measure adherence using indirect methods such as self-report, pill counts, pharmacy refills, electronic monitoring, and indicators of medication impact such as HIV-1 RNA viral load and CD4 lymphocyte count (Simoni et al. 2007; Usitalo et al. 2014). Direct measures of adherence gathered via bodily fluid (such as blood assays of active drug) can directly confirm drug ingestion, but are considered more costly and logistically complicated than indirect measures (Simoni et al. 2006). Accordingly, researchers often examine the association among subjective (i.e., self-report) or objective measures of medication dosage (i.e., pill count, pharmacy refills, and electronic monitoring) and variables indicating efficacy of medical treatment (i.e., viral load and CD4 count) to demonstrate the validity of adherence measurement methodologies (Farley et al. 2008; Usitalo et al. 2014). In a recent meta-analysis of adherence among youth, researchers found that even across different measurement methodologies, greater adherence was robustly related to decreased viral load outcomes (Kahana et al. 2013). When examining each method, it is important to recognize the unique benefits and limitations that may influence the practicality and feasibility of their use.

Self-report

Self-report measures of medication adherence from caregivers and youth involve single questions or questionnaires requiring caregivers and youth to recall missed medication doses over a specified time period. While measures vary across studies, common self-report assessments involve estimation of doses missed in the past few days, week, or month, as well as report of general adherence (e.g., over the last 6 months) using analog scales or percentages (Usitalo et al. 2014). Some researchers support the benefit of examining longer recall periods such as one month (Evans et al. 2015; Farley et al. 2008). For example, Farley et al. (2008) established that caregiver and youth recall of medication adherence in the last month was associated with viral load, while recall of missed doses in the last three days was not. This alludes to the increased benefit of extended time periods for recall, yet recall accuracy with longer time periods is important to consider, especially among youth with developing cognitive capacities.

Typically, self-report of child and adolescent adherence is obtained from both the caregiver and youth (Dolezal et al. 2003). Research supports discrepancy between caregiver and youth reports of missed medication doses (Dolezal et al. 2003; Evans et al. 2015), especially between caregivers and adolescents compared to caregivers and children (Dolezal et al. 2003). This highlights the importance of obtaining multiple sources of information when using self-report methodology for youth adherence. When examining the association between dosing recall and viral load based on the self-report source, Evans et al. (2015) found differences across youth development. During early middle childhood and early adolescence, parents may offer more accurate reports of adherence, and during later adolescence, youth may be better informants than their parents (Evans et al. 2015). This is consistent with parent–adolescent relationships in general, whereby as youth age, parental involvement, monitoring, and awareness of daily routines and behaviors decrease as youth rely more and have greater involvement with peers (Casey et al. 2008; Laursen and Collins 2009).

While some research utilizes self-report measures of adherence and data support the validity of this method given high associations with viral load (Usitalo et al.

2014), other studies have found self-report information to be less accurate, given its subjective nature, compared to objective measures (e.g., pill count) of medication adherence (Martin et al. 2009). Findings generally support several factors that may detrimentally influence the accuracy of self-report adherence measures. For example, caregivers and youth may be driven by social desirability to overestimate rates of adherence (Dolezal et al. 2003; Wagner and Miller 2004), a finding that may be even more pronounced among certain racial and ethnic minority groups owing to cultural and power differences in patient–provider relationships. Additionally, patients and families may have unintentional memory lapses when retrospectively recalling medication adherence rates (Wagner and Miller 2004). On the other hand, adherence experts have recommended strategies to reduce the impact of retrospective recall bias and social desirability when using self-report adherence measures. Specifically, recommendations such as using item phrasing that normalizes non-adherence, having question items focus on recent behavior, and anchoring reports to important life events have all been effective in improving self-report adherence measures (Simoni et al. 2006). Despite accuracy concerns associated with self-report measures, this remains a relevant and useful measure of adherence due to its ease of use, cost-effectiveness, and strong associations with viral load (Simoni et al. 2007; Usitalo et al. 2014).

Pill Count or Refills

Pill counts and pharmacy medication refill information are utilized as objective measures of adherence (Burack et al. 2010; Farley et al. 2008). Pill counts, which are often obtained during home visits or clinic visits when patients are asked to bring in medication bottles, compare the amount of medication remaining in the bottle to the amount that should be remaining based on daily dosage, the initial prescription, and the time since the medication was filled. This method provides researchers or clinicians with an objective measure of unused medication doses (Farley et al. 2008). Similarly, pharmacy refill records provide information on the timing and occurrence of medication refills, with delayed or missed refills indicating decreased adherence (Burack et al. 2010; Marhefka et al. 2006). Although study findings indicate associations between viral load and pill count (Intasan et al. 2014), as well as pharmacy refill records (Marhefka et al. 2006), such findings have not been consistent in the literature (Farley et al. 2008; Marhefka et al. 2006).

While monitoring adherence via pill counts or refill records is inexpensive and minimally complicated, these methods may be limited in the type of information they can provide. For example, neither pill count nor refill records measure the daily timing of the doses administered or missed (Martin et al. 2009) nor do these methods assess ingestion of the pills, as it is possible that youth may take medications out of the bottles without actually swallowing the pills. Additionally, youth may not begin taking the medication on the day the prescription was filled, thus resulting in potential overestimation of adherence (Farley et al. 2008). A specific limitation of refill records is that this method does not account for unused medications at the end of the prescription period (Marhefka et al. 2006). Specifically, while caregivers and patients may refill and receive their medications regularly, they may have doses or even unopened bottles remaining at the end of the prescription period, resulting in overestimation of adherence. This limitation of the refill record method, however, is addressed with the pill count method.

Electronic Monitoring

With advances in technology, electronic methods of monitoring medication adherence are more prevalent and considered to be the current gold standard of adherence assessment (Nichols et al. 2012; Usitalo et al. 2014). One such monitoring method is the Medication Event Monitoring System (MEMS) cap, which electronically registers and tracks the dates and times of all medication bottle openings (Martin et al. 2009). Adherence measured using the MEMS cap has been significantly associated with decreased viral load among youth (Farley et al. 2003; Martin et al. 2007; Muller et al. 2008). Additionally, compared to adherence monitoring methods such as self-report and pill counting, electronic monitoring is considered one of the most detailed and reliable assessments of adherence (Martin et al. 2009). This method allows for medication timing specificity, the lack of which is a major limitation of self-report, pill count, and pharmacy refill methods.

Despite the benefits in reporting accuracy, the cost of electronic monitoring methods may limit their use in both research and routine clinical care settings (Nichols et al. 2012; Usitalo et al. 2014). Further, similar to pill counting or refill record assessments, electronic monitoring may not accurately reflect whether or not the dose was actually ingested (Martin et al. 2009). Researchers have also reported problematic malfunction of the MEMS cap system, resulting in loss of data, as well as lack of consistent principles guiding data interpretation from the MEMS cap (Martin et al. 2009). The MEMS cap system may also be problematic for youth whose regimens involve more than one pill per day and thus may rely on pillboxes to aid their medication management (Berg and Arnsten 2006), making the use of MEMS cap in these situations more cumbersome. Additionally, youth may take out more than one pill when the cap is opened (e.g., when going to a friend's house or work and not wanting to take the bulky pill bottle), and thus, cap opening frequency does not necessarily equate pill ingestion. However, MEMS cap calculations allow for adjustments based on these types self-report issues. However, if youth lose the MEMS cap, the data are lost.

In addition to the use of MEMS cap, new forms of electronic monitoring (e.g., real-time monitoring via electronic recorders and smart phones) have emerged as potential adherence monitoring tools among adults with HIV (Lester et al. 2010; Pop-Eleches et al. 2011). It will be important for future research to evaluate the usefulness and effectiveness of these more novel methods among children, adolescents, and young adults (Kahana et al. 2013).

Viral Load or CD-4 Count

HIV-1 RNA viral load (VL) and CD4 lymphocyte count are medical indicators of ART impact (Simoni et al. 2007; Usitalo et al. 2014) that are measured through laboratory analysis of blood (AIDS Etc. National Resource Center 2014). VL and CD4 are indicators of disease progression that are highly related to the effectiveness of and adherence to ART, with elevated viral load and decreased CD4 associated with morbidity and mortality (Gibb 2008; Kahana et al. 2013). CD4 count is typically measured by counting the number of CD4 cells per microliter of blood, and VL is measured by counting the number of HIV-1 RNA per milliliter of plasma (AIDS Etc. National Resource Center 2014). As previously noted, VL and CD4 are frequently measured and compared to subjective and objective measures of adherence in the literature (Simoni et al. 2007; Usitalo et al. 2014).

Overall, research alludes to the importance of utilizing multiple markers of adherence for optimal assessment of adherence in youth. The level of accuracy needed likely depends on the reasons for medication monitoring. Specifically, research studies may require higher levels of reporting accuracy than routine clinical practice. Furthermore, the costs associated with more accurate devices (such as MEMS cap) may be prohibitive and too time-intensive for regular use in a clinic. Accordingly, providers and researchers should balance cost and specific needs when making decisions about the optimal adherence tool to be used.

Evidence-Based Interventions for Improving Adherence

There is currently no gold standard intervention for improving ART adherence among youth. However, researchers have identified several factors that individually contribute to or facilitate improved adherence, most of which were described above and in previous work (Lyon et al. 2003; MacDonell et al. 2013; Naar-King et al. 2013). The unique developmental concerns of children and adolescents underscore the need for tailored ART adherence interventions to meet their needs. Specifically, family and peer relationships are critical for positive youth development, and research has shown that interventions that include family members and/or peers have been effective in increasing adherence in youth (Lyon et al. 2003). The location where adherence interventions are administered is also critical with respect to issues of accessibility that affect engagement in adherence interventions. While most interventions tend to occur in clinic settings, interventions in patients' homes have also been shown to be effective in improving adherence (Berrien et al. 2004), and such interventions have the added benefit of increased accessibility for youth and their caregivers. With respect to intervention content, given variance in youth cognitive development, most adherence interventions incorporate strategies to increase HIV knowledge. This is especially important, given that poor HIV knowledge and low health literacy have been associated with decreased ART adherence in youth (Navarra et al. 2014). However, HIV literacy is only one piece of the adherence puzzle and is likely insufficient to improve overall ART adherence in youth alone.

The modality of intervention distribution has also been the focus of many HIV interventions. Over the past two decades, there has been a major shift in technology use, one that has been even more pronounced among youth. Approximately 78% of teenagers in the US have a personal cell phone, and 93% have a personal computer or access to one at home (Madden et al. 2013). The ubiquitous nature of technology coupled with research indicating that technology use can improve youth adherence (Shegog et al. 2012) has resulted in the increased use of various aspects of technology in ART adherence interventions. Researchers have developed Web-based interventions (Shegog et al. 2012) and incorporated text messaging (Dowshen et al. 2013; Haberer et al. 2010; Thurston et al. 2014) to increase adherence in youth via medication adherence monitoring, medication reminders, psychoeducation about HIV and medication regimens, as well as used technology to send motivational messages that encourage adherence (Dowshen et al. 2013; Puccio et al. 2006).

Given the varied aspects associated with improved adherence in youth, many ART interventions have taken a multicomponent approach, often addressing a wide range of factors shown to positively impact adherence among youth. Below, we provide more details about published interventions conducted in clinic-based settings and home-/community-based settings, as well as interventions that incorporate technology.

Clinic-Based Interventions

Lyon and colleagues conducted a family/peer group intervention in a clinic setting to increase adherence among youth living with HIV (Lyon et al. 2003). Specifically, the program consisted of six biweekly caregiver (or "treatment buddy") and youth education sessions and six biweekly youth-only education sessions. The sessions covered topics related to the dynamics of HIV, purpose of ART, medication choices and side effects, nutrition, exercise, alternative treatments, communication with doctors and healthcare providers, and separating fact and fiction in the media. Each session began with a thirty-minute dinner with the cofacilitators, youth, and treatment buddies; then, treatment buddies and youth had separate 60-min education sessions and rejoined each other for a 30-min interactive review of the material presented using a game show format. On alternate weeks, only youth met in a group therapy format to discuss concerns related to taking multiple medications. Each week a new device was introduced to help youth adhere to ART medications including pillboxes, beepers, calendars, wristwatches with multiple alarms, and gym bags. This intervention produced positive results, with 91% of youth reporting increased adherence after completing the program. Furthermore, four youth had significant reduction in their viral loads to the undetectable level during the program. Other benefits of the intervention to overall health included increase in hepatitis B and influenza immunizations, attending medical and dental appointments, and obtaining referrals for mental health and substance abuse treatment.

Garvie and colleagues examined the efficacy of pill-swallowing training in relation to improved adherence (Garvie et al. 2007). Adolescents engaged in individual training sessions in which a pediatric psychologist demonstrated how to appropriately swallow a pill. The adolescents then practiced swallowing placebos, which gradually increased in size. In order to move on to the next size, youth had to swallow two of each placebo size. If the adolescent was not successful on either of the two trials, the adolescent was given a third chance before regressing to the last placebo size that s/he was successfully able to swallow. This intervention produced positive results. Specifically, the pill-swallowing training was found to improve adherence six months after the training. Furthermore, immediate and long-term (six month) improvements in CD4 count and viral load were reported following the intervention.

Home-/Community-Based Interventions

Several interventions have been implemented to improve ART adherence in pediatric patients. Berrien and colleagues designed and tested a multicomponent intervention that targeted HIV knowledge and barriers to adherence during eight home visits over the span of three months by the same home care nurse (Berrien et al. 2004). Sessions were conducted with youth and their caregivers and covered basic HIV knowledge, ability to name medications, knowledge of how the medications work, knowledge of the proper dose for each medication, talking to medical providers about medication problems, interacting with the pharmacist, pill-swallowing training, overcoming identified barriers to adherence, and potential challenges from missing doses or not taking medications at all. Youth kept a journal to record completed medication doses and received incentives (such as pillboxes, pill crushers, diaries, and beepers) for taking medications. Youth and caregivers were taught how these devices could aid in adherence. The intervention resolved with a role reversal that required the youth to teach the nurse and his/her caregivers what the youth had learned. The intervention significantly improved youths' HIV/adherence knowledge and medication refill history. Medication adherence did improve in youth from baseline to follow-up, but was not statistically significant ($p = 0.07$).

Gaur and colleagues examined the feasibility and effectiveness of a community-based directly observed therapy (DOT) for non-adherent youth living with HIV (Gaur et al. 2010). Trained facilitators provided DOT once a day at the youth's choice of a community-based site, which could include their home. Across four sites in the US, 20 participants were enrolled. Participants completed an initial two-week period of daily DOT; this was then tapered to five days a week for six weeks and then reduced to self-administered therapy depending on the youth's adherence. Every youth enrolled in the study received at least 12 weeks of DOT before being transitioned to self-administered therapy (if they had at least 93% adherence). Monthly follow-up visits continued until week 24. Results indicated that only half of the participants maintained above a 90% medication adherence rate 12 weeks after discontinuing DOT, and thus, results were not maintained over time. However, youth with depression at baseline benefitted the most from the intervention.

Letourneau and colleagues examined the effectiveness of a multisystemic therapy (MST) intervention adapted to address adherence barriers in a pilot randomized controlled trial (RCT) for youth living with HIV (Letourneau et al. 2013). MST is a home and community-based intervention aimed at addressing multiple sources of youth problem behaviors (Henggeler et al. 2009). In this intervention, therapists used a variety of evidence-based intervention techniques including cognitive-behavioral therapy, parent training, behavioral family systems therapy, and communications skills training, to address barriers to ART adherence. Results indicated that the MST intervention resulted in significant viral load reduction and improved self-reported medication adherence among youth.

Interventions Incorporating Technology

A Web-based HIV medication adherence intervention, *+Click,* was piloted with 10 youth living with HIV for usability and psychosocial outcomes as a potential adjunct to traditional clinic-based, self-management education. Youths' reactions to the application and their psychosocial outcomes (including self-efficacy and ratings of importance of ART) were assessed (Shegog et al. 2012). *+Click* is a Web-based, tailored application that involves interactive activities addressing attitudes, knowledge, skills, and self-efficacy related to ART adherence; animation; and videos by peers and experts. It was designed for individual access during routine clinic visits. Youth start out with providing brief demographics, information on current adherence, barriers to adherence, predisposing factors (i.e., self-efficacy and adherence intentions), and self-reported viral load and CD4 count. Activities are then tailored based on this information. Findings indicated that *+Click* affected variables associated with adherence, but the study did not assess adherence directly. Specifically, there was a significant increase in the perceived importance of taking ART at consistent times, improved self-efficacy to adhere to medications, and increased HIV and adherence knowledge. Youth also found *+Click* to be relevant and useful, thus indicating openness to using technology for HIV medication adherence.

Dowshen et al. (2013) tested the feasibility and validity of a real-time adherence intervention for youth using text messaging. Specifically, they examined the practicality and validity of interactive text message response (ITR) as a way to assess adherence to ART in youth living with HIV. Each youth worked collaboratively with a research assistant to determine the time of day and frequency of receiving daily text message reminders. The reminder was personally crafted by each youth and then programmed by the research assistant to be sent out daily. A follow-up message was sent to youth one hour after they received their reminders to assess whether they had taken their medication. Findings indicated that youth responded to follow-up messages and reported their adherence 61% of the time. The feasibility of ITR as a valid measure of adherence was determined by calculating the proportion of positive responses where youth indicated that they had taken their medication divided by the total number of messages sent by researches requesting a response. This score was then compared to ratings on a visual analogue scale (VAS), a self-report adherence measure where respondents indicate their level of agreement or disagreement with statements along a continuous line between two end points (Crichton 2001). The overall mean ITR adherence rate was 57%. ITR and VAS scores were only moderately correlated during the first six weeks of the study. Thus, overall, this pilot study showed the ITR was moderately effective.

While technology has been the sole focus of many interventions, other studies have used technology to augment intervention content. For example, in their adherence intervention for AYA, Thurston and colleagues modified a well-established adult intervention, (Safren et al. 2009) for youth. This adapted intervention, Positive STEPS (Strategies To Enhance Problem-Solving Skills), incorporated text messaging as reminders to take ART (Thurston et al. 2014). Specifically, Positive STEPS was designed to address barriers to adherence among heterosexual and lesbian, gay, and bisexual (LGB) youth living with HIV. The intervention consisted of five one-hour sessions that involved problem-solving strategies to address adherence barriers and peer videos of patient testimonials addressing adolescent-specific adherence barriers, such as sticking to a medication schedule. Youth also learned positive coping skills for managing distress, which might impact adherence and learned about the importance of adherence via an interactive tool. Youth developed customized reminder text messages during the first session, which was then sent to them daily consistent with their medication dosing schedule. Each session ended with the clinician helping youth make a link between the medication adherence barriers covered in session to his/her life values as well as coming up with solutions to improve adherence over the following week. Findings indicated that Positive STEPS did maintain and improve adherence; however, gains were not consistently maintained over time.

This review of published adherence interventions for children and adolescents highlights numerous gaps. Many of the interventions described target the unique needs of youth but are still in their infancy with respect to being in the preliminary/early stages of testing, as most were pilot and feasibility studies. Accordingly, the lasting effects on adherence have yet to be proven. Given that adherence rates among youth remain suboptimal, strides should be made to develop efficacious interventions and move pilot-tested interventions forward via RCTs. Furthermore, the effectiveness of these interventions in the "real-world setting" needs to be evaluated.

Cultural Considerations in Working with Youth Living with HIV

Culture has a significant influence on medication adherence (Crespo-Fierro 1997; Penn et al. 2011). For instance, educational materials in physicians' offices may not address language and health literacy barriers, which may contribute to patients' misunderstanding or getting inaccurate information about medication regimens contributing to poor adherence. When a multicultural perspective (in general) and a patient's culture (specifically) are not taken into account by health providers, issues with medication adherence may ensue. Specifically, individuals from certain cultural groups are less likely to ask direct questions of those in authority (such as medical providers), and others have a tendency to avoid conflict or disappointing providers, while others still have a long history of poor health treatment and so may be distrustful of the individuals in authority, including health providers (Sue and Sue 2012). All of these cultural differences may contribute to poor patient–provider relationships and accordingly affect adherence (Chen et al. 2013; Dang et al. 2013; Gaston 2013). These cultural differences and their resultant impact on the patient–provider relationship should be considered in assessment, treatment, and research efforts given associations with HIV treatment adherence (Beach et al. 2006).

Notably, medical service providers serving youth living with HIV have often achieved higher education levels, are from higher SES backgrounds, and belong to majority (e.g., English-speaking, White, heterosexual) groups compared to their patients (Saha et al. 2013; Van Ryn 2002). Consequently, service providers and their patients are likely to differ with respect to race, ethnicity, sexual orientation, religious beliefs, gender, language, literacy level, SES, and access to resources. Taking a multicultural perspective, one that takes a stance of cultural humility and openness to other groups (Hook et al. 2013) can therefore improve the patient–provider relationship and accordingly medication adherence (Beach et al. 2006; Penn et al. 2011). Therefore, it is critical for providers to strive toward cultural humility by increasing their awareness of their own multicultural background, staying knowledgeable about issues relevant to the multicultural clients they serve, and maintaining relevant skills in culturally competent practice, especially those that have been adapted and shown to be effective with multicultural clients (Hook et al. 2013; Tervalon and Murray-Garcia 1998). All of these critical areas of multicultural practice can have a significant impact on medication adherence in pediatric populations in general and more specifically, among minority youth populations most impacted by HIV and poor adherence. For more information about the impact of culture, please refer to Rahill et al. (2017) chapter on cultural considerations for pediatric HIV research and practice.

Future Directions for Research and Practice

This chapter provided a detailed review of HIV medication adherence in children and AYA. With this knowledge in mind, there are several areas for moving the field forward with respect to research and practice. Future research needs to move away from a primary risk perspective to one of resilience by not only focusing on barriers to ART adherence but also exploring facilitators. Specifically, learning from youth who are successful with ART adherence and using this knowledge to develop interventions will be beneficial. Clinicians should explore periods of time when youth living with HIV are more adherent to ART. Thus, rather than thinking of youth's adherence dichotomously (i.e., adherent or not), clinicians should consider adherence on a continuum and use a strength-based approach that reinforces youth for these more adherent occurrences, which may lead to youth feeling more empowered and promote ongoing adherence.

There is a dearth of evidence-based interventions for improving ART adherence in pediatric populations. The majority of the published interventions are in early stages of assessment (i.e., pilot and feasibility testing), and it is notable that most of the pilot interventions did not have lasting effects even in pilot testing. Accordingly, long-term impact on youth adherence is not known. It is thus critical for future research efforts to advance intervention testing beyond initial trials to examine effects in RCT and then effectiveness trials in real-world settings. Additionally, none of the available interventions take multicultural considerations into account, despite significant disparities in rates of HIV and ART adherence among racial/ethnic minorities. Given research highlighting the value of multicultural considerations in treatment, incorporating cultural factors in intervention design and implementation may provide novel target areas for ART adherence interventions. In clinical settings, evidence indicates that taking multicultural considerations into account improves rapport and therapeutic alliance, factors relevant to improving ART adherence. Thus, clinicians should incorporate cultural values and beliefs into treatment. This may include involving the patient's community in treatment, using methods from other chronic illness conditions shown to engage minority youth, and addressing issues of intersecting stigma (e.g., HIV status, race, gender, and sexual orientation) that are especially prominent in minority youth and their families.

In conclusion, research on ART adherence among pediatric populations is still in its infancy with multiple avenues for advancing the field and clinically addressing adherence in developmentally and culturally responsive ways. It is our hope that this chapter has elucidated potential areas of focus for future research and clinical efforts.

Conclusion

Approximately 26% of all new HIV infections in the US occur among adolescents and young adults (AYA) aged 13–25. Due to advances in antiretroviral therapy (ART), HIV is now managed as a chronic illness. Current World Health Organization guidelines recommend starting ART as soon as individuals are diagnosed with HIV. However, the effectiveness of ART is only maximized when youth take their medications as prescribed (i.e., 90–95% of doses prescribed). Unfortunately, adherence to ART remains suboptimal among youth who typically have adherence rates between 28 and 69%. Notably, there are significant disparities in ART adherence with research indicating lower rates of adherence among racial/ethnic minorities, individuals from lower socioeconomic status, older adolescents, and female youth. Barriers to ART adherence among children and AYA include medication-related factors (e.g., side effects, medication fatigue, and pill burden) and psychosocial factors (e.g., psychopathology, fear of disclosure, and stigma). Barriers unique to children include caregiver factors (i.e., caregiver distress, quality of life, and cognitive functioning), and those unique to adolescents include developmental stage, poor transition to independent care, and peer relationships. Research on adherence facilitators is lacking; however, strong parent–child communication, higher life satisfaction, and increased understanding of HIV and benefits of ART among youth are related to better adherence. Assessment of adherence is maximized by utilizing multiple measurements (such as self-report, pill counts, refills, electronic monitoring, and/or viral load/CD4 count). Our review of published adherence interventions for children and AYA across clinic, home/community settings, and interventions involving technology highlights numerous gaps in the literature, with most interventions still being in the preliminary stages of pilot and feasibility testing. Considering the detrimental consequences of untreated/poorly managed HIV in youth, future research and practice efforts examining long-term outcomes and effectiveness of interventions in clinical settings are critically needed.

Acknowledgments Thanks to the CHANGE Laboratory and Research Assistant Dominic Ingram for helping to conduct the literature reviews for this chapter.

Annotated Bibliography

Berman, J. (2007). *Tools for building culturally competent HIV prevention programs: With CD-ROM*. Springer Publishing Company.

Berman's book, informed by the scientific literature, discusses culture and cultural competence within the context of HIV risk and prevention. The book offers a comprehensive guide to help researchers and practitioners create, implement, and evaluate culturally competent and effective HIV prevention programs in their local communities.

Kahana, S., Rohan, J., Allison, S., Frazier, T., & Drotar, D. (2013). A meta-analysis of adherence to antiretroviral therapy and virologic responses in HIV-infected children, adolescents, and young adults. *AIDS and Behavior, 17*(1), 41–60. doi:10.1007/s10461-012-0159-4

This meta-analysis examined potential factors that influence the relationship between antiretroviral therapy adherence and clinical outcomes (i.e., viral load) among children, adolescents, and young adults living with HIV. Particularly informative is the study's examination of a range of adherence measurement methodologies and their associations with clinical outcomes.

Reisner, M. S. L., Mimiaga, M. J., Skeer, M. M., Perkovich, M. B., Johnson, M. C. V., & Safren, S. A. (2009). A review of HIV antiretroviral adherence and intervention studies among HIV–infected youth. *Topics in HIV Medicine, 17(1),* 14–25.

Reisner and colleagues review all relevant US-based studies published between 1999 and 2008 focused on HIV medication adherence and interventions designed to increase adherence in youth living with HIV between the ages of 13–24. Findings highlighted the importance of broader contextual factors when studying adherence among youth.

Vreeman, R., Nyandiko, W., Liu, H., Tu, W., Scanlon, M., Slaven, J., et al. (2015). Comprehensive evaluation of caregiver-reported antiretroviral therapy adherence for HIV-infected children. *AIDS and Behavior, 19*(4), 626–634. doi:10.1007/s10461-015-0998-x

In this study, authors evaluated adherence rates and predictors of adherence among a large group of children ($N = 191$) aged 0–14 years and their caregivers over a 6 month time frame. Parent-report of adherence and parent-reported barriers to adherence were examined as well as their associations with an objective measure of ART adherence (i.e., Medication Event Monitoring System—MEMS).

References

AIDS Etc., National Resource Center. (2014). Guide for HIV/AIDS clinical care: CD4 and viral load monitoring. Retrieved November 6, 2015, from http://aidsetc.org/guide/cd4-and-viral-load-monitoring

AIDSInfo. (2014). Guidelines for the use of antiretroviral agents in HIV-1-infected adults and adolescents. Retrieved 2015, from https://aidsinfo.nih.gov/guidelines/html/1/adult-and-adolescent-arv-guidelines/10/initiating-art-in-treatment-naive-patients

AIDSInfo. (2015). Preventing mother-to-child transmission of HIV after birth: HIV/AIDS fact sheets. Retrieved 2015, from https://aidsinfo.nih.gov/education-materials/fact-sheets/24/71/preventing-mother-to-child-transmission-of-hiv-after-birth

Bartlett, J. A. (2002). Addressing the challenges of adherence. *JAIDS Journal of Acquired Immune Deficiency Syndromes, 29,* S2–S10. doi:10.1097/00126334-200202011-00002

Beach, M. C., Keruly, J., & Moore, R. D. (2006). Is the quality of the patient-provider relationship associated with better adherence and health outcomes for patients with HIV? *Journal of General Internal Medicine, 21*(6), 661–665. doi:10.1111/j.1525-1497.2006.00399.x

Becker, S., Dezii, C., Burtcel, B., Kawabata, H., & Hodder, S. (2002). Young HIV-infected adults are at greater risk for medication nonadherence. *MedGenMed: Medscape General Medicine, 4* (3), 21.

Berg, K. M., & Arnsten, J. H. (2006). Practical and conceptual challenges in measuring antiretroviral adherence. *Journal of Acquired Immune Deficiency Syndromes (1999), 43*(Suppl 1), S79–S87. doi:10.1097/01.qai.0000248337.97814.66

Berrien, V. M., Salazar, J. C., Reynolds, E., & McKay, K. (2004). Adherence to antiretroviral therapy in HIV-infected pediatric patients improves with home-based intensive nursing intervention. *AIDS Patient Care and STDS, 18*(6), 355–363. doi:10.1089/1087291041444078

Buchanan, A. L., Montepiedra, G., Sirois, P. A., Kammerer, B., Garvie, P. A., Storm, D. S., et al. (2012). Barriers to medication adherence in HIV-infected children and youth based on self- and caregiver report. *Pediatrics, 129*(5), 1244–1251. doi:10.1542/peds.2011-1740

Burack, G., Gaur, S., Marone, R., & Petrova, A. (2010). Adherence to antiretroviral therapy in pediatric patients with human immunodeficiency virus (HIV-1). *Journal of Pediatric Nursing, 25*(6), 500–504. doi:10.1016/j.pedn.2009.07.002

Casey, B. J., Jones, R. M., & Hare, T. A. (2008). The adolescent brain. *Annals of the New York Academy of Sciences, 1124*, 111–126. doi:10.1196/annals.1440.010

CDC. (2012). HIV among pregnant women, infants, and children in the United States. Retrieved 2015, from http://www.cdc.gov/hiv/group/gender/pregnantwomen/index.html

CDC. (2015a). HIV among pregnant women, infants, and children. Retrieved November 5, 2015, from http://www.cdc.gov/hiv/group/gender/pregnantwomen/index.html

CDC. (2015b). HIV among youth. Retrieved 2015, from http://www.cdc.gov/hiv/group/age/youth/index.html

Chandwani, S., Koenig, L. J., Sill, A. M., Abramowitz, S., Conner, L. C., & D'Angelo, L. (2012). Predictors of antiretroviral medication adherence among a diverse cohort of adolescents with HIV. *Journal of Adolescent Health, 51*(3), 242–251. doi:10.1016/j.jadohealth.2011.12.013. (S1054-139X(11)00676-8 [pii]).

Chen, W.-T., Wantland, D., Reid, P., Corless, I. B., Eller, L. S., Iipinge, S., et al. (2013). Engagement with health care providers affects self-efficacy, self-esteem, medication adherence and quality of life in people living with HIV. *Journal of AIDS and Clinical Research, 4*(11), 256.

Chenneville, T., Clutter, M. O., Hintz, S., Walsh, A., Emmanuel, P., Lujan-Zilberman, J., et al. (2015). Decisional capacity and medication adherence among youth with HIV. *AIDS Care, 27*(3), 338–341. doi:10.1080/09540121.2014.993582

Chesney, M. (2003). Adherence to HAART regimens. *Aids Patient Care and STDS, 17*(4), 169–177. doi:10.1089/108729103321619773

ChildHealth. (2011). Pediatric HIV and AIDS, from http://mchb.hrsa.gov/chusa11/hstat/hsc/pages/210pha.html

Crespo-Fierro, M. (1997). Compliance/adherence and care management in HIV disease. *Journal of the Association of Nurses in AIDS Care, 8*(4), 43–54. doi:10.1016/S1055-3290(97)80012-X

Crichton, N. (2001). Visual analogue scale (VAS). *Journal of Clinical Nursing, 10*(5), 706.

Cunningham, W. E., Markson, L. E., Andersen, R. M., Crystal, S. H., Fleishman, J. A., Golin, C., et al. (2000). Prevalence and predictors of highly active antiretroviral therapy use in patients with HIV infection in the United States. *JAIDS Journal of Acquired Immune Deficiency Syndromes, 25*(2), 115–123. doi:10.1097/00126334-200010010-00005

Dang, B. N., Westbrook, R. A., Black, W. C., Rodriguez-Barradas, M. C., & Giordano, T. P. (2013). Examining the link between patient satisfaction and adherence to HIV care: A structural equation model. *PLoS ONE, 8*(1), e54729. doi:10.1371/journal.pone.0054729

Dolezal, C., Mellins, C., Brackis-Cott, E., & Abrams, E. J. (2003). The reliability of reports of medical adherence from children with HIV and their adult caregivers. *Journal of Pediatric Psychology, 28*(5), 355–361. doi:10.1093/jpepsy/jsg025

Dowshen, N., Kuhns, L. M., Gray, C., Lee, S., & Garofalo, R. (2013). Feasibility of interactive text message response (ITR) as a novel, real-time measure of adherence to antiretroviral therapy for HIV+ youth. *AIDS and Behavior, 17*(6), 2237–2243. doi:10.1007/s10461-013-0464-6

Evans, S. D., Mellins, C. A., Leu, C.-S., Warne, P., Elkington, K. S., Dolezal, C., et al. (2015). HIV treatment adherence measurement and reporting concordance in youth with perinatally acquired HIV infection and their caregivers. *AIDS Patient Care and STDs, 29*(1), 43–51. doi:10.1089/apc.2014.0058

Farley, J., Hines, S., Musk, A., Ferrus, S., & Tepper, V. (2003). Assessment of adherence to antiviral therapy in HIV-infected children using the Medication Event Monitoring System, pharmacy refill, provider assessment, caregiver self-report, and appointment keeping. *Journal of Acquired Immune Deficiency Syndromes, 33*(2), 211–218. doi:10.1097/00126334-200306010-00016

Farley, J., Montepiedra, G., Storm, D., Sirois, P. A., Malee, K., Garvie, P., et al. (2008). Assessment of adherence to antiretroviral therapy in perinatally HIV-infected children and youth using self-report measures and pill count. *Journal of Developmental and Behavioral Pediatrics, 29*(5), 377–384. doi:10.1097/DBP.0b013e3181856d22

Fields, E. L., Bogart, L. M., Thurston, I. B., Wachman, M., Closson, E. F., Skeer, M. R., et al. (2012). Qualitative comparison of barriers to antiretroviral medication adherence among perinatally and behaviorally HIV-infected youth. *Journal of Adolescent Health, 50*(2), S8–S9. doi:10.1016/j.jadohealth.2011.10.036

Garvie, P. A., Lensing, S., & Rai, S. N. (2007). Efficacy of a pill-swallowing training intervention to improve antiretroviral medication adherence in pediatric patients with HIV/AIDS. *Pediatrics, 119*(4), e893–e899. doi:10.1542/peds.2006-1488

Gaston, G. B. (2013). African-Americans' perceptions of health care provider cultural competence that promote HIV medical self-care and antiretroviral medication adherence. *AIDS care, 25*(9), 1159–1165. doi:10.1080/09540121.2012.752783

Gaur, A. H., Belzer, M., Britto, P., Garvie, P. A., Hu, C., Graham, B., et al. (2010). Directly observed therapy (DOT) for nonadherent HIV-infected youth: Lessons learned, challenges ahead. *AIDS Research and Human Retroviruses, 26*(9), 947–953. doi:10.1089/aid.2010.0008

Gebo, K. A., Fleishman, J. A., Conviser, R., Reilly, E. D., Korthuis, P. T., Moore, R. D., et al. (2005). Racial and gender disparities in receipt of highly active antiretroviral therapy persist in a multistate sample of HIV patients in 2001. *JAIDS Journal of Acquired Immune Deficiency Syndromes, 38*(1), 96–103. doi:10.1097/00126334-200501010-00017

Gibb, D. M. (2008). Markers for predicting mortality in untreated HIV-infected children in resource-limited settings: A meta-analysis. *AIDS, 22*(1), 97–105. doi:10.1097/01.aids.0000302262.51286.a5

Haberer, J. E., Kiwanuka, J., Nansera, D., Wilson, I. B., & Bangsberg, D. R. (2010). Challenges in using mobile phones for collection of antiretroviral therapy adherence data in a resource-limited setting. *AIDS and Behavior, 14*(6), 1294–1301. doi:10.1007/s10461-010-9720-1

Hazra, R., Siberry, G. K., & Mofenson, L. M. (2010). Growing up with HIV: Children, adolescents, and young adults with perinatally acquired HIV infection. *Annual Review of Medicine, 61*, 169–185. doi:10.1146/annurev.med.050108.151127

Henggeler, S. W., Schoenwald, S. K., Borduin, C. M., Rowland, M. D., & Cunningham, P. B. (2009). *Multisystemic therapy for antisocial behavior in children and adolescents*. Guilford Press.

Hook, J. N., Davis, D. E., Owen, J., Worthington, E. L., Jr., & Utsey, S. O. (2013). Cultural humility: Measuring openness to culturally diverse clients. *Journal of Counseling Psychology, 60*(3), 353–366. doi:10.1037/a0032595

Hosek, S. G., Harper, G. W., & Domanico, R. (2005). Predictors of medication adherence among HIV-infected youth. *Psychology, Health and Medicine, 10*(2), 166–179. doi:10.1080/1354350042000326584

IAPAC. (2015). Guidelines for optimizing the HIV care continuum for adults and adolescents. *Journal of the International Association of Providers of AIDS Care*. doi:10.1177/2325957415613442

Intasan, J., Bunupuradah, T., Vonthanak, S., Kosalaraksa, P., Hansudewechakul, R., Kanjanavanit, S., et al. (2014). Comparison of adherence monitoring tools and correlation to virologic failure in a pediatric HIV clinical trial. *AIDS Patient Care and STDs, 28*(6), 296–302. doi:10.1089/apc.2013.0276

Kahana, S., Rohan, J., Allison, S., Frazier, T., & Drotar, D. (2013). A meta-analysis of adherence to antiretroviral therapy and virologic responses in HIV-infected children, adolescents, and young adults. *AIDS and Behavior, 17*(1), 41–60. doi:10.1007/s10461-012-0159-4

Koenig, L. J., & Bachanas, P. J. (2006). Adherence to medications for HIV: Teens say, 'too many, too big, too often'. In M. E. Lyon & L. J. D'Angelo (Eds.), *Teenagers, HIV, and AIDS: Insights from youths living with the virus* (pp. 45–65). Westport, CT, US: Praeger Publishers/Greenwood Publishing Group.

Koenig, L. J., Nesheim, S., & Abramowitz, S. (2011). Adolescents with perinatally acquired HIV: Emerging behavioral and health needs for long-term survivors. *Current Opinion in Obstetrics and Gynecology, 23*(5), 321–327. doi:10.1097/GCO.0b013e32834a581b

Laursen, B., & Collins, W. A. (2009). Parent-child relationships during adolescence. In R. M. Lerner & L. Steinberg (Eds.), *Handbook of adolescent psychology* (3rd ed., Vol. 2). Hoboken, NJ: Wiley. doi:10.1002/9780470479193.adlpsy002002

Lester, R. T., Ritvo, P., Mills, E. J., Kariri, A., Karanja, S., Chung, M. H., et al. (2010). Effects of a mobile phone short message service on antiretroviral treatment adherence in Kenya (WelTel Kenya1): A randomised trial. *The Lancet, 376*(9755), 1838–1845. doi:10.1016/S0140-6736(10)61997-6

Letourneau, E. J., Ellis, D. A., Naar-King, S., Chapman, J. E., Cunningham, P. B., & Fowler, S. (2013). Multisystemic therapy for poorly adherent youth with HIV: Results from a pilot randomized controlled trial. *AIDS Care, 25*(4), 507–514. doi:10.1080/09540121.2012.715134

Lyon, M. E., Trexler, C., Akpan-Townsend, C., Pao, M., Selden, K., Fletcher, J., et al. (2003). A family group approach to increasing adherence to therapy in HIV-infected youths: Results of a pilot project. *AIDS Patient Care and STDs, 17*(6), 299–308. doi:10.1089/108729103322108175

MacDonell, K., Naar-King, S., Huszti, H., & Belzer, M. (2013). Barriers to medication adherence in behaviorally and perinatally infected youth living with HIV. *AIDS and Behavior, 17*(1), 86–93. doi:10.1007/s10461-012-0364-1

Madden, M., Lenhart, A., Duggan, M., Cortesi, S., & Gasser, U. (2013). *Teens and technology 2013*. Pew Internet and American Life Project Washington, DC.

Malee, K., Williams, P., Montepiedra, G., McCabe, M., Nichols, S., Sirois, P. A., et al. (2011). Medication adherence in children and adolescents with HIV infection: Associations with behavioral impairment. *AIDS Patient Care and STDs, 25*(3), 191–200.

Marhefka, S. L., Tepper, V. J., Brown, J. L., & Farley, J. J. (2006). Caregiver psychosocial characteristics and children's adherence to antiretroviral therapy. *AIDS Patient Care and STDs, 20*(6), 429–437. doi:10.1089/apc.2006.20.429

Martin, S., Elliott-DeSorbo, D. K., Calabrese, S., Wolters, P. L., Roby, G., Brennan, T., et al. (2009). A comparison of adherence assessment methods utilized in the United States: Perspectives of researchers, HIV-infected children, and their caregivers. *AIDS Patient Care and STDs, 23*(8), 593–601. doi:10.1089/apc.2009.0021

Martin, S., Elliott-DeSorbo, D. K., Wolters, P. L., Toledo-Tamula, M. A., Roby, G., Zeichner, S., et al. (2007). Patient, caregiver and regimen characteristics associated with adherence to highly active antiretroviral therapy among HIV-infected children and adolescents. *Pediatr Infect Dis J, 26*(1), 61–67. doi:10.1097/01.inf.0000250625.80340.48

Mellins, C. A., Brackis-Cott, E., Dolezal, C., & Abrams, E. J. (2004). The role of psychosocial and family factors in adherence to antiretroviral treatment in human immunodeficiency virus-infected children. *Pediatric Infectious Disease Journal, 23*(11), 1035–1041 (doi:00006454-200411000-00012 [pii]).

Mellins, C. A., Tassiopoulos, K., Malee, K., Moscicki, A. B., Patton, D., Smith, R., et al. (2011). Behavioral health risks in perinatally HIV-exposed youth: Co-occurrence of sexual and drug use behavior, mental health problems, and nonadherence to antiretroviral treatment. *AIDS Patient Care STDS, 25*(7), 413–422. doi:10.1089/apc.2011.0025

Merzel, C., VanDevanter, N., & Irvine, M. (2008). Adherence to antiretroviral therapy among older children and adolescents with HIV: A qualitative study of psychosocial contexts. *AIDS Patient Care and STDs, 22*(12), 977–987. doi:10.1089/apc.2008.0048

Muller, A. D., Bode, S., Myer, L., Roux, P., & von Steinbuchel, N. (2008). Electronic measurement of adherence to pediatric antiretroviral therapy in South Africa. *The Pediatric Infectious Disease Journal, 27*(3), 257–262. doi:10.1097/INF.0b013e31815b1ad4

Murphy, D. A., Belzer, M., Durako, S. J., Sarr, M., Wilson, C. M., & Muenz, L. R. (2005). Longitudinal antiretroviral adherence among adolescents infected with human immunodeficiency virus. *Archives of Pediatrics and Adolescent Medicine, 159*(8), 764–770. doi:10.1001/archpedi.159.8.764

Murphy, D. A., Wilson, C. M., Durako, S. J., Muenz, L. R., & Belzer, M. (2001). Antiretroviral medication adherence among the REACH HIV-infected adolescent cohort in the USA. *AIDS Care, 13*(1), 27–40. doi:10.1080/09540120020018161

Naar-King, S., Arfken, C., Frey, M., Harris, M., Secord, E., & Ellis, D. (2006a). Psychosocial factors and treatment adherence in paediatric HIV/AIDS. *AIDS Care, 18*(6), 621–628. doi:10.1080/09540120500471895

Naar-King, S., Montepiedra, G., Garvie, P., Kammerer, B., Malee, K., Sirois, P. A., et al. (2013). Social ecological predictors of longitudinal HIV treatment adherence in youth with perinatally acquired HIV. *Journal of Pediatric Psychology, 38*(6), 664–674. doi:10.1093/jpepsy/jst017

Naar-King, S., Templin, T., Wright, K., Frey, M., Parsons, J. T., & Lam, P. (2006b). Psychosocial factors and medication adherence in HIV-positive youth. *Aids Patient Care and STDS, 20*(1), 44–47. doi:10.1089/apc.2006.20.44

Navarra, A.-M., Neu, N., Toussi, S., Nelson, J., & Larson, E. L. (2014). Health literacy and adherence to antiretroviral therapy among HIV-infected youth. *Journal of the Association of Nurses in AIDS Care, 25*(3), 203–213. doi:10.1016/j.jana.2012.11.003

Nichols, S. L., Montepiedra, G., Farley, J. J., Sirois, P. A., Malee, K., Kammerer, B., et al. (2012). Cognitive, academic, and behavioral correlates of medication adherence in children and adolescents with perinatally acquired HIV infection. *Journal of Developmental and Behavioral Pediatrics, 33*(4), 298–308. doi:10.1097/DBP.0b013e31824bef47

Paterson, D. L., Swindells, S., Mohr, J., Brester, M., Vergis, E. N., Squier, C., et al. (2000). Adherence to protease inhibitor therapy and outcomes in patients with HIV infection. *Annals of Internal Medicine, 133*(1), 21–30. doi:10.7326/0003-4819-133-1-200007040-00004

Penn, C., Watermeyer, J., & Evans, M. (2011). Why don't patients take their drugs? The role of communication, context and culture in patient adherence and the work of the pharmacist in HIV/AIDS. *Patient Education and Counseling, 83*(3), 310–318. doi:10.1016/j.pec.2011.02.018

Pop-Eleches, C., Thirumurthy, H., Habyarimana, J. P., Zivin, J. G., Goldstein, M. P., de Walque, D., et al. (2011). Mobile phone technologies improve adherence to antiretroviral treatment in a resource-limited setting: A randomized controlled trial of text message reminders. *AIDS, 25*(6), 825–834. doi:10.1097/QAD.0b013e32834380c1

Puccio, J. A., Belzer, M., Olson, J., Martinez, M., Salata, C., Tucker, D., et al. (2006). The use of cell phone reminder calls for assisting HIV-infected adolescents and young adults to adhere to highly active antiretroviral therapy: A pilot study. *AIDS Patient Care and STDs, 20*(6), 438–444. doi:10.1089/apc.2006.20.438

Radcliffe, J., Doty, N., Hawkins, L. A., Gaskins, C. S., Beidas, R., & Rudy, B. J. (2010). Stigma and sexual health risk in HIV-positive African American young men who have sex with men. *AIDS patient care and STDs, 24*(8), 493–499. doi:10.1089/apc.2010.0020

Rahill, G. J., Joshi, M., & Lescano, C. (2017). Cultural Considerations for Pediatric HIV Research and Practice. In T. Chenneville (Ed), *A Clinical Guide to Pediatric HIV*, 259–271. Dordrecht: Springer.

Rao, D., Kekwaletswe, T. C., Hosek, S., Martinez, J., & Rodriguez, F. (2007). Stigma and social barriers to medication adherence with urban youth living with HIV. *AIDS Care, 19*(1), 28–33. doi:10.1080/09540120600652303

Rapoff, M. A. (2010). *Adherence to Pediatric Medical Regimens* (2nd ed.). New York: Springer. doi:10.1007/978-1-4419-0570-3

Reisner, S. L., Mimiaga, M. J., Skeer, M., Perkovich, B., Johnson, C. V., & Safren, S. A. (2009b). A review of HIV antiretroviral adherence and intervention studies among HIV-infected youth. *Topics in HIV Medicine, 17*(1), 14–25.

Rudy, B. J., Murphy, D. A., Harris, D. R., Muenz, L., & Ellen, J. (2009). Patient-related risks for nonadherence to antiretroviral therapy among HIV-infected youth in the United States: A study of prevalence and interactions. *Aids Patient Care and STDS, 23*(3), 185–194. doi:10.1089/apc.2008.0162

Rudy, B. J., Murphy, D. A., Harris, D. R., Muenz, L., & Ellen, J. (2010). Prevalence and interactions of patient-related risks for nonadherence to antiretroviral therapy among perinatally infected youth in the United States. *Aids Patient Care and STDS, 24*(2), 97–104. doi:10.1089/apc.2009.0198

Safren, S. A., O'Cleirigh, C., Tan, J. Y., Raminani, S. R., Reilly, L. C., Otto, M. W., et al. (2009). A randomized controlled trial of cognitive behavioral therapy for adherence and depression (CBT-AD) in HIV-infected individuals. *Health Psychology, 28*(1), 1. doi:10.1037/a0012715

Saha, S., Korthuis, P. T., Cohn, J. A., Sharp, V. L., Moore, R. D., & Beach, M. C. (2013). Primary care provider cultural competence and racial disparities in HIV care and outcomes. *Journal of General Internal Medicine, 28*(5), 622–629. doi:10.1007/s11606-012-2298-8

Shegog, R., Markham, C. M., Leonard, A. D., Bui, T. C., & Paul, M. E. (2012). "+ CLICK": Pilot of a web-based training program to enhance ART adherence among HIV-positive youth. *AIDS Care, 24*(3), 310–318. doi:10.1080/09540121.2011.608788

Simoni, J. M., Kurth, A. E., Pearson, C. R., Pantalone, D. W., Merrill, J. O., & Frick, P. A. (2006). Self-report measures of antiretroviral therapy adherence: A review with recommendations for HIV research and clinical management. *AIDS and Behavior, 10*(3), 227–245. doi:10.1007/s10461-006-9078-6

Simoni, J. M., Montgomery, A., Martin, E., New, M., Demas, P. A., & Rana, S. (2007). Adherence to antiretroviral therapy for pediatric HIV infection: A qualitative systematic review with recommendations for research and clinical management. *Pediatrics, 119*(6), e1371–e1383. doi:10.1542/peds.2006-1232 (peds.2006-1232 [pii]).

Sue, D. W., & Sue, D. (2012). *Counseling the culturally diverse: Theory and practice* (6th ed.). Hoboken, NJ: Wiley.

Tervalon, M., & Murray-Garcia, J. (1998). Cultural humility versus cultural competence: A critical distinction in defining physician training outcomes in multicultural education. *Journal of Health Care for the Poor and Underserved, 9*(2), 117–125. doi:10.1353/hpu.2010.0233

Thurston, I. B., Bogart, L. M., Wachman, M., Closson, E. F., Skeer, M. R., & Mimiaga, M. J. (2014). Adaptation of an HIV medication adherence intervention for adolescents and young adults. *Cognitive and Behavioral Practice, 21*(2), 191–205. doi:10.1016/j.cbpra.2013.11.001

Usitalo, A., Leister, E., Tassiopoulos, K., Allison, S., Malee, K., Paul, M. E., et al. (2014). Relationship between viral load and self-report measures of medication adherence among youth with perinatal HIV infection. *AIDS Care, 26*(1), 107–115. doi:10.1080/09540121.2013.802280

Valenzuela, J. M., Buchanan, C. L., Radcliffe, J., Ambrose, C., Hawkins, L. A., Tanney, M., et al. (2011). Transition to adult services among behaviorally infected adolescents with HIV—A qualitative study. *Journal of Pediatric Psychology, 36*(2), 134–140. doi:10.1093/jpepsy/jsp051

Van Ryn, M. (2002). Research on the provider contribution to race/ethnicity disparities in medical care. *Medical care, 40*(1), I-140–I-151. doi:10.1097/00005650-200201001-00015

Vreeman, R., Nyandiko, W., Liu, H., Tu, W., Scanlon, M., Slaven, J., et al. (2015). Comprehensive evaluation of caregiver-reported antiretroviral therapy adherence for HIV-infected children. *AIDS and Behavior, 19*(4), 626–634. doi:10.1007/s10461-015-0998-x

Wagner, G., & Miller, L. G. (2004). Is the influence of social desirability on patients' self-reported adherence overrated? [Letter]. *Journal of Acquired Immune Deficiency Syndrome, 35*, 203–204. doi:10.1097/00126334-200402010-00016

Williams, P. L., Storm, D., Montepiedra, G., Nichols, S., Kammerer, B., Sirois, P. A., et al. (2006). Predictors of adherence to antiretroviral medications in children and adolescents with HIV infection. *Pediatrics, 118*(6), e1745–e1757. doi:10.1542/peds.2006-0493 (peds.2006-0493 [pii]).

Woolston, C. (2015). Children and HIV. Retrieved 2015, from http://consumer.healthday.com/encyclopedia/diseases-and-conditions-15/misc-diseases-and-conditions-news-203/children-and-hiv-648452.html

World Health Organization. (2013). Global update on HIV treatment 2013: Results, impact and opportunities. Retrived from http://www.who.int/hiv/data/global_treatment_report_presentation_2013.pdf

World Health Organization. (2015). Global health sector response to HIV, 2000–2015: Focus on innovations in Africa. Retrieved from http://apps.who.int/iris/bitstream/10665/198065/1/9789241509824_eng.pdf

Wrubel, J., Moskowitz, J. T., Richards, T. A., Prakke, H., Acree, M., & Folkman, S. (2005). Pediatric adherence: Perspectives of mothers of children with HIV. *Social Science and Medicine, 61*(11), 2423–2433. doi:10.1016/j.socscimed.2005.04.034

Chapter 8
HIV Disclosure in Pediatric Populations: Who, What, When to Tell, and then What?

Stephanie L. Marhefka, DeAnne E. Turner and Tiffany Chenneville

Introduction

In pediatric HIV, disclosure of HIV-positive status is a critical component of care for youth affected by and living with HIV. Disclosure is multifaceted and complex; thus, a clear definition is warranted. In this chapter, we refer to disclosure as a process, during which Person A tells Person B *at least some information* about the HIV-positive status of Person A or Person B. In the scientific literature, the term disclosure typically implies "full disclosure"; that is, a process or event that involves sharing the fact that someone is living with HIV. "Partial disclosure" describes a process that involves relaying information about an illness or a condition, without labeling it "HIV" or "AIDS" (Dorrell and Katz 2014); in some cases, false information may be given (i.e., children may be told they have asthma, a stomach problem, malaria, etc.; Dorrell and Katz 2014; Instone 2000; Namasopo-Oleja et al. 2015). This can create "a context of confusion and mistrust" (Abadía-Barrero and LaRusso 2006, pp 36). We will discuss three main HIV disclosure-related situations that involve children:

S.L. Marhefka (✉) · D.E. Turner
University of South Florida, Tampa, FL, USA
e-mail: smarhefk@health.usf.edu

D.E. Turner
e-mail: dturner@health.usf.edu

T. Chenneville
University of South Florida, St. Petersburg, FL, USA
e-mail: chennevi@mail.usf.edu

T. Chenneville (ed.), *A Clinical Guide to Pediatric HIV*,
DOI 10.1007/978-3-319-49704-4_8

- Parents confront decisions about when and how to tell their children they (the parents) are living with HIV.
- Parents/primary caregivers and the healthcare team face the problem of when and how to tell the child living with perinatally acquired HIV about the child's positive HIV status.
- Children and adolescents living with HIV experience decision-making regarding who to tell about their own status, and how and when disclosure should take place.

Over time, the broader context of HIV-positive status disclosure has become somewhat less intimidating, as HIV infection has largely been transformed from a "death sentence" to a chronic illness (Matic et al. 2006). Moreover, antiretroviral treatment (ART) regimens have improved substantially, resulting in more consistently positive health outcomes, in addition to less complicated regimens involving fewer pills/formulations. Despite these advances, families affected by HIV often have difficulty making disclosure decisions.

Ultimately, parents/primary caregivers and healthcare providers share a common goal—to provide both a physically and emotionally supportive environment for young people affected by and living with HIV. While there is no universal reason for disclosure or "right" way in which to disclose, research can help us understand the antecedents, correlates, processes and outcomes of disclosure, and can provide guidance on best practices for HIV disclosure to children. In the sections to follow, we address each type of disclosure noted above and, within these disclosure types, the patterns and correlates affecting disclosure, and known outcomes. We end with a review of available guidance and best practices related to each type of disclosure described.

Disclosure of Parental HIV Status to Children

Parents living with HIV face challenges in disclosing their own HIV-positive status to their children, regardless of the child's HIV status. Such challenges include deciding *whether* to tell their children about their HIV-positive status, *when* and *how* such information should be shared, and concerns regarding how disclosure of parental HIV-positive status may *affect* their children.

What Are the Patterns and Correlates of Parental HIV Status Disclosure?

Globally rates of parental HIV-positive status disclosure to children are low (Armistead et al. 2001; Corona et al. 2006; Murphy et al. 2001; Nöstlinger et al. 2004; Qiao et al. 2013; Simoni et al. 2000). Studies suggest disclosure to children is uncommon, with rates as low as 10% in some populations (Nöstlinger et al. 2004). Approximately one-third (Armistead et al. 2001; Murphy et al. 2001) to one-half (Qiao et al. 2013; Simoni et al. 2000) of study participants generally report disclosure to at least one child, with most studies focused on disclosure to minor (rather than adult) children. Disclosure is further complicated, as parents may disclose to some, but not all of their children, due to differences between children such as age or maturity (Corona et al. 2006; Lee and Rotheram-Borus 2002; Rwemisisi et al. 2008; Simoni et al. 2000). Overwhelmingly, parents share one primary concern regarding disclosure: *How do I protect the emotional and physical well-being of my children?* (Hawk 2007).

Parents describe a myriad of reasons to disclose and not disclose their HIV-positive status to a child; these reasons are generally similar to the reasons for and against telling a child that he or she is living with HIV (see next section). For example, the rationale for telling a child includes not wanting the child to be told by other people (Kennedy et al. 2010; Ostrom Delaney et al. 2008; Rwemisisi et al. 2008) and believing the child has a right to know (Ostrom Delaney et al. 2008). In cases where the child is living with HIV, parental disclosure also has been used to explain the child's illness (Nam et al. 2009); disclosure of a parent's HIV-positive status may be conducted before, during, or after telling the child he or she is living with HIV (Rwemisisi et al. 2008).

Reasons for non-disclosure of parental HIV-positive status are also similar to the reasons for not telling a child about his or her own HIV-positive status. A major concern regarding disclosure is the emotional and psychological impact on the child, both short- and long-term (Corona et al. 2006; Hawk 2007; Nam et al. 2009; Nöstlinger et al. 2004; Ostrom Delaney et al. 2008). Another concern is that disclosure of a parent's HIV-positive status may change the parent–child dynamic, resulting in rejection or loss of respect from the child (Corona et al. 2006; Rwemisisi et al. 2008). Parents also express concerns that the child will act out or may disclose the parent's HIV-positive status to others (Corona et al. 2006). Moreover, some parents fear their children will want to know *how* their parents acquired HIV, and parents may be uncomfortable talking with their children about previous sexual behavior and/or substance use (Wiener et al. 2007).

When parents do consider disclosure, they are often unsure of the appropriate age for disclosure and often feel ill-equipped to navigate the disclosure process (Nam et al. 2009; Nöstlinger et al. 2004; Rwemisisi et al. 2008). They may also have difficulty determining what exactly to tell their children. Research shows that the level of detail shared with a child during disclosure varies, ranging from partial disclosure of illness—telling the child that the parent is ill, has a chronic disease, or is dying—to specific disclosure, using the terms "HIV" or "AIDS" (Corona et al. 2006; Lee and Rotheram-Borus 2002).

Research suggests parental attributes (such as parental race, ethnicity, or gender) and parental concerns (such as fear that the child will have questions or guardianship concerns) may play a role in parents' decisions to disclose their

HIV-positive status to their children. Similarly, child characteristics such as age, maturity, and gender also are considered important when deciding to disclose a parent's HIV-positive status. These are described in more detail below.

Parental Attributes Associated with Disclosure

There are conflicting findings regarding how the severity of a parent's illness may affect disclosure patterns. Many studies have found that the sicker a parent is, the more likely he or she is to disclose their HIV-positive status to their child (Armistead et al. 1997; Armistead et al. 2001; Hawk 2007; Lee and Rotheram-Borus 2002; Nam et al. 2009). Some have suggested that changes in a parent's health may raise questions from children, thus prompting the disclosure event (Kennedy et al. 2010), while other studies have found that disclosure was not related to illness in the case of mothers living with HIV (Simoni et al. 2000). These conflicting findings may be due to the variety of indicators that have been used to measure illness. For example, among mothers, self-reported sickness was found to predict disclosure, but not medical measures of disease progression (Armistead et al. 2001; Nam et al. 2009). In one study, mothers on antiretroviral medication were more likely to disclose that their HIV infection may lead to death; this same study revealed that mothers' level of detail during the disclosure was higher when their T cell counts were higher (Kirshenbaum and Nevid 2002).

A parent's illness is not the only parental attribute that is associated with disclosure. Income also has been associated with disclosure, where parents with a lower income were less likely to disclose to their children (Armistead et al. 2001; Corona et al. 2006; Nam et al. 2009). Some research also suggests that the route of transmission may impact parental HIV disclosure. Parents who contracted HIV through injection drug use were more likely than those who contracted HIV through heterosexual intercourse to disclose their HIV-positive status to their children (Corona et al. 2006). In a US-based study, mothers living with HIV were more likely to disclose to their children than fathers living with HIV, and they did so at earlier developmental points (Lee and Rotheram-Borus 2002).

Child Attributes Associated with Disclosure

The most common factor parents consider when deciding whether to disclose their HIV-positive status is the child's age. Overwhelmingly, across contexts, research shows parents are more likely to disclose to older children compared to younger children (Armistead et al. 1997, 2001; Hawk 2007; Kirshenbaum and Nevid 2002; Lee and Rotheram-Borus 2002; Rwemisisi et al. 2008; Simoni et al. 2000). Although research suggests teenage years are the most common years for a child to learn about a parent's HIV-positive status (Kennedy et al. 2010), some studies suggest this process begins much earlier. A study of Ugandan parents found that children were often told about their parent's HIV-positive status at age eight years or older (Rwemisisi et al. 2008). A US study found that the first age of disclosure of any information related to a parent's HIV-positive status was age seven years (Kirshenbaum and Nevid 2002). That same study suggests the amount of detail provided during disclosure also varies based on age. While older children were told directly about the HIV-positive status of their parent (i.e., received *full disclosure*), younger children were more likely to be told that their parent was sick (i.e., received *partial disclosure*; Kirshenbaum and Nevid 2002). In a US-based study of parents living with HIV and their children, reasons for non-disclosure also varied based on age. For younger children, age was a reason for non-disclosure. Among older children, reasons for non-disclosure included the parent lacking the skill set needed to disclose to their child, and fear of the child rejecting or losing respect for the parent living with HIV (Kennedy et al. 2010). Beyond age, parents often consider the developmental level of the child (Hawk 2007; Kennedy et al. 2010; Qiao et al. 2013) and agree it is important to ensure disclosure is developmentally appropriate. However, level of maturity is largely subjective and difficult to measure.

Child gender may play an important role in parental HIV-positive status disclosure. Studies have shown that daughters are more likely to be disclosed to than sons (Armistead et al. 2001; Hawk 2007; Kirshenbaum and Nevid 2002; Lee and Rotheram-Borus 2002). Moreover, daughters are often provided a greater amount of detail during the disclosure process than their male counterparts (Hawk 2007; Kirshenbaum and Nevid 2002).

What Outcomes of Parental HIV Status Disclosure Do Children Experience?

Research shows the outcome of disclosure can be both positive and negative (Kennedy et al. 2010); yet typically, the disclosure of a parent's HIV-positive status is helpful for both parents and children (Qiao et al. 2013). Parents have reported that, despite initial reservation, outcomes of disclosure were not as negative as they anticipated (Kennedy et al. 2010). In fact, most parents have indicated they did not regret disclosing their HIV-positive status to their children (Ostrom Delaney et al. 2008).

During disclosure, some children are told not to share their parent's HIV-positive status with others (Corona et al. 2006; Kirshenbaum and Nevid 2002) or are asked to keep their parent's HIV-positive status a secret (Murphy et al. 2002). The reasons for encouraging secrecy include a fear of stigma and resulting harm to the child (Murphy et al. 2002). However, research indicates that encouraging the child to keep the parent's HIV-positive status a secret may result in poorer mental health for the child (Murphy et al. 2002; Nam et al. 2009). Some parents have found middle ground by explaining to the child it is safe to tell certain people about the parent's HIV-positive status, and talking with the child about who are safe people with whom to have these discussions (Murphy et al. 2002).

Immediately after learning about a parent's HIV-positive status, children have responded with encouragement, hugs, and questions (Corona et al. 2006; Kennedy et al. 2010; Ostrom et al. 2006). Children also have expressed concern regarding the health of their parents (Kennedy et al. 2010). Negative immediate responses from children have included fear of catching the virus from the parent, anger, or feeling overwhelmed (Corona et al. 2006; Kennedy et al. 2010).

Several studies have corroborated findings suggesting that disclosing a parent's HIV-positive status to a child does not negatively affect the child's behavior (Armistead et al. 2001; Cree et al. 2006); however, other factors related to a parent's HIV-positive status—such as parental stress brought on by the infection (Murphy et al. 2010)—may affect the child's behavior. In some cases, disclosure of a parent's HIV-positive status has been associated with child depression (Armistead et al. 1997), especially among those who were told to keep the status of their parent confidential (Kirshenbaum and Nevid 2002) or who felt stigmatized due to their parent's HIV-positive status (Murphy et al. 2006).

Research suggests the relationship between disclosure and academic well-being may be positive or negative. Findings from the 1990s revealed poorer school performance after disclosure of a parent's HIV-positive status (Armistead et al. 1997). In the school setting, children seek normalcy from teachers and classmates (Cree et al. 2006) and have experienced negative feelings during HIV and school-based sexual health programming (Cree et al. 2006). Although some children experienced negative reactions from other children (such as teasing and bullying), one study found peers were more likely to provide emotional support than to respond in a negative manner (Corona et al. 2006).

Knowledge about parental HIV-positive status disclosure is still rather limited. Practitioners who hope to translate research findings into practice should note that the majority of research on this topic has focused on maternal HIV and has been conducted in the US; less information is known about disclosure of paternal HIV-positive status and disclosure of any parental HIV in other settings. It is important to note that the context of disclosure matters; social norms and stigma may change over time and will likely vary across settings. With those changes, new considerations for disclosure may emerge.

What Guidance and Assistance is Available for Disclosure of Parental HIV-Positive Status?

Given the low rates of disclosure of parental HIV-positive status and parents' concerns regarding parental HIV disclosure, counseling and behavioral interventions are recommended to support parents who wish to disclose to their children (Qiao et al. 2013). The World Health Organization (2011) has provided this "key recommendation" regarding disclosure of parental HIV-positive status to children: "Children of school age should be told the HIV status of their parents or caregivers; younger children should be told this incrementally to accommodate their cognitive skills and emotional maturity" (World Health Organization 2011, pp 12). Yet the World Health Organization (WHO) acknowledges that this recommendation is not well supported by evidence.

Unfortunately, comprehensive guidelines to assist healthcare teams or parents with this process are lacking. Some advocacy and government Web sites addressing HIV do provide limited guidance for parental HIV-positive status disclosure (AIDSmap 2015; Positive Women's Network n.d.; U.S. Department of Health & Human Services 2009, 2011); although helpful, these recommendations have not been consistently updated or rigorously tested.

Parents considering disclosure may benefit from understanding some general information about child development. As discussed in one review (Murphy 2008), young children tend to have concrete views of illness and incomplete understanding of the meaning of death. Yet this tends to change around age 9, when children are capable of understanding how some encounters with people living with HIV do not pose transmission risks (e.g., hugs) but others do (e.g., touching their blood) and they comprehend the finality of death, as well. As children reach the teenage years, they develop the ability to grasp the complexities of HIV (i.e., that there are multiple transmission risks, that not everyone exposed to HIV will become infected, that some people are able to live a long life despite having HIV disease). Parents should know that these are generalizations, and children who experience developmental delays and those who are precocious may have different capabilities at the ages discussed here.

Given the lack of formal guidelines for parents who wish to disclose their own HIV-positive status, we propose the following recommendations, derived largely from the literature and guidelines on parent disclosure of a child's HIV status. Programs serving adults living with HIV may wish to share these recommendations with their staff and/or create parent handouts that communicate this information. When possible, staff could be trained to support parents in considering and preparing for disclosure. Yet healthcare staff may not always have the time to counsel parents about disclosure (Alemu et al. 2013). Alternatively, peer counselors could be trained to share these recommendations with parents living with HIV.

1. Parents living with HIV should be encouraged to provide developmentally (Wilfert et al. 1999; Lesch et al. 2007; New York State Department of Health AIDS Institute 2009) and culturally (Clifford et al. 2013; Lesch et al. 2007) appropriate information to their child about the parent's HIV-positive status. Parents may need assistance in determining what is developmentally appropriate (Murphy 2008).
2. When children ask questions about the parent's condition, parents should be discouraged from reporting mistruths (Lester et al. 2002; Vreeman et al. 2015; e.g., if they are not going to inform the child the parent is living with HIV, they

could tell them their blood needs some special medicine to keep it working well, rather than tell them they have another condition, like asthma).

3. Parents should consider the potential value of telling their children they (parents) are living with HIV before the child is likely to engage in sexual behavior, as child knowledge of the parent's HIV-positive status may help reduce the likelihood that the child will engage in behaviors that put them at substantial risk for HIV (i.e., unprotected sex and injection drug use; note that this recommendation is theoretical but has not been well tested).
4. Parents who have multiple children must consider that whatever information they share with one child may be shared with the other children; depending on the circumstances, telling the children together may be the best way to ensure that all children get the correct information. However, not all of their children may be ready to receive the diagnosis at the same time (Murphy 2008).
5. Parents may want to discuss with their children who is "safe" to talk with about the parent's HIV-positive status, as research suggests that when children are asked to keep a "secret," the children may suffer psychological distress (Murphy et al. 2002; Nam et al. 2009; Tompkins 2007). Most parents will not want the children to share information about a parent's HIV-positive status widely, but it may help the children if they have one or more people other than the parents with whom they can discuss it (Murphy et al. 2002).
6. Once parents have informed a child of the parent's HIV-positive status, they should be encouraged to follow up with the child and create opportunities for additional discussion; questions and concerns may arise as the child processes the disclosure (Dorrell and Katz 2014; Mburu et al. 2014).

The above recommendations are based on the research literature, but the strategies have not been rigorously tested. Moreover, the recommendations do not account for all of the unique circumstances that may arise, which may warrant special considerations. For example, disclosure of a parent's HIV-positive status when children are of mixed serostatus (i.e., one child is HIV-positive; one child is not) can make decision-making especially complex (Gachanja et al. 2014). Where available, parents in this and other unique situations may benefit from counseling assistance to determine the best strategies for their family.

Unfortunately, there are limited counseling recommendations available to assist parents with HIV-positive status disclosure. The paucity of evidence-based counseling recommendations has been blamed for inconsistent counseling in countries such as Uganda (Rwemisisi et al. 2008). Parents who have already disclosed to their children have suggested creating a disclosure plan with a counselor prior to disclosing their HIV-positive status to their child (Kennedy et al. 2010). Others have suggested group counseling may benefit the children of parents living with HIV, alleviating fears and allowing a safe place to talk through concerns (Reyland et al. 2002). Such support may be beneficial in assisting youth post disclosure, although as noted, a shortage of counselors, healthcare workers, and time among existing healthcare staff in many regions with substantial HIV epidemics (Alemu et al. 2013) means such programs will not be feasible everywhere.

Structured Behavioral Interventions

Many researchers have suggested that a family-centered context may be important for the disclosure of a parent's HIV-positive status to a child (Armistead et al. 1997, 2001; DeMatteo et al. 2002; Nam et al. 2009). One such family-centered intervention was a randomized controlled trial (RCT) of an intervention in the late 1990s focused on parents and their adolescent children aged 11–18 (Rotheram-Borus et al. 1997, 2001). This intervention aimed to reduce risky behaviors among parents living with HIV and their adolescent children, as well as increase emotional coping skills of participants. The first of the three modules of this intervention is directed at parents and includes education and support for decision-making related to parental HIV status disclosure to children (Rotheram-Borus et al. 2001). Adolescents who knew of the parent's HIV-positive status joined their parents in the second part of the intervention, which focused on adolescents coping with their parent's diagnosis, reduction of risky sexual behaviors, and guardianship concerns. At 4-year follow-up, intervention participants were less likely to experience problem behaviors and teenage pregnancies than those in the control group, with the positive effect from the intervention decreasing over time; although disclosure (having disclosed or not disclosed the parent's HIV-positive serostatus) was also assessed, the findings were not significant (Rotheram-Borus et al. 2003). Despite the intervention not having effects on disclosure rates, the intervention provided a safe place to discuss related disclosure outcomes and concerns.

More recently, a study in South Africa evaluated "Amagugu," a HIV-positive status disclosure intervention for mothers of children aged 6–10 years (Rochat et al. 2014). Lay counselors were trained to deliver this 6-session, home-based, structured intervention to mothers. The first, third, and fourth sessions occur with the mother and counselor only, and involve preparing the mother for disclosure, providing her with a 5-step strategy for disclosing to the child. The second session includes family members, takes a strengths-based approach, and teaches the family how to use play as a way to communicate. The mother undertakes disclosure to the child independently from the counselor and then meets with the counselor individually for session 5 to discuss the disclosure and ways of moving forward. The last session includes the mother, counselor, and the child, reinforces the benefits of communication with play and rewards both mothers and children for the work they have done. Only 10 of the 291 mothers who enrolled in this quasi-experimental project failed to complete the six sessions. Of the 281 who completed, the majority (61%) engaged in full disclosure to the child; the remainder engaged in partial disclosure. Maternal and child mental health benefits were found in pre–post testing, suggesting that the intervention was beneficial for both parties. It is noteworthy that only 28 of the eligible participants chose not to enroll in the intervention project, suggesting that the program was welcomed by the vast majority of eligible mothers. With the use of lay counselors, an added benefit of this intervention is the potential for widespread feasibility.

One US-based longitudinal pilot study tested the Teaching, Raising, And Communicating with Kids (TRACK) program among English- and Spanish-speaking mothers living with HIV and their 6–12-year-old children (Murphy et al. 2011). Based on Integrative Disclosure Theory (Derlega et al. 2004) and building on Family Systems Theory (Alexander et al. 2002), the program involved three individual in-person sessions with caregivers one week apart and one follow-up phone call. Sessions focused on: (1) child development, family life, and pros and cons of disclosure; (2) improving mother-child communication; and (3) practicing disclosure. Mothers in the TRACK (versus treatment as usual control) condition were six times more likely to disclose their HIV-positive status to the child. Emotional benefits were found for both mothers and children. A larger randomized controlled efficacy trial is currently underway to examine the impact of the TRACK program over time (Allison and Siberry 2015).

Other studies are ongoing to test the effectiveness of several parental HIV disclosure interventions (Allison and Siberry 2015). Many of these interventions also focus on a family-centered approach. One such study involves testing a culturally adapted parental HIV disclosure to children intervention for parents in Guangxi, China. This study focuses on children aged 6–15 years, and aims to assist in disclosure decisions and improve psychosocial outcomes in both parents and children. This large, cluster randomized trial will follow children and parents for 3 years (Li 2015). Currently underway in Zimbabwe is a RCT testing a three-session parental disclosure (of a parent's HIV-positive status) intervention against an attention-matched nutrition intervention; uniquely, the effects of the intervention on disclosure of child HIV-positive serostatus to the child will also be examined (Lightfoot 2015). This intervention focuses on making decisions about when to disclose a parent's HIV-positive status, the reactions of the child, and how disclosure affects the family.

Disclosure of Child HIV-Positive Status to Child

A major challenge in pediatric HIV remains disclosing the child's HIV-positive status to the child. Advances in care and treatment have dramatically improved the landscape of HIV infection (Matic et al. 2006). Yet despite these tremendous developments, the process of informing a child that he or she is living with HIV is often wrought with substantial anxiety on the part of parents/primary caregivers, as well as medical providers. The following paragraphs describe what is known about patterns and correlates of disclosure, the impact of disclosure on children and the caregiver-child relationship, and specific approaches for facilitating the disclosure process.

What Are the Patterns and Correlates of Child HIV-Positive Status Disclosure to the Child?

Great variations in the timing and processes of disclosure have been documented. Before the advent and widespread availability of highly active antiretroviral therapy, the need to disclose to children who were perinatally infected with HIV was perceived to be lower because there was no expectation that they would survive into adolescence or adulthood. At that time, children living with HIV were often infantilized and told mistruths or partial truths about their illness—ranging from "you have stomach problems" (and they often did have gastrointestinal side effects of the medication) to "there is a problem with your blood" (Funck-Brentano et al. 1997; Oberdorfer et al. 2006). Naturally, as it became clear that these children would likely grow into adolescents and adults, the perceived importance of disclosure increased, as did the incidence of informing these children of their HIV-positive status (Forsyth 2003). In 1999, the American Academy of Pediatrics (AAP) published guidelines suggesting that children living with HIV should be provided with developmentally appropriate information about their condition. The authors strongly encouraged disclosure to "school-aged children" and firmly stated that "adolescents should know their HIV status." (Wilfert et al. 1999). Since those guidelines emerged, there has developed a substantial body of literature.

Numerous systematic reviews have been conducted regarding disclosure of pediatric HIV infection to children. Those reviews have concluded that the majority of children are informed about their HIV-positive status between the ages of 10 and 15. One review reported that the mean age of disclosure ranged from age 7.0 to 13.7 years, with the disclosure age range lower in high-income (7–11 years) versus low- or middle-income countries (8.1–15.0 years; Pinzon-Iregui et al. 2013). Yet it is difficult to derive a meaningful average age of disclosure, as many research studies on the topic have focused on families in which disclosure had already occurred, creating a bias toward younger ages because those who are older at the age of disclosure are less likely to be captured in such studies. Although much of the literature suggests disclosure should be a process rather than a single event, there is generally an implicit consensus that "age of disclosure" is the age at which a child first is informed they are living with HIV.

Outside of age, few factors have been consistently associated with perinatal HIV infection disclosure across a large number of studies. There is a lack of substantial evidence that disclosure timing differs based on gender (Vreeman et al. 2013). In high-income countries, educational level is highly correlated with age and thus is less informative for understanding disclosure determinants. However, in low- and middle-income countries, where school attendance might be a more meaningful determinant, there is some evidence that children enrolled in school are substantially more likely to have experienced disclosure (Alemu et al. 2013; Bhattacharya et al. 2011; Myer et al. 2006) and that children with a higher level of education are more likely to have experienced disclosure (Kallem et al. 2011). Also in low- and middle-income countries, children on ART (compared to those not on ART) are more likely to have experienced disclosure (Menon et al. 2007), as are those who have been on ART for a longer (versus shorter) duration (Alemu et al. 2013; Bhattacharya et al. 2011; Kallem et al. 2011). There is some evidence that caregiver and family level factors are associated with greater likelihood of child disclosure, including urban (versus rural) residence (Alemu et al. 2013), not having a biological father as a primary caregiver (Kallem et al. 2011; Oberdorfer et al. 2006), and having a caregiver who is also living with HIV and has self-disclosed their own HIV-positive status (Moodley et al. 2006). Having a caregiver with a higher level of educational achievement (Bhattacharya et al. 2011; Biadgilign et al. 2011) and who is employed (Alemu et al. 2013) also is associated with greater likelihood of disclosure. While religious and spiritual beliefs and practices have not been well studied in relation to disclosure, one study found Orthodox Christians were more likely to disclose to their children than caregivers of other faiths, possibly due to beliefs about God's ability to heal (Alemu et al. 2013; Moore and Williamson 2011). Other potential correlates that warrant additional study include, but are not limited to, living with more family members, having siblings who are not living with HIV, and having a primary caregiver who is HIV-uninfected and having financial challenges.

When Should Children Be Informed of Their Status?

Although the American Academy of Pediatrics recommends that "adolescents" should be informed of their HIV-positive status (Wilfert et al. 1999), definitions of "adolescents" vary widely—with some suggesting adolescence begins as early as nine years. Some studies in low- or middle-income countries have found a caregiver preference for disclosing at age 14 and older (Pinzon-Iregui et al. 2013). Children and caregivers who have experienced disclosure vary in their opinions about when disclosure should occur (Pinzon-Iregui et al. 2013). Evidence suggests in some cases, children who are living with HIV but have not been informed of their HIV-positive status understand that something is amiss and experience substantial anxiety, sometimes worrying about what is wrong and why nobody is telling them (Dorrell and Katz 2014). Although it is not well studied, disclosing to children in "pre-adolescence" may be ideal, in that most children at that age are able to comprehend the basic components of HIV as an illness without conceptualizing the impact that living with HIV may have on their future sexual relationships (Blasini et al. 2004). Thus, telling a child they are living with HIV prior to adolescence may allow them to more gradually accept the more complex realities of their illness than if they are informed later. Regardless of when the child is informed, the information they receive should be developmentally appropriate to the child (Wiener et al. 2007; Wilfert et al. 1999).

Often, disclosure is prompted by: (a) desire for the child to assume greater responsibility for, or investment in, adherence to ART; (b) concerns that the child is reaching, or has hit, puberty and needs to know his status to ensure that he protects others from [primarily sexual] HIV transmission; (c) illness-related questions posed by the child; (d) belief that the child has “a right to know”; (e) guilt about the child not knowing her HIV-positive status; or (f) concerns that she will learn about her HIV-positive status in another way (Krauss et al. 2013; Pinzon-Iregui et al. 2013). In developing countries, attending school sometimes prompts disclosure as well (Bhattacharya et al. 2011; Myer et al. 2006; Vaz et al. 2011).

Who Should Disclose?

The literature shows a preference for parents/primary caregivers (versus healthcare providers or both caregivers and healthcare providers) to inform children they are living with HIV (Pinzon-Iregui et al. 2013; Vreeman et al. 2013). However, in some cases, the healthcare provider has been the preferred choice of both providers and caregivers (Moodley et al. 2006; Myer et al. 2006). In most studies in which disclosure of child HIV-positive status to the child has occurred, the primary agent of disclosure (i.e., the one who tells the child) has been the caregiver (Vreeman et al. 2013).

Parents/primary caregivers and healthcare providers sometimes experience conflict over disclosure decisions (Klitzman et al. 2008). This may be most common when the primary caregiver is a parent who is living with HIV and is concerned that the child will blame them for the HIV transmission (Beima-Sofie et al. 2014). Such parents often have tremendous guilt about their role in the child acquiring HIV and fear their relationship with the child will be deeply scarred by disclosure (Vreeman et al. 2015). Ironically, the children in these situations are sometimes much angrier at the parents for lying about the child’s HIV infection or failing to disclose at an earlier time than they are angry about transmission itself (Lester et al. 2002). Another concern parents may have is that the child will tell others about the child’s *and* parent’s HIV-positive status (Pinzon-Iregui et al. 2013)—something that could lead to substantial stigmatization of the parent, child, and family. Conflict between caregivers and healthcare providers can occur also when caregivers are not emotionally prepared to have disclosure discussions with the child, or lack skills or self-efficacy related to disclosure (Brandt et al. 2015). There is some evidence to suggest that this can be addressed with a clinic-based disclosure process that is systematic, gradual, non-threatening, and occurs in collaboration between clinic staff, primary caregiver(s), and the child, or with group or individual-based counseling for caregivers (Blasini et al. 2004).

What Outcomes Do Children and Adolescents Experience After Learning They Are Living with HIV?

Limited studies have explored health outcomes as they relate to disclosing a child's HIV-positive status to the child. One study (Ferris et al. 2007) did find a significantly decreased risk of death among children who had experienced disclosure, which may be due to a shift in medication adherence following disclosure. However, the causal mechanism is difficult to determine because data were derived from medical record review.

In terms of mental health, generally, outcomes of disclosure are more positive than parents/caregivers anticipate. Parents/caregivers are often concerned that their children will be devastated upon learning their HIV-positive status and will face substantial psychological sequelae (Chew et al. 2012; Mellins et al. 2002; Pinzon-Iregui et al. 2013; Vreeman et al. 2010). In some cases, this may happen, although few studies have reported significant psychosocial negative outcomes from disclosure to children (New et al. 2007; Wiener et al. 2007). Other studies have found no significant relationship between disclosure and mental health (Lester et al. 2002; Mellins et al. 2002; Wiener et al. 1996). In fact, some research has shown that children who know their HIV-positive status experience lower levels of mental health problems than children who have not experienced disclosure (Krauss et al. 2013). This is not to suggest that it is easy for a child to learn they have a highly stigmatized life-threatening disease that may require them to take medication for the remainder of his or her life. A recent review of four studies reporting on initial reactions to disclosure found some children experienced sadness or worry (36%), shock (16%), anger (15%), or confusion (8%), although others reported feeling normal or neutral (28%) or experiencing relief (6%; Krauss et al. 2013). Children who do experience negative initial reactions—and those who do not—will likely benefit from continued communication with a trusted source (i.e., parent/caregiver, healthcare provider), during which they can ask questions and receive additional support (Dorrell and Katz 2014). Fortunately, one study suggests that six months following disclosure, many of the initial negative reactions dissipate and more positive emotions increase (Blasini et al. 2004). Post-disclosure, children who already suspected they had a serious illness may even experience increased self-confidence and become closer to parents (Blasini et al. 2004).

There is some conflicting evidence regarding the impact of disclosure on medication adherence (Blasini et al. 2004; Cluver et al. 2015; Hammami et al. 2004; Marhefka et al. 2006; Mellins et al. 2002). Some studies suggest disclosure may increase the commitment children have to taking their medication (Cluver et al. 2015). However, disclosure may also lead parents/primary caregivers to completely shift responsibility for remembering medication-taking to their child, because they believe the child will now ensure full adherence (Vaz et al. 2011). In some cases, this may not be developmentally appropriate and may not be successful (Marhefka et al. 2008). Furthermore, some children may "act out" in response to learning their diagnosis and may actually refuse to take their ART medications or lie about taking them—at least for a time (Merzel et al. 2008).

As noted, a major consideration regarding the timing of disclosure is preventing young people living with HIV from unwittingly passing HIV to others via sexual intercourse. To our knowledge, there is little research suggesting that disclosure prevents—or does not prevent—young people living with HIV from engaging in risky sexual behavior (i.e., engaging in unprotected vaginal or anal intercourse), although there is some evidence that youth who are living with HIV and know their HIV-positive status are more likely to use condoms consistently than youth not living with HIV (Belzer et al. 2001; Sturdevant et al. 2001). Certainly, if someone does not know they are living with HIV, they are unlikely to be concerned about passing HIV to a sexual partner; thus, disclosure is a necessary condition for young people living with HIV to purposefully prevent transmitting the virus to their partners.

What Guidance and Assistance Is Available for Disclosure of Child HIV-Positive Status to the Child?

Recommendations, Tools, and Strategies

Not all families will desire help in navigating disclosure, but many may. Despite the largely unmet need for resources to help parents/primary caregivers disclose to their children, there are some evidence-based tools and strategies available—although few have been evaluated in randomized controlled trials. General recommendations (Table 8.1) often focus on the importance of providing developmentally appropriate information and stress that disclosure should be approached as a process rather than a single event. As children have time to cognitively process the information regarding their HIV-positive status, new questions and concerns are likely to arise; parents/primary caregivers and healthcare workers should create a relationship with the child that facilitates ongoing opportunities for children and adolescents to ask questions and receive answers, as well as support (Dorrell and Katz 2014; Mburu et al. 2014). For example, a child who initially learns they are living with HIV at age nine may not be thinking about the implications for child-bearing or sexual behavior. Yet as the child becomes older, it will be important for him or her to have opportunities to discuss such implications with a trusted information source.

Perhaps the most well-known intervention for pediatric HIV disclosure was developed and tested in a quasi-experimental study conducted at a Puerto Rican pediatric HIV clinic (Blasini et al. 2004). In this approach, the healthcare team (i.e., psychologists, social workers, pediatricians, and nurses) plays a key role in facilitating disclosure. The team is taught to consider disclosure as a process and to respect the parent/caregiver's preference regarding when disclosure will occur. Disclosure during a medical crisis/acute illness is discouraged. The team is also

Table 8.1 Guidelines and recommendations for disclosing a child's HIV status to the child

	Chew et al. (2012)	WHO (2011)	Wiener et al. (2007)	AAP (1999)
Who Should Know and What They Should Know				
– School age children should know they have HIV		✓		[a]
– Adolescents (to participate in treatment decisions and to make informed decisions about sexual behaviors) should know they have HIV			✓	✓
– Young children do not need to know the name of the illness but symptomatic children should be informed in some way			✓	✓
– Young children should be informed incrementally		✓	[b]	[b]
– Information should be tailored to developmental level, cognitive abilities, and other child circumstances		✓	✓	✓
– Decisions should consider the child's well-being	[b]	✓	[b]	[b]
Role of the Healthcare Team				
– Receive training in pediatric HIV disclosure	✓			
– Counsel caregivers regarding disclosure				✓
– Engage caregivers in a "collaborative process of information gathering and trust building" in preparation for disclosure	✓			
– Assess caregivers' abilities (i.e., mental health, social support, and feelings regarding disclosing HIV-related "family secrets")			✓	
– Identify sources of support for caregivers and children	✓		✓	
– Assess caregiver and child knowledge continuously	✓		✓	
– Support caregivers to disclose through role-playing disclosure scenarios	✓		✓	
– Negotiate with the caregivers regarding when to disclose, balancing parent needs vs. patient rights	✓			
– Maintain open communication with the family, including post-disclosure follow-up and informational and emotional support	✓		✓	
Role of Caregivers				
– Negotiate with the healthcare team regarding when to disclose, balancing parent needs vs. patient rights	✓			

(continued)

Table 8.1 (continued)

	Chew et al. (2012)	WHO (2011)	Wiener et al. (2007)	AAP (1999)
– Decide when and where disclosure occurs and who is present	✓			
– Prepare to manage the child's reaction	✓			
– Encourage open dialogue with the child throughout the disclosure process			✓	

Notes ✓source provided this guideline or recommendation
[a]Source strongly encourages this
[b]We believe this was implied by the source but it was not explicitly listed as a guideline or recommendation

taught to be mindful about their own feelings regarding disclosure—this is intended to minimize "vicarious trauma" healthcare staff may experience (Blasini et al. 2004, p. 183).

Parents/caregivers and children meet individually with healthcare staff to build rapport. Three to six parent/caregiver sessions prepare parents/caregivers for the disclosure experience, including how to address "embarrassing questions" (i.e., *how did I get HIV?*). The disclosure process proceeds when the child indicates on a questionnaire that he or she is "ready to learn more" about the illness and when the parent/caregiver is also ready. The healthcare team presents parents/caregivers with two options regarding disclosure, both of which involve substantial support from the healthcare team. In option 1, parents/caregivers ultimately inform the child of his or her HIV-positive status. In option 2, parents/caregivers and the healthcare team work together to disclose to the child. The healthcare team encourages the use of visual materials to support the disclosure, especially a cartoon book about HIV. After the primary disclosure occurs (i.e., after the child is told he or she is living with HIV), the healthcare team checks in with the family in two to four weeks and meets monthly with the family, or child, as needed to provide support. Ultimately, children are encouraged to engage in an open dialogue with family members and the healthcare team, asking questions about their HIV-positive status as they arise. This is especially important as children become older and have questions regarding sexual behavior and child-bearing. Research on this approach has demonstrated positive impacts for healthcare providers (i.e., reduced insecurity around disclosure) and parents/caregivers (i.e., increased feelings of relief, self-confidence and security, and positive views of the process). Although some children did report immediate negative reactions to learning their HIV-positive status, the majority did not report negative emotions related to disclosure at six months, and 85% evaluated their disclosure experience positively (Blasini et al. 2004).

The Blasini intervention has been adapted for use in Haiti and the Dominican Republic (Beck-Sagué et al. 2015). In addition to being translated from Spanish into

Haitian Creole, adaptations included adding a multimedia training and retraining session for healthcare workers, as well as a video that shows young people living with and managing a variety of chronic conditions. Preliminary data on this adapted intervention suggest general acceptability and higher-than-expected retention. However, investigators reported one instance of severe depression and one instance of a child found preparing to hang himself. While this is alarming, it is worth noting that there is little evidence in the literature that suicidal behavior is common in response to disclosure. This finding should serve as a reminder for those of us involved in disclosure work that careful assessment of the child's emotional state as well as close supervision and monitoring by caregivers should be in place following disclosure.

O'Malley and colleagues (2015) evaluated a model of disclosure designed by the Namibia Ministry of Health and Social Services, which is in many ways consistent with the Blasini model. Like the Blasini model, the disclosure process takes place in the context of a provider–parent partnership. A key component is the use of a cartoon book to guide the disclosure process (O'Malley et al. 2015). Healthcare workers are trained to guide families through the process. The process begins when a healthcare worker starts disclosure sessions with the family—generally when the child is six years old—and works through the process over a period of months or years with the goal of full disclosure (i.e., naming the illness "HIV") by age 10. In the five-chapter cartoon book, HIV is named "the bad guy" and "body soldiers" work to fight him off; each chapter builds on the next, with the final chapter revealing the name of "the bad guy" (i.e., "HIV") and the "soldiers" (i.e., "CD4 cells"). Consistent with the Blasini model, a healthcare provider completes a child and caregiver assessment tool that dictates the speed and approach to disclosure. A "disclosure form" tracks the knowledge the youth obtain throughout the disclosure process. With these procedures, all members of the healthcare team are able to identify how much of the process has been completed and how ready the child is for the next step. In one evaluation, healthcare workers reported that the book "simplifies the disclosure process" and "reduces caregiver resistance." Research on this intervention demonstrated improved confidence among healthcare workers with regard to their ability to work with families to address disclosure (O'Malley et al. 2015). However, implementation challenges were noted, including the fact that not all healthcare workers completed the training, at times healthcare workers were too busy to complete the process, and the forms had components that were not applicable with certain families (O'Malley et al. 2015). Related recommendations have been adopted by the WHO (2011; Table 8.2).

Numerous other disclosure intervention trials are ongoing, including those recently funded by the US National Institute of Mental Health Office of AIDS Research (Allison and Siberry 2015). In Kenya, Vreeman et al. (2015) are conducting a RCT testing a patient-centered child HIV-positive status disclosure intervention against a usual care disclosure approach that has been implemented in that setting for over 10 years. In Ghana, Paintsil (2015) and others are testing an approach using an "adherence and disclosure specialist" familiar with community norms to work with the families, guided by the Information, Motivation, Behavioral

Table 8.2 Disclosing child HIV-positive status to the child: Recommendations for healthcare workers (HCW) providing assistance

Recommendations from Blasini et al. (2004)	Broader recommendations from the World Health Organization (2011)
1. Train healthcare workers	
2. Establish partnerships between caregivers/family and HCWs as well as between children living with HIV and healthcare workers to facilitate a trusting, collaborative process	
3. Conduct numerous family meetings and individual sessions with children living with HIV to prepare for disclosure "event" (typically over 4–6 months)	Provide information about HIV and related treatment to caregivers and children Choose culturally appropriate and available resources to assist in the process
4. Tailor communication to needs and concerns of family and to developmental/cognitive level of child	Tailor communication to child age
5. Prepare family members for handling "embarrassing questions"	Prepare caregivers to answer children's questions
6. Only name the illness when the child is curious and both the child and the family are "ready" (approximately 6–8 months from starting the process)	
7. Provide post-disclosure support for child and family members, in which focus is on coping and living with HIV as a chronic illness	Prepare caregivers for child reactions (short and long term) Develop a plan for caregiver and child disclosure to others Identify "safe" people with whom child and caregiver can discuss HIV Help caregivers engage in life-planning with the child

Skills Model. This child HIV-positive status disclosure intervention will be tested against usual care in a RCT. Results of these studies will be important for enhancing our knowledge of how to best support caregivers in the disclosure process.

An Alternative Approach: Developmental Illness Models

It is important to note that not everyone advocates for "disclosure models" for children living with perinatally acquired HIV. For example, Abadía-Barrero and LaRusso (2006), in response to results of interviews focused on the lived experience of children living with HIV/AIDS in Brazil, argue that children should be provided with "developmentally appropriate information about HIV/AIDS … at all ages," which they believe "would eliminate the need for *disclosure* and reduce children's emotional distress." (Abadía-Barrero and LaRusso 2006, pp 36). These authors seem to suggest that standard practice should be to gradually provide the child more detailed information about the child's illness—something that would be very similar to what the literature shows many caregivers already do when they engage in *partial disclosure* (for example, by telling them "you need medication because you have a problem in your blood") on the way to *full disclosure* (i.e., revealing that the "problem in their blood" is actually HIV). There may be subtleties in their argument that are worth considering. For example, rather than wait until a child is deemed "old enough" to begin the disclosure process, or wait until the family has already told the child mistruths about her illness, what if healthcare teams started working with caregivers to make a disclosure plan shortly after birth? Caregivers of children living with HIV could meet every six months with a counselor to envision and unfold a plan for gradually informing the child of his HIV-positive status—creating a culture that, intentionally and from the beginning, balances respect for the child's right to know, the child's developmental capabilities, and the potential unintended consequences of the child knowing (e.g., stigma). In the case of the child experiencing a change in caregiver(s), the plan could then be shared with the new caregiver(s) via the healthcare team. Currently, when it is expected that many children born with perinatal HIV infection will live well into adulthood, a proactive approach such as this may be warranted and could reduce the emotional burden of undisclosed perinatal HIV on both caregivers and children. Related research is warranted.

Child Disclosure to Family, Friends, Romantic, and Sexual Partners

Once they have learned they are living with HIV, children and adolescents must choose to whom to disclose their HIV-positive status—including family, friends, acquaintances, coworkers, and romantic and sexual partners. They also face decisions about disclosing within the school environment (Hosek et al. 2008). Much like other forms of disclosure, and as noted by researchers (Lee et al. 2015), HIV-positive status disclosure to others is often a long-term process that occurs over time.

What are Key Developmental Considerations?

It is important to acknowledge that children and adolescents make decisions about self-disclosure in the context of a developing brain. Research has illuminated particular aspects of the developing adolescent brain that may uniquely affect disclosure decision-making and outcomes. Perhaps most important is the "asynchronous maturation of prefrontal and limbic systems," which has been associated with impulsiveness and risk-taking in adolescents in general (Bava and Tapert 2010 pp 408). For youth, this could manifest in engaging in impulsive and risky disclosure (e.g., they may disclose to someone who may be inclined to react with violence or to indiscriminately tell others) or it could manifest in the failure to disclose to others when non-disclosure may be unethical and/or illegal (e.g., nondisclosure to someone with whom they may have unprotected sex)—although these are just hypotheses, as brain development among youth living with HIV has not been specifically studied in relation to disclosure. Of course, despite the challenges associated with the developing adolescent brain, some youth make thoughtful, informed decisions about who to tell, when to tell, and how to tell their friends, family members, and romantic and sexual partners.

What are the Patterns and Correlates of Disclosure?

To Whom Do Youth Disclose?

A large study of over 400 young people in the US reported that 82.7% of 12–24-year-olds had disclosed their HIV positive serostatus to at *least one person*—be it a friend, sexual partner, or family member (Lee et al. 2015). Similar results have been found over the last two decades, with 80% or more of youth sampled indicating they had disclosed their HIV-positive status to at least one person (Hightow-Weidman et al. 2013; Lam et al. 2007; Lee et al. 1999; Rongkavilit et al. 2010). The frequency of disclosure varied based on the type of relationship the young person had with the person to whom they were disclosing. For example, in several studies and countries, youth were most likely to disclose to family members, compared to friends or others (Lam et al. 2007; Lee et al. 1999, 2015; Michaud et al. 2009), with three-fourths of youth disclosing to family. However, studies have found that about half of youth also disclose to close friends (Lam et al. 2007; Lee et al. 1999).

Why Do Youth Disclose?

As with adults living with HIV, youth with HIV may disclose their HIV-positive status to others for a variety of reasons, including: (a) social support (Siu et al. 2012); (b) to increase closeness with others (Gillard and Roark 2012, 2013; Hogwood et al. 2013); (c) to avoid lying or deceiving (Gillard and Roark 2013); and (d) to prevent sexual transmission of HIV or relieve the burden of guilt related to potential transmission (Marhefka et al. 2011).

Fear of stigma is commonly the primary reason for non-disclosure. Indeed, most other reasons for non-disclosure can be linked to fear of stigma. As with adults, to avoid disclosure to someone who may highly stigmatize them for HIV, savvy youth may "test" the person by engaging in jokes related to HIV or bringing up a scenario about someone who has HIV to gauge the response of their peers before they decide it is "safe" to disclose (Siu et al. 2012). Some may have other people who do the disclosing on their behalf in order to distance themselves from potential stigma. For example, during a research interview with the first author of this chapter (Marhefka 2007), one young woman with perinatally acquired HIV explained:

> I used to have my sister tell them [about my HIV] because usually I went out with her best friends. And you know, they were cool people so I usually had, you know, her tell them and if they didn't like it [the fact that I have HIV], you know, I guess we would have broke up or—but it never happened like that; they really didn't care.

Of note, particularly among youth who acquired HIV horizontally, the stigma fear is not always of HIV-related stigma; some youth may refrain from disclosing their HIV-positive status due to fear of stigma associated with sexual abuse (Clum et al. 2013), engaging in premarital sex (Kyaddondo et al. 2013), unintended pregnancy (Crankshaw et al. 2014), or same-sex encounters (D'Angelo et al. 2001). Inevitably, when youth disclose, they will be asked about the transmission route; this presumptive need for double disclosure may pose a formidable barrier. Youth may lack the cognitive and interpersonal maturity to navigate these concerns and consequently avoid disclosure altogether.

How Does Self-disclosure Vary Based on Characteristics of Youth Living with HIV?

Youth's self-disclosure has been studied with respect to many youth characteristics, including: sexual orientation and behavior, age, race, relationship status, and education. However, results reflect mixed disclosure findings related to many of these characteristics.

A recent study in the US found that sexual orientation was not associated with familial knowledge of a young person's HIV-positive status (Lee et al. 2015). However, earlier findings suggest sexual orientation may play a role. Disclosure to mothers was not related to sexual orientation, but disclosure to fathers was more common among heterosexual youth than homosexual youth—including both males and females (D'Angelo et al. 2001). This possible shift in association between sexual orientation and disclosure to family members over time may be reflective of a cultural shift toward greater openness in discussing sexual orientation in the US.

The relationship between sexual orientation and disclosure may be largely dependent upon cultural and geographical factors. For example, studies of Latino men in the US show disclosure is common between gay men; this may be due to cultural norms in the Hispanic community (Marks et al. 1992; Mason et al. 1995).

Internationally, sexual orientation may also play a role in whom a young person chooses to disclose their HIV status. In at least one study of men who have sex with men (MSM) in Thailand, disclosure was more common to friends than to family members (Rongkavilit et al. 2010).

The seriousness of a romantic or sexual relationship has been associated with disclosure in several studies based in the US (Batterham et al. 2005; D'Angelo et al. 2001; Wiener and Battles 2006) as has the number of sexual partners (Dempsey et al. 2012). However, the findings are somewhat inconsistent. Research suggests main partners are disclosed to more often than casual partners (Batterham et al. 2005; D'Angelo et al. 2001). One study found that young people living with HIV who had only one sexual partner in a 90-day period were more likely to have disclosed their HIV-positive status to their sexual partner than those with more than one sexual partner in a 90-day period (Dempsey et al. 2012). Conversely, in another study a greater number of sexual encounters were associated with more frequent disclosure (D'Angelo et al. 2001).

While some research has shown that age is not associated with disclosure to others (D'Angelo et al. 2001; Lee et al. 1999), other research has shown that disclosure increases with age (Wiener and Battles 2006). Researchers have explained this potential difference based on a number of factors, including developmental stages—where younger youth reflected their parents' attitudes of disclosure patterns, and older youth searched for their own rationale for disclosure (Michaud et al. 2009).

Demographic factors such as race and ethnicity (D'Angelo et al. 2001; Lee et al. 2015) and educational attainment (D'Angelo et al. 2001; Lee et al. 2015) do not appear to play a role in disclosure in the US, but the literature on the role of gender shows conflicting findings. Studies have shown gender does not affect disclosure to family members (Lee et al. 1999) or sexual partners (D'Angelo et al. 2001), except that young women have been found to be more likely to disclose to their fathers than young men (D'Angelo et al. 2001). Additionally, young men may disclose to friends more often than young women (Lee et al. 1999; Rongkavilit et al. 2010), perhaps due to a sense of comradery surrounding HIV in the LGBT community.

What Youth HIV Illness-Related Characteristics are Associated with Self-disclosure?

Several characteristics specific to disease progression and timing have been studied in relation to disclosure, primarily in the US. Some research indicates the age a young person learns of their diagnosis may not be directly associated with disclosing to romantic partners, although in one study those who knew their diagnosis for longer disclosed to more people, and those who had disclosed to more people were more likely to have disclosed to romantic or sexual partners (Wiener and Battles 2006). A study specific to MSM found disclosure to sexual partners was more frequent when the length of time since diagnosis was longer (Batterham et al. 2005). Among a sample that included a broad range of sexual orientations and preferences, one study found that disclosure to sexual partners was more common when the HIV status of the sexual partner was known (Dempsey et al. 2012) with disclosure more common to HIV-positive partners than to HIV-negative partners (Batterham et al. 2005; D'Angelo et al. 2001). Being engaged in HIV care and receiving counseling has been associated with disclosure (Lam et al. 2007; Lee et al. 1999; Wiener and Battles 2006). Stage of HIV infection (Lee et al. 1999), CD4 count and transmission mode (Wiener and Battles 2006) have not been associated with disclosure.

What Parental Characteristics are Associated with Self-disclosure?

Research demonstrates parental support and parent–child relationships play a role in disclosure. In a study based in Switzerland, adoptive and foster parents were more likely than biological parents to promote disclosure among youth who primarily acquired HIV through perinatal transmission (Michaud et al. 2009), perhaps because they have less at stake, since adoptive parents are typically not living with HIV and thus their child disclosing to others will not involve disclosure of the parents' HIV-positive status. The younger the adolescent, the more likely they are to share the same disclosure views as their parent (Michaud et al. 2009). Regardless of gender, youth appear to be more likely to disclose their HIV-positive status to their mothers than their fathers (D'Angelo et al. 2001).

What are the Outcomes of Self-disclosure?

Social Support

In cases of a young person disclosing their HIV-positive status to a parent, research suggests youth ages 14–19 years are likely to perceive the social support from their parents as high (D'Angelo et al. 2001). These findings are consistent with research conducted in Tanzania and Botswana, where disclosure was associated with increased ART use and social support among peers (Midtbo et al. 2012). Not surprisingly, perceived social support may be low when family and friends limit communication with a young person after disclosure (Lee et al. 2015).

Relationship Dynamics and Stigma

Rejection by family and friends is the most commonly researched negative outcome of self-disclosure among young people living with HIV. Participants in various studies within high-income countries have reported feeling rejected by family (Hosek et al. 2008; Rao et al. 2007; Travers and Paoletti 1999), sexual partners (Leonard et al. 2010; Michaud et al. 2009; Travers and Paoletti 1999) and friends

(Hosek et al. 2008). Some youth have reported that such negative experiences resulted in them choosing not to disclose their status to others (Michaud et al. 2009). This is an important finding, as it suggests that early experiences with disclosure may dictate future decisions about disclosure. Assisting youth with identifying the right time and place for disclosure as well as strategies for disclosure, and preparing youth for the potential outcomes of disclosure, may have important long-term consequences, as disclosure is critical to HIV-specific social support, which has been associated with adherence to care and treatment (Leonard et al. 2010; Siu et al. 2012). Moreover, disclosure to sexual partners may, in some cases, increase condom use (Hightow-Weidman et al. 2013; Leonard et al. 2010) or pre-exposure prophylaxis (PrEP) use of those partners in the case of serodiscordance, although this has not been well studied—especially among youth.

Self-disclosure, Secondary Prevention, and Sexual Relationships

Youth living with HIV have reported a fear of intimacy and new relationships due to the barrier of having to address disclosure with new partners (Busza et al. 2013). In a study based in Tanzania, the anxiety of some perinatally infected youth caused them to avoid sexual relationships completely (Busza et al. 2013). Avoidance of sexual relationships to avoid disclosure has been found in the US as well (Marhefka et al. 2011).

There have been mixed findings regarding the relationship between disclosure, condom use, and safer sex behaviors. Unfortunately, data show many youth living with HIV are not disclosing *and* not using condoms during sexual intercourse (Dempsey et al. 2012). Similarly, Sturdevant et al. (2001) reported that young people who had not disclosed their HIV-positive status were less likely to use condoms than their peers who had disclosed their status. Disclosure has been associated with increased condom use among young women aged 13–23 (Lee et al. 1999), and among young men who have sex with men aged 13–24 (Hightow-Weidman et al. 2013). One should not assume that disclosure automatically leads to condom use, however. If the partner living with HIV shifts the responsibility of condom use to the partner, condom use may actually decrease in some cases (Marhefka et al. 2011; Leonard et al. 2010).

Other Physical and Psychological Outcomes

As noted, there are positive outcomes associated with disclosure. For example, adolescents have reported that disclosure improved relationships (Hogwood et al. 2013; Leonard et al. 2010). Despite concerns regarding rejection, disclosure to family and friends is not typically associated with poor mental health (Lam et al. 2007). On the contrary, disclosure to family and friends has been associated with increased support and engagement in care (Leonard et al. 2010; Siu et al. 2012). Among young children (aged 8–13), one study found self-disclosure to friends was associated with positive health outcomes, including increased CD4 counts (Sherman et al. 2000). Contrary to parental concerns, child's behavior and self-concept were not found to be affected by the disclosure event (Sherman et al. 2000). Similarly, among adolescents in Botswana and Tanzania, disclosure to others led to less internalized stigma, even when external stigma occurred (Midtbo et al. 2012). Additionally, fear of disclosure has been associated with poor ART adherence both in the US (Rao et al. 2007) and in international settings (Cluver et al. 2015; Midtbo et al. 2012); thus, removing the barrier of disclosure may increase adherence and overall health.

What Available Guidance and Assistance Exists to Help Youth Disclose to Family, Friends, and Sexual Partners?

Recommendations, Tools, and Strategies

Many researchers note the need for interventions and guidance to help youth with self-disclosure of HIV-positive status (Hosek et al. 2008; Lee et al. 1999, 2015; Michaud et al. 2009; Greenhalgh et al. 2015; Evangeli and Foster 2014), but there is currently a dearth of recommendations, tools, and strategies to assist youth with self-disclosure. Researchers recommend social support, especially utilizing peers who have already disclosed their status to others (Thoth et al. 2014), and yet youth may benefit from more structured education and guidance. Midtbo et al. (2012) described some of the benefits youth received from support groups in Tanzania and Botswana, including: a place to seek advice from healthcare professionals, peer support, theme-based seminars, and age-appropriate activities with youth who were aware of the young person's HIV-positive status. Although not well tested among youth, counseling and structured interventions that include disclosure planning and practice of disclosure-related skills (i.e., determining who to tell, determining the best time to disclose, determining what to reveal during the disclosure, and identifying strategies for coping with negative outcomes) may help (Kalichman et al. 2001; Serovich et al. 2009). Counseling and other interventions should consider the role of the family in decision-making and support for disclosure to friends and sexual partners (Thoth et al. 2014), but note that family input may be highly valued for some youth but could be destructive for others. Opportunities for disclosure education, skills building, and support should also involve imparting information about local and national HIV disclosure laws where applicable (Chenneville et al. 2015; Fernet et al. 2011).

One particular issue that may be important for counseling and related programs to address is how to talk about HIV to sexual partners in a way that communicates the seriousness of the condition and the risk of sexual transmission but also communicates "hope for the future," including a long life for people living with HIV (Greenhalgh et al. 2013, pp 449). Youth are often rightfully concerned about rejection from [potential] sexual partners, who fear they will contract HIV if they remain in the relationship (Greenhalgh et al. 2013). Fortunately, this may be easier with the increasing availability of Truvada® (tenofovir/emtricitabine) as pre-exposure prophylaxis (PrEP), which dramatically reduces the risk of HIV transmission when a HIV-negative partner consistently takes the once-daily pill (Baeten et al. 2012). For now, however, we are a long way from universal access to Truvada® as PrEP for people in mixed serostatus relationships (Centers for Disease Control and Prevention, Health Resources and Services Administration & National Institutes of Health 2014). Research is also limited, albeit ongoing, regarding the use of PrEP for adolescents under the age of 18, further limiting its reach among young people.

Youth living with HIV have provided feedback on strategies they have used during the disclosure process. Suggested strategies generally relate to establishing or testing the presence of trust in the relationship, thus determining who is a "safe" person to tell (Fair and Albright 2012; Hogwood et al. 2013). For example, some youth recommend first telling other (non-HIV-related) sensitive information to friends and partners, to see if they can be trusted, prior to revealing their HIV status (Blake et al. 2012). Similarly, youth encourage peers to mention HIV in a less serious fashion initially, to gauge the person's response; if the person responds positively, that is a sign that they could be accepting of a partner who is living with HIV (Siu et al. 2012; Greenhalgh et al. 2015). When building a relationship, youth living with HIV advise taking it slowly and knowing that supportive relationships are possible (Fair and Albright 2012).

Potential for Peer-Based Approaches

Given the lack of interventions designed to help youth make decisions about self-disclosure of their HIV-positive status, peer mentorship may be an avenue worth considering. Slightly older peers who have known their HIV-positive status for several years, have experienced self-disclosure, and are willing to undergo training and follow guidance may be good candidates for lay health counseling regarding youth disclosure. As noted elsewhere in this chapter, a shortage of healthcare providers for youth living with HIV in much of the world means relying on paraprofessionals or trained peer counselors may be the best option for providing assistance to these youth (Alemu et al. 2013). Models that use existing evidence to create peer training programs should be explored and tested.

Ethical Considerations

In this chapter, we have described three scenarios related to HIV disclosure: (1) disclosure of parental HIV status to child; (2) disclosure of child's HIV status to child; and (3) child's disclosure of HIV status to family, friends, and sexual partners. There are moral, ethical, and legal considerations in at least two of these three scenarios, namely, disclosure of child's HIV status to child and child's disclosure of HIV status to sexual partners. In the case of the former, the issues relate to children's rights, whereas in the case of the latter, issues relate to preventing harm to others. Broadly speaking, both situations involve the principles of beneficence, nonmaleficence, autonomy, and justice (Klitzman et al. 2008). The complexities of ethical decision-making in each of these scenarios are described more fully below.

Disclosure of Child's HIV Status to Child

The potential benefits and importance of disclosing to a child his/her HIV status were described earlier in this chapter. Aside from these potential benefits are moral and ethical concerns related to a child's right to know she is living with a chronic illness. Complicating these concerns are questions about age, maturity, and decisional capacity. For example, at what age does a child have a right to know he is living with HIV? Beyond age, how can you assure a child is mature enough or otherwise has the capacity to comprehend and make use of an HIV diagnosis? These are important questions because children are considered vulnerable and in need of protection. It is the responsibility of adults, including parents, to ensure children are physically and emotionally protected, and it is assumed that parents act in the best interests of their children. Legally, parents' right to autonomy trumps the child's right to autonomy. However, over protection may actually cause harm to children. Therefore, balancing protection with autonomy is imperative when working with children with HIV. Chenneville et al. (2010) present a model for trying to achieve this balance, which requires a case-by-case analysis and involves an assessment of decisional capacity. Klitzman et al. (2008) also advocate for a case-by-case analysis and encourage a thorough dissection of the principles of beneficence, nonmaleficence, autonomy, and justice. A goodness-of-fit ethical (GFE) framework, which draws on relational ethics and emphasizes the importance of finding a fit between the characteristics of the child and the context, also may be useful when thinking about how best to balance protection and autonomy (Fisher 2017; Masty and Fisher 2008; Fisher and Goodman 2009). Originally designed to address ethical dilemmas arising in research settings, the GFE framework also has clinical implications.

Disclosure of HIV Status to Sexual Partners

For clinicians working with youth with HIV, disclosure of status to sexual partners presents its own unique moral, ethical, and legal dilemmas. Health professionals, including mental health professionals, have both an ethical and legal duty to maintain the confidentiality of their clients. They also have an ethical and legal duty to protect others from harm as established in the landmark Tarasoff case (Tarasoff v.

Regents of the University of California 1976, 1974). However, the extent to which Tarasoff applies to situations where someone with HIV knowingly engages in sexual behavior with an unknowing partner is unclear. While state laws do not provide clear guidance on how to address these types of situations, professional organizations offer definitive positions on this topic. For example, the American Psychological Association (APA 1991) clearly opposes a legal duty to protect third parties from HIV infection, advocating instead for strict client confidentiality. Meanwhile, taking a utilitarian approach, the American Medical Association (AMA) allows for exceptions to confidentiality in cases where attempts to persuade the patient to cease the endangering behavior are unsuccessful (Lin and Liang 2005). Specifically, physicians are encouraged to notify authorities and, if authorities do not act, are permitted to notify a third party.

A separate but closely related issue of relevance to situations involving youth who fail to disclose their HIV status to sexual partners is the controversy over HIV criminalization laws, which make it illegal for someone with HIV to engage in sexual behavior with an unknowing partner. Such laws exist in at least 24 states in the US (Lehman et al. 2014) and in 63 countries (Levine 2012; National AIDS Manual 2010). It is well accepted among HIV professionals that such laws defy wisdom. Not only are they ineffective for curtailing endangering sexual behavior, but they contribute to HIV-related stigma and, thus, create barriers to HIV testing, treatment, and retention in care. In addition, these laws are considered a violation of human rights. In support of this opinion, the APA (2016) recently issued a resolution opposing HIV criminalization.

Legal implications aside, health professionals do have a moral and ethical obligation to help youth prevent the spread of HIV to third parties. In addition to providing education about transmission, health professionals can explore with their clients barriers to protective behavior and engage in joint problem solving. Mental health professionals are likely to be particularly well suited to work with youth with HIV who are struggling to modify behaviors that put sexual partners at risk for HIV transmission.

Future Directions

In general, the literature on pediatric HIV disclosure is relatively young and under-developed. Important work has been done—especially demonstrating that disclosure generally does not lead to long-term mental health challenges and can, in some cases, even lead to positive outcomes such as relief, decreased anxiety, improved relationships, and improved ART adherence. Yet there are many gaps in our knowledge about disclosure. Fathers and other male caregivers have been infrequently studied, and it is not known whether this is because fathers are seldom involved in the disclosure process or because studies have not focused on their perspectives. Little has been written about how the view of "treatment as prevention" or how the emergence of Truvada® as PrEP affects: (a) the decisions parents make to disclose to the child; (b) the child's reaction; or (c) the child's disclosure to sexual partners. Also, there is substantial need for well-designed trials assessing the efficacy of disclosure interventions and understanding the impact of disclosure over time. In addition to understanding how disclosure affects mental health and well-being over time, research is needed to understand how the experiences of learning about a parent's HIV-positive status and one's own pediatric HIV-positive status affects one's future disclosure to others. Additionally, we need interventions to help youth with HIV make decisions about disclosing their own HIV-positive status—especially to sexual partners—and to understand how and if those interventions should be different for youth with perinatally acquired HIV and behaviorally acquired HIV, as well as how or if they should be different from those for adults. Studies should illustrate how family composition, the cultural context, HIV prevalence, and HIV treatment successes within a child's community affect disclosure experiences and intervention needs.

Conclusion

This chapter covered pediatric HIV disclosure, including disclosure of a caregiver/parent's HIV-positive status to a child, disclosure of a child's HIV-positive status to the child; and disclosure of a child's HIV-positive status to friends, families, and sexual partners. Many factors have been associated with pediatric HIV disclosure, including child age and maturity. Generally, the outcomes associated with disclosure have been positive, although some negative experiences have been documented. Much of the literature regarding disclosure to children as well as youth's self-disclosure largely represents high-income countries, although the literature base from low- and middle-income countries is expanding. Evidence-based disclosure counseling guidelines and structured interventions for pediatric HIV disclosure are limited, and the need for them is substantial. Disclosure interventions should appropriately engage the numerous stakeholders and consider the "complex, dynamic influences on HIV status disclosure," including cultural context (Li et al. 2015, pp. s2). Models that involve peer mentors or other paraprofessionals may be the most feasible, given a shortage of healthcare workers in many regions. There is much work to be done to assist parents, caregivers, healthcare teams, and youth with disclosure decision-making and disclosure processes.

Annotated Bibliography

Krauss, B. J., Letteney, S., De Baets, A. J., Baggaley, R., & Okero, F. A. (2013). Caregiver's HIV disclosure to children 12 years and under: a review and analysis of the evidence. AIDS Care, 25(4), 415–429. doi:10.1080/09540121.2012.712664

Krauss and colleagues conducted a systematic literature review to examine the disclosure of a caregiver HIV-positive status to a child under the age of 12. Major findings highlight the importance of child age and maturity during the disclosure process. Age-appropriate disclosure is also discussed.

Qiao, S., Li, X., & Stanton, B. (2013). Disclosure of parental HIV infection to children: a systematic review of global literature. AIDS Behav, 17(1), 369–389. doi:10.1007/s10461-011-0069-x

Qiao and colleagues conducted a systematic review of literature published prior to 2011 examining disclosure of a parental HIV-positive status to a child. Disclosure rates were often low, and tended to be higher in the United States than internationally. Reasons for disclosure, non-disclosure, and related outcomes are discussed.

Vreeman, R. C., Gramelspacher, A. M., Gisore, P. O., Scanlon, M. L., & Nyandiko, W. M. (2013). Disclosure of HIV status to children in resource-limited settings: a systematic review. J Int AIDS Soc, 16, 18466. doi:10.7448/IAS.16.1.18466

Vreeman and colleagues conducted a systematic review to examine the disclosure of a child's HIV-positive status to the child in resource limited areas. Major findings indicate that disclosure rates varied from 0 to 69% and anti-retroviral adherence improved post disclosure. Correlates, barriers, and outcomes related to disclosure are discussed.

References

Abadía-Barrero, C. E., & LaRusso, M. D. (2006). The disclosure model versus a developmental illness experience model for children and adolescents living with HIV/AIDS in Sao Paulo, *Brazil AIDS Patient Care & STDs, 20*(1), 36–43. doi:10.1089/apc.2006.20.36

AIDSmap. (2015). Talking to your child about your own or other family members' HIV. Retrieved from http://www.aidsmap.com/Talking-to-your-child-about-HIV/page/1374807/#item2955640

Alemu, A., Berhanu, B., & Emishaw, S. (2013). Challenges of caregivers to disclose their children s HIV positive status receiving highly active anti retroviral therapy at pediatric antiretroviral therapy clinics in Bahir dar, North West Ethiopia. *Journal of AIDS & Clinical Research, 2013.*

Alexander, J. F., Sexton, T. L., & Robbins, M. S. (2002). The developmental status of family therapy in family psychology intervention science.

Allison, S. M., & Siberry, G. K. (2015). National Institutes of Health investment in studies of HIV disclosure to children. *Aids, 29,* S109–S118. doi:10.1097/qad.0000000000000663

American Academy of Pediatrics Committee on Pediatric AIDS. (1999). Disclosure of illness status to children and adolescents with HIV infection. Pediatrics, 103(1), 164–166.

American Psychological Association. (1991). *Legal liability related to confidentiality and the prevention of HIV transmission.* Retrieved from http://www.apa.org/about/policy/confidentiality.aspx.

American Psychological Association. (2016). *Resolution opposing HIV criminalization.* Retrieved from: http://www.apa.org/about/policy/hiv-criminalization.aspx

Armistead, L., Klein, K., Forehand, R., & Wierson, M. (1997). Disclosure of parental HIV infection to children in the families of men with hemophilia: Description, outcomes, and the role of family processes. *Journal of Family Psychology, 11*(1), 49. doi:10.1037/0893-3200.11.1.49

Armistead, L., Tannenbaum, L., Forehand, R., Morse, E., & Morse, P. (2001). Disclosing HIV status: Are mothers telling their children? *Journal of Pediatric Psychology, 26*(1), 11–20. doi:10.1093/jpepsy/26.1.11

Baeten, J. M., Donnell, D., Ndase, P., Mugo, N. R., Campbell, J. D., Wangisi, J., et al. (2012). Antiretroviral prophylaxis for HIV prevention in heterosexual men and women. *New England Journal of Medicine, 367*(5), 399–410. doi:10.1056/NEJMoa1108524

Batterham, P., Rice, E., & Rotheram-Borus, M. J. (2005). Predictors of serostatus disclosure to partners among young people living with HIV in the pre- and post-HAART eras. *AIDS and Behavior, 9*(3), 281–287. doi:10.1007/s10461-005-9002-5

Bava, S., & Tapert, S. F. (2010). Adolescent brain development and the risk for alcohol and other drug problems. *Neuropsychology Review, 20*(4), 398–413. doi:10.1007/s11065-010-9146-6

Beck-Sagué, C. M., Dévieux, J., Pinzón-Iregui, M. C., Lerebours-Nadal, L., Abreu-Pérez, R., Bertrand, R., … & Halpern, M. (2015). Disclosure of their HIV status to perinatally infected youth using the adapted Blasini disclosure model in Haiti and the Dominican Republic: preliminary results. *AIDS (London, England), 29*(0 1), S91. doi:10.1097/QAD.0000000000000665

Beima-Sofie, K., John-Stewart, G., Shah, B., Wamalwa, D., Maleche-Obimbo, E., & Kelley, M. (2014). Using health provider insights to inform pediatric HIV disclosure: A qualitative study and practice framework from Kenya. *AIDS patient care and STDs, 28*(10), 555–564. doi:10.1089/apc.2014.0040

Belzer, M., Rogers, A. S., Camarca, M., Fuchs, D., Peralta, L., Tucker, D.,… & Adolescent Medicine HIV/AIDS Research Network. (2001). Contraceptive choices in HIV infected and HIV at-risk adolescent females. *Journal of Adolescent Health, 29*(3), 93–100. doi:10.1016/S1054-139X(01)00282-8

Bhattacharya, M., Dubey, A. P., & Sharma, M. (2011). Patterns of diagnosis disclosure and its correlates in HIV-Infected North Indian children. *Journal of Tropical Pediatrics, 57*(6), 405–411. doi:10.1093/tropej/fmq115

Biadgilign, S., Deribew, A., Amberbir, A., Escudero, H. R., & Deribe, K. (2011). Factors associated with HIV/AIDS diagnostic disclosure to HIV infected children receiving HAART: A multi-center study in Addis Ababa. *Ethiopia. PLoS One, 6*(3), e17572. doi:10.1371/journal.pone.0017572

Blake, B., Robley, L., & Taylor, G. (2012). A lion in the room: Youth living with HIV. *Pediatric nursing, 38*(6), 311.

Blasini, I., Chantry, C., Cruz, C., Ortiz, L., Salabarria, I., Scalley, N., et al. (2004). Disclosure model for pediatric patients living with HIV in Puerto Rico: Design, implementation, and evaluation. *Journal of Developmental and Behavioral Pediatrics, 25*(3), 181–189. doi:10.1097/00004703-200406000-00007

Brandt, L., Beima-Sofie, K., Hamunime, N., Shepard, M., Ferris, L., Ingo, P., et al. (2015). Growing-up just like everyone else: Key components of a successful pediatric HIV disclosure intervention in Namibia. *Aids, 29*, S81–S89. doi:10.1097/qad.0000000000000667

Busza, J., Besana, G. V., Mapunda, P., & Oliveras, E. (2013). 'I have grown up controlling myself a lot.' Fear and misconceptions about sex among adolescents vertically-infected with HIV in Tanzania. *Reproductive health matters, 21*(41), 87–96.

Centers for Disease Control and Prevention, Health Resources and Services Administration, & National Institutes of Health. (2014). Recommendations for HIV prevention with adults and adolescents with HIV in the United States, 2014.

Chenneville, T., Lynn, V., Peacock, B., Turner, D., & Marhefka, S. L. (2015). Disclosure of HIV status among female youth with HIV. *Ethics and Behavior, 25*(4), 314–331. doi:10.1080/10508422.2014.934371

Chenneville, T., Sibille, K., & Bendell-Estroff, D. (2010). Decisional capacity among minors with HIV: A model for balancing autonomy rights with the need for protection. *Ethics and Behavior, 20*(2), 83–94. doi:10.1080/10508421003595901

Chew, J., Beng, A. L., & Mun, S. (2012). Parental concerns about disclosure of a child's HIV/AIDS status in Singapore. *Social Work in Health Care, 51*(1), 5–21. doi:10.1080/00981389.2011.622624

Clifford, G., Craig, G. M., McCourt, C., & Barrow, G. (2013). What are the benefits and barriers of communicating parental HIV status to seronegative children and the implications for Jamaica? In *A Narrative Review of the Literature in Low/Middle Income Countries*.

Clum, G. A., Czaplicki, L., Andrinopoulos, K., Muessig, K., Hamvas, L., Ellen, J. M. & the Adolescent Medicine Trials Network for HIV/AIDS Interventions, J. M. (2013). Strategies and outcomes of HIV status disclosure in HIV-positive young women with abuse histories. *AIDS Patient Care and STDs, 27*(3), 191–200. doi:10.1089/apc.2012.0441

Cluver, L. D., Hodes, R. J., Toska, E., Kidia, K. K., Orkin, F. M., Sherr, L., & Meinck, F. (2015). HIV is like a tsotsi. ARVs are your guns: Associations between HIV-disclosure and adherence to antiretroviral treatment among adolescents in South Africa. *Aids, 29 Suppl 1*, S57–65. doi:10.1097/QAD.0000000000000695

Corona, R., Beckett, M. K., Cowgill, B. O., Elliott, M. N., Murphy, D. A., Zhou, A. J., et al. (2006). Do children know their parent's HIV status? Parental reports of child awareness in a nationally representative sample. *Ambulatory Pediatrics, 6*(3), 138–144. doi:10.1016/j.ambp.2006.02.005

Crankshaw, T. L., Voce, A., King, R. L., Giddy, J., Sheon, N. M., & Butler, L. M. (2014). Double disclosure bind: Complexities of communicating an HIV diagnosis in the context of unintended pregnancy in Durban. *South Africa. AIDS and Behavior, 18*(1), 53–59. doi:10.1007/s10461-013-0521-1

Cree, V., Kay, H., Tisdall, E., & Wallace, J. (2006). Listening to children and young people affected by parental HIV: Findings from a Scottish study. *AIDS Care, 18*(1), 73–76. doi:10.1080/09540120500161793

D'Angelo, L. J., Abdalian, S. E., Sarr, M., Hoffman, N., Belzer, M., & Network, A. M. H. A. R. (2001). Disclosure of serostatus by HIV infected youth: the experience of the REACH study. *Journal of Adolescent Health, 29*(3), 72–79. doi:10.1016/S1054-139X(01)00285-3

DeMatteo, D., Wells, L. M., Salter Goldie, R., & King, S. M. (2002). The 'family' context of HIV: A need for comprehensive health and social policies. *AIDS Care, 14*(2), 261–278. doi:10.1080/09540120120076940

Dempsey, A. G., MacDonell, K. E., Naar-King, S., Lau, C. Y., & Adolescent Medicine Trials Network for, H. I. V. A. I. (2012). Patterns of disclosure among youth who are HIV-positive: a multisite study. *Journal of Adolesc Health, 50*(3), 315–317. doi:10.1016/j.jadohealth.2011.06.003

Derlega, V. J., Winstead, B. A., Greene, K., Serovich, J., & Elwood, W. N. (2004). Reasons for HIV disclosure/nondisclosure in close relationships: Testing a model of HIV–disclosure decision making. *Journal of Social and Clinical Psychology, 23*(6), 747–767. doi:10.1521/jscp.23.6.747.54804

Dorrell, J., & Katz, J. (2014). You're HIV positive: Perinatally infected young people's accounts of the critical moment of finding out their diagnosis. *AIDS Care, 26*(4), 454–458. doi:10.1080/09540121.2013.841833

Evangeli, M., & Foster, C. (2014). Who, then what? The need for interventions to help young people with perinatally acquired HIV disclose their HIV status to others. *Aids, 28*, S343–S346. doi:10.1097/qad.0000000000000334

Fair, C., & Albright, J. (2012). Don't tell him you have HIV unless he's 'the one': Romantic relationships among adolescents and young adults with perinatal HIV infection. *AIDS patient care and STDs, 26*(12), 746–754. doi:10.1089/apc.2012.0290

Fernet, M., Wong, K., Richard, M. E., Otis, J., Lévy, J. J., Lapointe, N., et al. (2011). Romantic relationships and sexual activities of the first generation of youth living with HIV since birth. *AIDS care, 23*(4), 393–400. doi:10.1080/09540121.2010.516332

Ferris, M., Burau, K., Schweitzer, A., Mihale, S., Murray, N., Preda, A., et al. (2007). The influence of disclosure of HIV diagnosis on time to disease progression in a cohort of Romanian children and teens. *AIDS Care, 19*(9), 1088–1094. doi:10.1080/09540120701367124

Fisher, C. B. (2017). *Decoding the ethics code: A practical guide for psychologists* (4th ed.). Los Angeles, CA: Sage Publications.

Fisher, C. B., & Goodman, S. J. (2009). Goodness-of-fit ethics for non-Intervention research involving dangerous and illegal behaviors. In D. Buchanan, C. B. Fisher, & L. Gable (Eds.), *Research with high-risk populations: Balancing science, ethics, and law* (pp. 25–46). Washington, DC: APA Books.

Forsyth, B. W. (2003). Psychological aspects of HIV infection in children. *Child and adolescent psychiatric clinics of North America, 12*(3), 423–437. doi:10.1016/S1056-4993(03)00023-3

Funck-Brentano, I., Costagliola, D., Seibel, N., Straub, E., Tardieu, M., & Blanche, S. (1997). Patterns of disclosure and perceptions of the human immunodeficiency virus in infected elementary school—age children. *Archives of Pediatrics and Adolescent Medicine, 151*(10), 978–985. doi:10.1001/archpedi.1997.02170470012002

Gachanja, G., Burkholder, G. J., & Ferraro, A. (2014). HIV-positive parents, HIV-positive children, and HIV-negative children's perspectives on disclosure of a parent's and child's illness in Kenya. *PeerJ, 2*, e486. doi:10.7717/peerj.486

Gillard, A., & Roark, M. F. (2012). Older Adolescents' Self-Determined Motivations to Disclose Their HIV Status. *Journal of Child and Family Studies, 22*(5), 672–683. doi:10.1007/s10826-012-9620-2

Gillard, A., & Roark, M. F. (2013). Older adolescents' self-determined motivations to disclose their HIV status. *Journal of Child and Family Studies, 22*(5), 672–683. doi:10.1007/s10826-012-9620-2

Greenhalgh, C., Evangeli, M., Frize, G., Foster, C., & Fidler, S. (2013). Intimate relationships in young adults with perinatally acquired HIV: Partner considerations. *AIDS care, 25*(4), 447–450. doi:10.1080/09540121.2012.712671

Greenhalgh, C., Evangeli, M., Frize, G., Foster, C., & Fidler, S. (2015). Intimate relationships in young adults with perinatally acquired HIV: A qualitative study of strategies used to manage HIV disclosure. *AIDS Care*, 1–6.

Hammami, N., Nöstlinger, C., Hoerée, T., Lefèvre, P., Jonckheer, T., & Kolsteren, P. (2004). Integrating adherence to highly active antiretroviral therapy into children's daily lives: A qualitative study. *Pediatrics, 114*(5), e591–e597. doi:10.1542/peds.2004-0085

Hawk, S. T. (2007). Disclosures of maternal HIV infection to seronegative children: A literature review. *Journal of Social and Personal Relationships, 24*(5), 657–673. doi:10.1177/0265407507081453

Hightow-Weidman, L. B., Phillips, G., II, Outlaw, A. Y., Wohl, A. R., Fields, S., Hildalgo, J., et al. (2013). Patterns of HIV disclosure and condom use among HIV-infected young racial/ethnic minority men who have sex with men. *AIDS and Behavior, 17*(1), 360–368. doi:10.1007/s10461-012-0331-x

Hogwood, J., Campbell, T., & Butler, S. (2013). I wish I could tell you but I can't: Adolescents with perinatally acquired HIV and their dilemmas around self-disclosure. *Clinical Child Psychology Psychiatry, 18*(1), 44–60. doi:10.1177/1359104511433195

Hosek, S. G., Harper, G. W., Lemos, D., & Martinez, J. (2008). An ecological model of stressors experienced by youth newly diagnosed with HIV. *Journal of HIV/AIDS Prevention in Children and Youth, 9*(2), 192–218. doi:10.1080/15538340902824118

Instone, S. L. (2000). Perceptions of children with HIV infection when not told for so long: Implications for diagnosis disclosure. *Journal of pediatric health care, 14*(5), 235–243. doi:10.1067/mph.2000.107338

Kalichman, S. C., Rompa, D., Cage, M., DiFonzo, K., Simpson, D., Austin, J., et al. (2001). Effectiveness of an intervention to reduce HIV transmission risks in HIV-positive people. *American Journal of Preventive Medicine, 21*(2), 84–92. doi:10.1016/S0749-3797(01)00324-5

Kallem, S., Renner, L., Ghebremichael, M., & Paintsil, E. (2011). Prevalence and pattern of disclosure of HIV status in HIV-infected children in Ghana. *AIDS and Behavior, 15*(6), 1121–1127. doi:10.1007/s10461-010-9741-9

Kennedy, D. P., Cowgill, B. O., Bogart, L. M., Corona, R., Ryan, G. W., Murphy, D. A., et al. (2010). Parents' disclosure of their HIV infection to their children in the context of the family. *AIDS and Behavior, 14*(5), 1095–1105. doi:10.1007/s10461-010-9715-y

Kirshenbaum, S. B., & Nevid, J. S. (2002). The specificity of maternal disclosure of HIV/AIDS in relation to children's adjustment. *AIDS Education and Prevention, 14*(1), 1–16. doi:10.1521/aeap.14.1.1.24331

Klitzman, R., Marhefka, S., Mellins, C., & Wiener, L. (2008). Ethical issues concerning disclosures of HIV diagnoses to perinatally infected children and adolescents. *The Journal of clinical ethics, 19*(1), 31.

Krauss, B. J., Letteney, S., De Baets, A. J., Baggaley, R., & Okero, F. A. (2013). Caregiver's HIV disclosure to children 12 years and under: A review and analysis of the evidence. *AIDS Care, 25*(4), 415–429. doi:10.1080/09540121.2012.712664

Kyaddondo, D., Wanyenze, R. K., Kinsman, J., & Hardon, A. (2013). Disclosure of HIV status between parents and children in Uganda in the context of greater access to treatment. *SAHARA-J: Journal of Social Aspects of HIV/AIDS, 10*(supl), S37–S45. doi:10.1080/02664763.2012.755323

Lam, P. K., Naar-King, S., & Wright, K. (2007). Social support and disclosure as predictors of mental health in HIV-positive youth. *AIDS Patient Care STDS, 21*(1), 20–29. doi:10.1089/apc.2006.005

Lee, M., Rotheram-Borus, M. J., & O'Hara, P. (1999). Disclosure of serostatus among youth living with HIV. *AIDS and Behavior, 3*(1), 33–40. doi:10.1023/A:1025415418759

Lee, M. B., & Rotheram-Borus, M. J. (2002). Parents' disclosure of HIV to their children. *Aids, 16* (16), 2201–2207. doi:10.1097/00002030-200211080-00013

Lee, S., Yamazaki, M., Harris, D. R., Harper, G. W., & Ellen, J. (2015). Social support and human immunodeficiency virus-status disclosure to friends and family: Implications for human immunodeficiency virus-positive youth. *Journal of Adolescent Health, 57*(1), 73–80. doi:10.1016/j.jadohealth.2015.03.002

Lehman, J. S., Carr, M. H., Nichol, A. J., Ruisanchez, A., Knight, D. W., Langford, A. E., et al. (2014). Prevalence and public health implications of state laws that criminalize potential HIV exposure in the United States. *AIDS and Behavior, 18*(6), 997–1006.

Leonard, A. D., Markham, C. M., Bui, T., Shegog, R., & Paul, M. E. (2010). Lowering the risk of secondary HIV transmission: Insights from HIV-positive youth and health care providers. *Perspect Sex Reprod Health, 42*(2), 110–116. doi:10.1363/4211010

Lesch, A. I. D. S., Swartz, L., Kagee, A., Moodley, K., Kafaar, Z., Myer, L., et al. (2007). Paediatric HIV/AIDS disclosure: Towards a developmental and process-oriented approach. *AIDS care, 19*(6), 811–816. doi:10.1080/09540120601129301

Lester, P., Chesney, M., Cooke, M., Whalley, P., Perez, B., Petru, A., et al. (2002). Diagnostic disclosure to HIV-infected children: How parents decide when and what to tell. *Clinical child psychology and psychiatry, 7*(1), 85–99. doi:10.1177/1359104502007001007

Levine, J. (2012). *Fact sheet on HIV and the law: Risks, rights and health*. Retrieved from http://www.hivlawcommission.org/resources/report/HIV&Law-Factsheet-EN.pdf

Li, X. (2015) *Theory-based hiv disclosure intervention for parents supported by Eunice Kennedy Shriver National Institute of Child Health and Human Development of the National Institutes of Health under award number 7R01HD074221-05*. Retrieved from https://projectreporter.nih.gov/project_info_description.cfm?aid=9135005&icde=28899635&ddparam=&ddvalue=&ddsub=&cr=1&csb=default&cs=ASC

Li, X., de Wit, J., Qiao, S., & Sherr, L. (2015). HIV disclosure to children in low-and middle-income countries: Towards effective interventions. *AIDS (London, England), 29*(0 1), S1. doi:10.1097/QAD.0000000000000730

Lightfoot, M. (2015). *Disclosure Intervention for Zimbabwean Parents, supported by Eunice Kennedy Shriver National Institute of Child Health and Human Development of the National Institutes of Health under award number 5R01HD074243-04*. Retrieved from https://projectreporter.nih.gov/project_info_description.cfm?aid=8869015&icde=28899718&ddparam=&ddvalue=&ddsub=&cr=4&csb=default&cs=ASC

Lin, L., & Liang, B. A. (2005). HIV and health law: Striking the balance between legal Mandates and medical ethics. *Virtual Mentor, 7*(10).

Marhefka, S. (2007). Disclosure experiences of young women living with perinatal HIV disease. In *Unpublished raw data*.

Marhefka, S. L., Koenig, L. J., Allison, S., Bachanas, P., Bulterys, M., Bettica, L., et al. (2008). Family experiences with pediatric antiretroviral therapy: responsibilities, barriers, and strategies for remembering medications. *AIDS Patient Care and STDs, 22*(8), 637–647. doi:10.1089/apc.2007.0110

Marhefka, S. L., Tepper, V. J., Brown, J. L., & Farley, J. J. (2006). Caregiver psychosocial characteristics and children's adherence to antiretroviral therapy. *AIDS Patient Care & STDs, 20*(6), 429–437. doi:10.1089/apc.2006.20.429

Marhefka, S. L., Valentin, C. R., Pinto, R. M., Demetriou, N., Wiznia, A., & Mellins, C. A. (2011). "I feel like I'm carrying a weapon". Information and motivations related to sexual risk among girls with perinatally acquired HIV. *AIDS Care, 23*(10), 1321–1328. doi:10.1080/09540121.2010.532536

Marks, G., Bundek, N. I., Richardson, J. L., Ruiz, M. S., Maldonado, N., & Mason, H. R. C. (1992). Self–disclosure of HIV infection: Preliminary results from a sample of Hispanic men. *Health Psychology, 11*, 300–306. doi:10.1037/0278-6133.11.5.300

Mason, H. R. C., Marks, G., Simoni, J. M., Ruiz, M. S., & Richardson, J. L. (1995). Culturally sanctioned secrets? Latino men's nondisclosure of HIV infection to family, friends, and lovers. *Health Psychology, 14*, 6–12. doi:10.1037/0278-6133.14.1.6

Masty, J., & Fisher, C. B. (2008). A goodness of fit approach to parent permission and child assent pediatric intervention research. *Ethics and Behavior, 13*, 139–160. doi:10.1080/10508420802063897

Matic, S., Lazarus, J. V., & Donoghoe, M. C. (2006). *HIV/AIDS in Europe: Moving from death sentence to chronic disease management*. World Health Organization.

Mburu, G., Hodgson, I., Kalibala, S., Haamujompa, C., Cataldo, F., Lowenthal, E. D., et al. (2014). Adolescent HIV disclosure in Zambia: barriers, facilitators and outcomes. *Journal of the International AIDS Society, 17*, 18866. doi:10.7448/IAS.17.1.18866

Mellins, C. A., Brackis-Cott, E., Dolezal, C., Richards, A., Nicholas, S. W., & Abrams, E. J. (2002). Patterns of HIV status disclosure to perinatally HIV-infected children and subsequent mental health outcomes. *Clinical Child Psychology and Psychiatry, 7*(1), 101–114. doi:10.1177/1359104502007001008

Menon, A., Glazebrook, C., Campain, N., & Ngoma, M. (2007). Mental health and disclosure of HIV status in Zambian adolescents with HIV infection: Implications for peer-support programs. *Journal of Acquired Immune Deficiency Syndromes, 46*(3), 349–354. doi:10.1097/QAI.0b013e3181565df0

Merzel, C., VanDevanter, N., & Irvine, M. (2008). Adherence to antiretroviral therapy among older children and adolescents with HIV: A qualitative study of psychosocial contexts. *AIDS Patient Care and STDs, 22*(12), 977–987. doi:10.1089/apc.2008.0048

Michaud, P. A., Suris, J. C., Thomas, L. R., Kahlert, C., Rudin, C., & Cheseaux, J. J. (2009). To say or not to say: A qualitative study on the disclosure of their condition by human immunodeficiency virus-positive adolescents. *Journal of Adolescent Health, 44*(4), 356–362. doi:10.1016/j.jadohealth.2008.08.004

Midtbo, V., Shirima, V., Skovdal, M., & Daniel, M. (2012). How disclosure and antiretroviral therapy help HIV-infected adolescents in sub-Saharan Africa cope with stigma. *Afr J AIDS Res, 11*(3), 261–271. doi:10.2989/16085906.2012.734987

Moodley, K., Myer, L., Michaels, D., & Cotton, M. (2006). *Paediatric HIV disclosure in South Africa-caregivers' perspectives on discussing HIV with infected children*.

Moore, A. R., & Williamson, D. (2011). Disclosure of Children's Positive Serostatus to Family and Nonfamily Members: Informal Caregivers in Togo, West Africa. *AIDS research and treatment*, 2011. doi:10.1155/2011/595301

Murphy, D. A. (2008). HIV-positive mothers' disclosure of their serostatus to their young children: A review. *Clinical Child Psychology and Psychiatry, 13*(1), 105–122. doi:10.1177/1359104507087464

Murphy, D. A., Armistead, L., Marelich, W. D., Payne, D. L., & Herbeck, D. M. (2011). Pilot trial of a disclosure intervention for HIV + mothers: The TRACK program. *Journal of Consulting and Clinical Psychology, 79*(2), 203. doi:10.1037/a0022896

Murphy, D. A., Austin, E. L., & Greenwell, L. (2006). Correlates of HIV-related stigma among HIV-positive mothers and their uninfected adolescent children. *Women and Health, 44*(3), 19–42. doi:10.1300/J013v44n03_02

Murphy, D. A., Marelich, W. D., Armistead, L., Herbeck, D. M., & Payne, D. L. (2010). Anxiety/stress among mothers living with HIV: Effects on parenting skills and child outcomes. *AIDS Care, 22*(12), 1449–1458. doi:10.1080/09540121.2010.487085

Murphy, D. A., Roberts, K. J., & Hoffman, D. (2002). Stigma and ostracism associated with HIV/AIDS: Children carrying the secret of their mothers' HIV + serostatus. *Journal of Child and Family Studies, 11*(2), 191–202. doi:10.1023/A:1015177609382

Murphy, D. A., Steers, W. N., & Dello Stritto, M. E. (2001). Maternal disclosure of mothers' HIV serostatus to their young children. *Journal of Family Psychology, 15*(3), 441. doi:10.1037/0893-3200.15.3.441

Myer, L., Moodley, K., Hendricks, F., & Cotton, M. (2006). Healthcare providers' perspectives on discussing HIV status with infected children. *Journal of Tropical Pediatrics, 52*(4), 293–295. doi:10.1093/tropej/fml004

Nam, S. L., Fielding, K., Avalos, A., Gaolathe, T., Dickinson, D., & Geissler, P. W. (2009). Discussing matters of sexual health with children: what issues relating to disclosure of parental HIV status reveal. *AIDS Care, 21*(3), 389–395. doi:10.1080/09540120802270276

Namasopo-Oleja, S. M., Bagenda, D., & Ekirapa-Kiracho, E. (2015). Factors affecting disclosure of serostatus to children attending Jinja Hospital Paediatric HIV clinic, Uganda. *African Health Sciences, 15*(2), 344–351. doi:10.4314/ahs.v15i2.6

National AIDS Manual. (2010, September). *Where HIV is a crime, not just a virus*. Retrieved from: http://www.aidsmap.com/Where-HIV-is-a-crime-not-just-a-virus/page/1509846/

New, M. J., Lee, S. S., & Elliott, B. M. (2007). Psychological adjustment in children and families living with HIV. *Journal of Pediatric Psychology, 32*(2), 123–131. doi:10.1093/jpepsy/jsj121

New York State Department of Health AIDS Institute. (2009). *Disclosure of HIV to perinatally infected children and adolescents*. New York: New York State Department of Health.

Nöstlinger, C., Jonckheer, T., de Belder, E., van Wijngaerden, E., Wylock, C., Pelgrom, J., et al. (2004). Families affected by HIV: Parents' and children's characteristics and disclosure to the children. *AIDS Care, 16*(5), 641–648. doi:10.1080/09540120410001716432

Oberdorfer, P., Puthanakit, T., Louthrenoo, O., Charnsil, C., Sirisanthana, V., & Sirisanthana, T. (2006). Disclosure of HIV/AIDS diagnosis to HIV-infected children in Thailand. *Journal of Paediatrics and Child Health, 42*(5), 283–288. doi:10.1111/j.1440-1754.2006.00855.x

O'Malley, G., Beima-Sofie, K., Feris, L., Shepard-Perry, M., Hamunime, N., John-Stewart, G.,… Group, M. S. (2015). If I take my medicine, I will be strong: Evaluation of a pediatric HIV disclosure intervention in Namibia. *JAIDS Journal of Acquired Immune Deficiency Syndromes, 68*(1), e1–e7. doi:10.1097/QAI.0000000000000387

Ostrom, R. A., Serovich, J. M., Lim, J. Y., & Mason, T. L. (2006). The role of stigma in reasons for HIV disclosure and non-disclosure to children. *AIDS Care, 18*(1), 60–65. doi:10.1080/09540120500161769

Ostrom Delaney, R., Serovich, J. M., & Lim, J.-Y. (2008). Reasons for and against maternal HIV disclosure to children and perceived child reaction. *AIDS Care, 20*(7), 876–880. doi:10.1080/09540120701767158

Paintsil, E. (2015) *A bioecological pediatric HIV disclosure intervention in Ghana, supported by Eunice Kennedy Shriver National Institute of Child Health and Human Development of the National Institutes of Health under award number 5R01HD074253-04*. Retrieved from https://projectreporter.nih.gov/project_info_description.cfm?aid=8867043&icde=28899295&ddparam=&ddvalue=&ddsub=&cr=1&csb=default&cs=ASC.

Pinzon-Iregui, M. C., Beck-Sague, C. M., & Malow, R. M. (2013). Disclosure of their HIV status to infected children: A review of the literature. *Journal of Tropical Pediatrics, 59*(2), 84–89. doi:10.1093/tropej/fms052

Positive Women's Network. (n.d.). *HIV disclosure to children*. Retrieved from http://pwn.bc.ca/hiv-community/disclosing-your-hiv-status/hiv-disclosure-to-children/

Qiao, S., Li, X., & Stanton, B. (2013). Disclosure of parental HIV infection to children: A systematic review of global literature. *AIDS and Behavior, 17*(1), 369–389. doi:10.1007/s10461-011-0069-x

Rao, D., Kekwaletswe, T. C., Hosek, S., Martinez, J., & Rodriguez, F. (2007). Stigma and social barriers to medication adherence with urban youth living with HIV. *AIDS Care, 19*(1), 28–33. doi:10.1080/09540120600652303

Reyland, S. A., Higgins-D'Alessandro, A., & McMahon, T. J. (2002). Tell them you love them because you never know when things could change: Voices of adolescents living with HIV-positive mothers. *AIDS Care, 14*(2), 285–294. doi:10.1080/09540120120076977

Rochat, T. J., Arteche, A. X., Stein, A., Mkwanazi, N., & Bland, R. M. (2014). Maternal HIV disclosure to young HIV-uninfected children: an evaluation of a family-centred intervention in South Africa. *AIDS, 28*, S331–S341.

Rongkavilit, C., Wright, K., Chen, X., Naar-King, S., Chuenyam, T., & Phanuphak, P. (2010). HIV stigma, disclosure and psychosocial distress among Thai youth living with HIV. *International Journal of STD and AIDS, 21*(2), 126–132. doi:10.1258/ijsa.2009.008488

Rotheram-Borus, M. J., Lee, M., Leonard, N., Lin, Y. Y., Franzke, L., Turner, E., et al. (2003). Four-year behavioral outcomes of an intervention for parents living with HIV and their adolescent children. *Aids, 17*(8), 1217–1225. doi:10.1097/01.aids.0000060337.12269.1d

Rotheram-Borus, M. J., Lee, M. B., Gwadz, M., & Draimin, B. (2001). An intervention for parents with AIDS and their adolescent children. *American Journal of Public Health, 91*(8), 1294–1302. doi:10.2105/AJPH.91.8.1294

Rotheram-Borus, M. J., Murphy, D. A., Miller, S., & Draimin, B. H. (1997). An intervention for adolescents whose parents are living with AIDS. *Clinical Child Psychology and Psychiatry, 2* (2), 201–219. doi:10.1177/1359104597022003

Rwemisisi, J., Wolff, B., Coutinho, A., Grosskurth, H., & Whitworth, J. (2008). 'What if they ask how I got it?' Dilemmas of disclosing parental HIV status and testing children for HIV in Uganda. *Health Policy Plan, 23*(1), 36–42. doi:10.1093/heapol/czm040

Serovich, J. M., Reed, S., Grafsky, E. L., & Andrist, D. (2009). An intervention to assist men who have sex with men disclose their serostatus to casual sex partners: Results from a pilot study. *AIDS Education and Prevention: Official Publication of the International Society for AIDS Education, 21*(3), 207. doi:10.1521/aeap.2009.21.3.207

Sherman, B. F., Bonanno, G. A., Wiener, L. S., & Battles, H. B. (2000). When children tell their friends they have AIDS: Possible consequences for psychological well-being and disease progression. *Psychosomatic Medicine, 62*(2), 238–247. doi:10.1097/00006842-200003000-00016

Simoni, J. M., Davis, M. L., Drossman, J. A., & Weinberg, B. A. (2000). Mothers with HIV/AIDS and their children: Disclosure and guardianship issues. *Women and Health, 31*(1), 39–54. doi:10.1300/J013v31n01_03

Siu, G. E., Bakeera-Kitaka, S., Kennedy, C. E., Dhabangi, A., & Kambugu, A. (2012). HIV serostatus disclosure and lived experiences of adolescents at the Transition Clinic of the Infectious Diseases Clinic in Kampala, Uganda: A qualitative study. *AIDS Care, 24*(5), 606–611. doi:10.1080/09540121.2011.630346

Sturdevant, M. S., Belzer, M., Weissman, G., Friedman, L. B., Sarr, M., Muenz, L. R., & Adolescent Medicine HIV/AIDS Research Network. (2001). The relationship of unsafe sexual behavior and the characteristics of sexual partners of HIV infected and HIV uninfected adolescent females. *Journal of Adolescent Health, 29*(3), 64–71. doi:10.1016/S1054-139X(01)00286-5

Tarasoff, V., & Regents of the University of California (1976, 1974). 17 Cal.3d 425, 551 P.2d 334.

Thoth, C. A., Tucker, C., Leahy, M., & Stewart, S. M. (2014). Self-disclosure of serostatus by youth who are HIV-positive: A review. *Journal of Behavioral Medicine, 37*(2), 276–288. doi:10.1007/s10865-012-9485-2

Tompkins, T. L. (2007). Disclosure of maternal HIV status to children: to tell or not to tell… that is the question. *Journal of Child and Family Studies, 16*(6), 773–788. doi:10.1007/s10826-006-9124-z

Travers, R., & Paoletti, D. (1999). Responding to the support needs of HIV positive lesbian, gay and bisexual youth. *Canadian Journal of Human Sexuality, 8*(4), 271–284.

U.S. Department of Health & Human Services (2009, August 24). *Children: How do you tell your child you have HIV*. Retrieved from https://www.aids.gov/hiv-aids-basics/just-diagnosed-with-hiv-aids/talking-about-your-status/children/.

U.S. Department of Health & Human Services, Office on Women's Health (2011, July 1). *HIV/AIDS: Telling people you are HIV-positive*. Retrieved from http://womenshealth.gov/hiv-aids/living-with-hiv-aids/telling-people-you-are-hiv-positive.html.

Vaz, L. M., Maman, S., Eng, E., Barbarin, O. A., Tshikandu, T., & Behets, F. (2011). Patterns of disclosure of HIV status to infected children in a Sub-Saharan African setting. *Journal of Developmental and Behavioral Pediatrics, 32*(4), 307–315. doi:10.1097/DBP.0b013e31820f7a47

Vreeman, R. C. (2015). *Patient-centered disclosure intervention for HIV-infected Children National Institute of Mental Health*.

Vreeman, R. C., Gramelspacher, A. M., Gisore, P. O., Scanlon, M. L., & Nyandiko, W. M. (2013). Disclosure of HIV status to children in resource-limited settings: a systematic review. *Journal of International AIDS Society, 16*(1). doi:10.7448/IAS.16.1.18466

Vreeman, R. C., Nyandiko, W. M., Ayaya, S. O., Walumbe, E. G., Marrero, D. G., & Inui, T. S. (2010). The perceived impact of disclosure of pediatric HIV status on pediatric antiretroviral therapy adherence, child well-being, and social relationships in a resource-limited setting. *AIDS Patient Care and STDs, 24*(10), 639–649. doi:10.1089/apc.2010.0079

Vreeman, R. C., Scanlon, M. L., Inui, T. S., McAteer, C. I., Fischer, L. J., McHenry, M. S., et al. (2015). 'Why did you not tell me?': Perspectives of caregivers and children on the social environment surrounding child HIV disclosure in Kenya. *Aids, 29*, S47–S55. doi:10.1097/qad.0000000000000669

Wiener, L., Battles, H., Heilman, N., Sigelman, C., & Pizzo, P. (1996). Factors associated with disclosure of diagnosis to children with HIV/AIDS. *Pediatric AIDS and HIV Infection, 7*(5), 310–324.

Wiener, L., Mellins, C. A., Marhefka, S., & Battles, H. B. (2007). Disclosure of an HIV diagnosis to children: history, current research, and future directions. *Journal of Developmental and Behavioral Pediatrics: JDBP, 28*(2), 155. doi:10.1097/01.DBP.0000267570.87564.cd

Wiener, L. S., & Battles, H. B. (2006). Untangling the web: A close look at diagnosis disclosure among HIV-infected adolescents. *Journal of Adolescent Health, 38*(3), 307–309. doi:10.1016/j.jadohealth.2005.03.024

Wilfert, C., Beck, D., Fleischman, A., Mofenson, L., Pantell, R., Schonberg, S., et al. (1999). Disclosure of illness status to children and adolescents with HIV infection. *Pediatrics, 103*(1), 164–166. doi:10.1542/peds.103.1.164

World Health Organization. (2011). *Guideline on HIV disclosure counselling for children up to 12 years of age*.

Chapter 9
Goodness-of-Fit Ethics for Practice and Research Involving Children and Adolescents with HIV

Celia B. Fisher, Miriam R. Arbeit and Tiffany Chenneville

Introduction

Treating pediatric HIV involves certain ethical challenges due to the complexity of children and adolescents' developmental processes and family contexts (Fisher et al. 1999). In addition, social, political, and economic inequities impact both individual health and the delivery of health services. As such, this chapter addresses four major ethical issues facing those who provide clinical care to, or conduct clinical research with, children and adolescents with HIV: (1) clinical decision-making through informed consent procedures, (2) communicating appropriately with families through confidentiality procedures, (3) addressing racial and ethnic health inequities through organizational access and multicultural competence, and (4) sexual health counseling for adolescents, with particular attention to the needs and experiences of sexual and gender minority youth (SGMY).

We draw upon relational ethics (Fisher 1999, 2000) within a goodness-of-fit ethical framework (GFE; Fisher 2017), which emphasizes the importance of empirical studies of participant consent strengths and vulnerabilities to design procedures that reflect a "fit" between participant characteristics and the unique demands of the research context (Fisher 2003a, 2005, 2015; Fisher and Masty 2006; Fisher and Goodman 2009; Fisher and Ragsdale 2006; Masty and Fisher 2008). Thus far, GFE has been mostly applied to ethical decisions in human subjects'

C.B. Fisher (✉)
Fordham University, Bronx, NY, USA
e-mail: fisher@fordham.edu

M.R. Arbeit
University of Virginia, Charlottesville, VA, USA
e-mail: mimi.arbeit@gmail.com

T. Chenneville
University of South Florida St. Petersburg, St. Petersburg, FL, USA
e-mail: chennevi@mail.usf.edu

T. Chenneville (ed.), *A Clinical Guide to Pediatric HIV*,
DOI 10.1007/978-3-319-49704-4_9

research. In recent years, Fisher's GFE has been applied to ethical issues involving clinical practice. We expand on this model in the present chapter by applying it to clinical practice involving pediatric HIV treatment, and as well, we note at several points how GFE can inform clinical research involving children and adolescents with HIV. We intend these guidelines to be used in ways that are responsive to the continuously evolving nature of intervention and prevention goals in treatment and research.

These ethical guidelines have been developed in the context of historical shifts in cultural norms regarding both medical practice and the personhood of children. Medical practice is shifting away from medical paternalism, in which physicians are considered the primary decision-makers for their patients, to a model of collaborative decision-making facilitated by doctors along with their patients (Pustilnik and Henry 2012). However, when patients are below the age of majority, it is generally expected, and in many cases legally required, that parents or legal guardians are involved in medical decision-making. Here, there have also been recent cultural shifts in the extent to which children are enabled and expected to make decisions about their own health. Children used to be considered the property of their parents, with parents having the right and responsibility to make decisions about their children's well-being (McCabe 1996; Ross 1997). However, children are increasingly being understood as morally autonomous persons, with the accordant rights and responsibilities (Fisher 2002, 2003b, 2005). With these two historical shifts, children, guardians, and physicians are now part of a relational system in which to navigate the ethical questions involved in HIV treatment and research.

Relational Ethics and Goodness of Fit

Relational ethics are an integration of justice-based approaches that prioritize respect, beneficence, and fairness (Kohlberg 1984) with care-based approaches that account for the interpersonal context of ongoing relationships (Gilligan 1982). The context of care delivery is characterized by the professional relationship between the child and the clinician, as well as by the child's age and health status. This context creates the child's vulnerability, which can be understood as a situation in which one person's individual welfare (e.g., the child) is dependent upon the actions of another (e.g., the clinician). This dependency creates a moral obligation on behalf of the clinician to plan and enact ethical procedures in such a way as to reduce or eliminate vulnerability (Fisher 1999). Within this dynamic relationship, the vulnerability of the child is thus defined not simply in terms of age, but in terms of the goodness of fit between the ethical procedures and children and adolescents' developing abilities and needs (Fisher 1999, 2017).

Relational ethics entails consideration of multiple aspects of the child's developmental context. Children with HIV have specific biomedical needs and side effects of related treatments that need to be considered. The family context in which children develop is also critically important, including the parent–child relationship and the family's cultural values and sociopolitical standing. Ethical procedures thus need to be fitted to the child's developmental level, health, and family context (Fisher 1999). These ethical procedures must be designed to address the inherent power differential in both treatment and research, taking into account social conditions and responsiveness to individual awareness of boundaries, competencies, and obligations (Fisher 1999; Fisher et al. 2002).

The ethical guidelines in this chapter are thus focused on facilitating goodness of fit (GFE) between the clinical context of the treatment and the developmental context of the child (Fisher 2017; Fisher and Masty 2006). The clinical context, including the organizational context of the medical care and the sociopolitical context of the HIV epidemic, can create or exacerbate different sources of patient vulnerability to risk. The individual clinician can also create or exacerbate patient vulnerability through the design and implementation of treatment. The youth developmental context includes the decisional capacity of the child, the guardian's comprehension of the medical information, and their personal and cultural norms and values.

GFE can be enacted through co-learning, which is a process of collaborating with families and communities about the best ways to approach ethical questions (Fisher 1999, 2002). Co-learning involves ethical contextualism, which requires that the clinicians maintain commitment to their own moral values while considering the context, cultural values, and lived experience of the patient (Fisher 2014). Clinicians may find that families differ in both their moral goals (e.g., their conception of what is good) and their moral processes (e.g., weighing risks and benefits). Co-learning is a process of collaboration in order to gain mutual understanding and build partnerships toward shared goals. However, the process is focused specifically on learning, not on making a decision. The clinician still has the ultimate responsibility for ethical practice, which can be informed by this learning about the moral goals and moral processes endorsed by their patients and families.

In the sections to follow, we apply GFE ethics to discussions about informed consent procedures, confidentiality and disclosures, addressing health inequities, and providing sexual health counseling. Within each of these sections, we highlight the aspects of the developmental and family context that need to be considered in relation to the context of the clinician and the clinical care being provided. When relevant, we add comments regarding additional questions that may arise when applying GFE to clinical research, in particular.

Informed Consent

Moral and Legal Frameworks

Both moral perspectives and legal regulations frame approaches around whether and how to involve children and their parents in decisions about HIV-related treatment and research. The central questions involve whether and how to solicit the child's input regarding the direction of treatment or participation in research, whether and how to solicit input from the parent or guardian, and whether the child or the parent should be the primary decision-maker.

Hein et al. (2015) propose an age-graded system for determining a child's role in joint medical decision-making, by drawing on the assessments of decisional competence with a sample of children and youth eligible for clinical research across several medical units in the Netherlands (Hein et al. 2015). The authors propose that before age 10, children do not demonstrate sufficient decisional competence, and they recommend that responsibility for providing consent remains with the parents. They recommend children and parents engage in a dual consent process, with separate child and parent consent forms, after age 12 and until the child reaches the age of majority (Hein et al. 2015). However, such a dual consent process would still need to carefully consider the child's illness status and other factors. For children ages 10–12, and for children older than 12 with limited mental capacity due to medical or developmental reasons, Hein et al. (2015) recommend a case-by-case assessment of child consent capacity.

Even if children under 10 are not giving informed consent, they can still be involved in medical decision-making in various ways and deserve access to developmentally appropriate medical information. Eliciting children's feedback about different treatment options shows respect and preserves their dignity (Walker 2002). Directly gathering information about a child's experience can both inform the resulting treatment decision and strengthen the child's investment in and compliance with the medical regimen selected, while mitigating the feelings of helplessness or confusion related to the medical situation (Alderson et al. 2006). For example, children and youth may work harder on adherence to taking pills regularly if they have had input into what the regimen is (e.g., which pills to take and when to take them). Indeed, children as young as four have been shown to have the capacity to understand and take responsibility for their own chronic health conditions (Alderson et al. 2006). There are also indirect benefits from fostering open communication with the child, such as strengthening parent–child and physician–child relationships and promoting child adjustment (McCabe 1996). But in some cases, the child may not want to be involved in decision-making or may choose to defer to their parents (Alderson et al. 2006; McCabe 1996).

Parents are considered the best proxy to advocate for the needs of the child and for how to best address and protect the child's health. It can be argued that parents have authority over their own children, including the right to knowledge about their child's medical situation and the right to decide about any medical interventions their child undergoes, or that parental decision-making preserves the integrity and autonomy of the family unit (e.g., Ross 1997).[1] However, from the perspective of treatment, arguments about parents' obligations to protect the health of their

[1]From a legal perspective, it is important to note that in the cases of divorce, a non-custodial parent retains parental rights unless parental rights have been explicitly terminated.

children are more ethically justified than arguments about parental rights (Mustanski and Fisher 2016). Therefore, when in rare circumstances healthcare practitioners acquire a legal decision that parents are not the best proxy (e.g., if parents do not want their child to receive a potentially life-saving treatment, or in cases of abuse or neglect), parents' decision-making can be legally overturned (Department of Health and Human Services 1990; Committee on Bioethics 2013).

Sharing the burden of decision-making with a parent can protect children from the emotional consequences of information they may not be prepared to understand and of bearing the responsibility for their own health, for example, if a treatment is not effective or has negative side effects (McCabe 1996). Child involvement is particularly important when there is no clear or obvious choice and when the outcome of the decision depends on a value judgment and a subjective assessment of issues affecting quality of life (McCabe 1996). As children gain the capacity to understand and process the information, they can then develop decision-making skills through child assent processes. These processes can involve shared collaboration and goal setting about both the treatment and the decision-making process (McCabe 1996).

Authoritative parenting approaches in which children's perspectives are regularly taken into account within the context of guidelines and boundaries set by adults will best facilitate the child's engagement in autonomous decision-making in the context of parental support and guidance (Hein et al. 2015). One study with healthy youth addressing hypothetical medical situations indicated that adolescents would prefer to make medical decisions for themselves (Ruggeri et al. 2014). However, this study used hypotheticals with adolescents who were not themselves facing a diagnosis. Within a dual consent approach, adolescents would be able to turn to their parents for advice and collaboration should they so choose (Hein et al. 2015). However, under circumstances in which children and adolescents do not have the legal right to refuse treatment, they must be clearly informed of these limits and not given the opportunity to refuse if it will be overridden (McCabe 1996; Ross 1997).

In other cases, adolescents can access treatment without parent permission or knowledge. State laws vary in the extent to which adolescents can get HIV testing or treatment on their own: 46 states have laws in which adolescents can consent to HIV-related care (English et al. 2010). However, some of these states only allow minor consent for HIV testing, but if they test positive, they are not allowed to obtain HIV treatment without parent permission. This creates a double standard and thus requires greater sensitivity from HIV testing counselors—both in pretest and in post-test counseling—to explain to the young person what the restrictions would be in the case of a positive result. Emancipated minors are people under the age of 18 who have obtained the legal rights of adults and can therefore consent to any of their own medical treatment. Situations under which minors can become emancipated include marriage, military service, and other forms of living independently, although a court order may be required to obtain this legal status (English et al. 2010).

In some situations, the state and the general public may be considered stakeholders in decisions about individual health care (Pustilnik and Henry 2012). The treatment of HIV is a public health concern, addressed through the use of treatment as prevention. People who are effectively treated for HIV and who thus have an undetectable viral load are less likely to transmit the virus to others, including their sexual partners. When someone does not want or is not compliant with treatment, questions are raised about whether and how to urge adherence. The criminalization of HIV is a potential pitfall to this line of argument. HIV criminalization laws, which exist in many states in the US and in countries around the world, make it illegal for someone who is aware of their status to expose others to HIV. It is important to emphasize that within the framework of public health concerns, the criminalization of HIV is a significant barrier to testing, treatment, and general health care for people living with HIV (Bernard 2006). Understanding the general public as stakeholders in the effectiveness of treatment as prevention is neither a moral nor a public health justification for using the state legal system to compel compliance.

Ethics in research are guided by the Belmont Report principles of respect for persons, beneficence, and justice (the National Commission for the Protection of Human Subjects of Biomedical and Behavioral Research 1979). With regard to the participation of children and adolescents in HIV-related research, a waiver of the requirement to obtain permission from parents can be solicited if requiring parent permission for research participation is not reasonable, or if it is not feasible. Parent permission is not reasonable when it is determined that it does not effectively protect the child, for example, if the parent is abusive or neglectful. Parent permission is not feasible if it is not practical or possible to conduct the study without it, for example, for youth who are not living with their parents or who are homeless. Some young people also may fear talking to their parents about their HIV status due to a risk of family rejection or homelessness (directly in response to the HIV status or in response to the disclosure of related factors such as sexual identity, sexual activity, or drug use). When parent permission is waived, the researchers must take steps to enhance the consent capacity of the research participants or, if additional protections are needed, to integrate a patient advocate into the research protocol who would be responsible for protecting the rights and interests of the children during the decision-making process.

The person soliciting a child's consent to participate in research needs to be clear about the separation between the clinician's role and the researcher's role. Researchers have something to gain from recruiting participants for their studies. Potential research participants need to understand that participation is voluntary and that they will continue to receive care regardless of whether they participate.

When parent permission is required for research, the child is still engaged in giving assent or agreement with the permission granted by the parent, which is legally distinct from the concept of consent. However, as noted above in the case of treatment, it is important to be clear about what the child's rights are in the event that the child does not want to participate in the research, even after parent permission has been obtained. For research that does not have treatment benefits (e.g., social behavioral research, or research about the child's experience and perspectives), child assent is required, and thus, the child has the right to refuse (McCabe 1996). Federal guidelines allow for a waiver of child assent and thus an override of child's dissent to participate, if the research would provide a benefit to the child that is not available elsewhere. For example, if the child has not responded to the standard treatments and participating in the research offers an opportunity for the child to access a new treatment, the parent could decide that the child will participate despite dissent.

Developmental and Family Factors

Developmental competencies are important for finding the right balance between protection and autonomy when thinking about informed consent and assent. Although age can serve as a guide for developmental maturity, developmental competencies vary widely among children even of the same age. As Meaux and Bell (2001) point out, children with developmental disabilities may be less able to make informed decisions than children with chronic illnesses. However, in the case of HIV, developmental delays and/or deterioration associated with the disease may complicate informed decision-making. Chenneville et al. (2010) stress the importance of assessing the decisional capacity of youth with HIV and using these data to respect autonomy without undue harm. Decisional capacity involves four components—understanding, appreciation, reasoning, and ability to express a choice—and is an important construct when thinking about capacity to provide informed consent for both treatment and research (Dunn et al. 2006; Grisso and Appelbaum 1998; Grisso et al. 1997). In a study of the decisional capacity for treatment among youth with HIV aged 13–24, Chenneville et al. (2014b) found deficits in the areas of understanding and reasoning. In another study, these researchers found a significant relationship between understanding and self-reported adherence (Chenneville et al. 2015) providing support for the importance of decisional capacity when thinking about informed decision-making related to treatment and research.

Family factors to include parents' strengths and vulnerabilities should be considered when thinking about informed consent and assent. Family dynamics also are important. Specifically, the relationships between parent–child and parent–parent should be examined to ensure that a child's assent is not coerced (Meaux and Bell 2001). This is particularly important in family situations where parents are divorced or separated. Clinicians and researchers must be aware of requirements for obtaining consent from one or both parents. As a general rule, minimal risk procedures and research require permission from one parent, while procedures and research posing greater-than-minimal risk typically require permission from both parents.

Best Practices: Goodness-of-Fit Ethics for Informed Consent for HIV Intervention and Research Involving Children and Youth

The unique characteristics of children and adolescents with or at risk for HIV create special informed consent challenges for practitioners and investigators because minors do not have the legal status to independently consent to treatment or research, and depending on the age of the child, they may lack the cognitive maturity or experience to make an informed participation decision. Fisher has called for a research ethic that conceptualizes informed consent for pediatric treatment and research in terms of the goodness of fit (GFE) among child, guardian, and treatment/research characteristics (Fisher and Masty 2006; Masty and Fisher 2008). The GFE framework shifts judgments regarding pediatric informed consent procedures away from an exclusive focus on assumed child or guardian vulnerabilities to an examination of those aspects of the clinical or experimental setting that can reduce or facilitate informed choice. The GFE model requires professionals to design informed consent procedures that reflect an understanding of (1) developmental and health-related factors influencing minors' ability to provide an informed, rationale, and voluntary choice to participate in an intervention or research; (2) guardians' comprehension of the child's health condition and their general HIV health literacy; (3) the cultural context and preferred modes of family healthcare decision-making; and (4) the unique characteristics of the specific treatment or research context (Fisher 2003a, b).

Extending the GFE framework, Fisher and Masty (2006) and Masty and Fisher (2008) propose the following "family-fitted" consent considerations for medical and mental health treatment and research involving children and adolescents with or at risk for HIV:

Fitting Assent Procedures to the Child's Cognitive and Emotional Readiness

Truly "informed" assent rests on children's ability to comprehend information presented during the consent conference and their emotional preparedness to process facts about their condition. The empirical literature is quite consistent in demonstrating that by age 14 consent comprehension of children without neuropsychological impairments approaches adult levels (Field and Behrman 2004). Parents' and children's opinions on the age at which youth should be given greater consent autonomy parallel empirical findings (Fisher 2002, 2003b; Masty and Fisher 2008; Masty et al. 2006). However, assent content tailored to the developmental level of the child may not be well fitted to the current cognitive or emotional deficiencies that children with HIV and other related health problems or mental disorders may develop. For example, newly diagnosed pediatric cancer patients demonstrate a decreased ability to comprehend clinical trials' information compared to children of the same age who were diagnosed with diabetes (Broome et al. 2001; Crisp et al. 1996).

As argued by Masty and Fisher (2008), the growing commitment among healthcare professionals to involve children in intervention and research decisions has advanced more rapidly than empirical examination of the mental health consequences on health and responsivity to treatment of placing this decisional responsibility on children with medical or mental disorders. HIV sero-positive status or other HIV-related mental health problems that bring families to the consent conference for medical or HIV behavioral preventive intervention might yield different reactions to the consent conference, especially when the disorder to be treated has been associated with HIV stigma or family conflict. In addition, for young children, certain aspects of HIV treatment research may potentially jeopardize the patient/practitioner therapeutic alliance. For example, asking children for a participation decision for a randomized control trial in which neither they nor their doctor will choose their treatment may be confusing to younger children who have not yet obtained the ability to think recursively and may be perceived as disingenuous by younger adolescents. At the same time, there is some evidence suggesting that involving children in the consent process can have both short- and long-term benefits by increasing children's feelings of self-worth, their ability to cope with anxiety regarding illness and treatments, their sense of self-efficacy, and their long-term emotional and social adjustment (Grodin and Burton 1988; Hall et al. 2012; Varni et al. 1996). Recognize that the informed consent process serves more than one purpose including importantly helping the child to be comfortable with procedures, the potential side effects that will be experienced, and behavioral adherence to health regimens that may be required.

Fitting Parental Permission to Parent Characteristics and Information Needs

HIV professionals working within the GFE framework will consider how to tailor the consent conference to the consent strengths and vulnerabilities of the parents or guardians who are legally responsible for the treatment or research participation decision. This can include parents' educational background, language, familiarity, and experience with medical aspects of pediatric HIV, treatment, or research relevant comorbid disorders or HIV risk behaviors and their knowledge of the distinctions between clinical research and treatment (Kodish et al. 2004). The GFE framework also demands sensitivity to the degree of emotional distress parents are experiencing at the time treatment or research decisions must be made. This is especially true when parents have just learned their child tested positive for HIV or when their children have been non-responders to standard treatments (Masty and Fisher 2008). Under the pressure of such stressful circumstances, parents are often unsure about their child's diagnosis and prognosis. Empirical studies on guardian's reactions to informed consent conferences for pediatric cancer (Eiser et al. 2005; Kodish et al. 2004; Kupst et al. 2003; Marshall et al. 2012) suggest that during the consent conferences for HIV clinical trials, guardian anxiety may interfere with understanding the nature of random assignment to treatment conditions or the ability to ask questions about the research and their child's illness.

Investigators also need to be sensitive to cultural differences that may affect parents' comfort in asking questions during the consent conference (Fisher 2005). The type of information investigators provide, in addition to their presentation style, may interact with culturally derived communication preferences and impact parents' comfort level (Fisher et al. 2002). For example, Miller et al. (2005) found that parents of racial minority and low socioeconomic status asked fewer questions and were more likely to miss or misunderstand consent information for pediatric cancer trials. They also learned that investigators provided less information to these families and made fewer partnership building statements.

The Family's History of Shared Decision-Making for the Child's Health-Related Matters

A family's history of cooperative discussion and shared decision-making should also be considered when "fitting" the consent conference to the child's needs. In general, when the child is older and more mature, when the disorder is not posing a serious threat to the child's physical or mental well-being, and when parents have included children in prior decisions about their health, there will be a greater propensity for HIV treatment or clinical research decisions to be made together as a family (Geller et al. 2003). On the other hand, if the family culture is such that the child's input is not sought on a regular basis, the child may not be accustomed to or wish to make health decisions and may choose to have their parents make the treatment decision either because that is what is customarily done, because they trust their parents to make decisions in their best interest, or because they do not want the pressure of making critical health decisions. Finally, parents of children with life-threatening conditions such as HIV and/or comorbid disorders such as depression or substance abuse (among older youth) may have found themselves frequently in the position of making healthcare decisions for their child to include decisions that the child may not have agreed to or been unable to make, but were nevertheless necessary for the child's well-being.

The Child's Autonomy Strivings Balanced With Parents' Duty and Responsibility to Make Decisions in Their Child's Best Interest

When conducting the consent conference, HIV practitioners and investigators working within the GFE framework face the dual task of supporting children's developing autonomy and parents' responsibility to make decisions in their children's best interest. Investigators routinely seek input from children during the consent process. But the degree and weight of pediatric participation in HIV treatment and clinical trial entry and withdrawal decisions will vary depending upon the child and family factors. Engaging children in discussions about their engagement in HIV treatment or research can help promote children's well-being as well as their developing autonomy and personal agency in communicating concerns and desires (Young et al. 2010).

At the same time, parents are responsible for determining what is in their child's best interest and for protecting their child against undue harm that may arise when consent participation is developmentally inappropriate (Melton 1999). Given some children's limited world experience and lack of a well-formulated life plan, investigators should be wary of reflexively giving child autonomy privileged status over parents' responsibilities to direct the autonomy strivings of their children

(Childress 1990; Fisher and Masty 2006; Ross 1997). In some contexts, parents may be justifiably concerned that assent procedures may increase their child's fear of the disorder, pessimism about the treatment, or anxiety about treatment risks (Barfield and Kane 2008). On the other hand, in some instances, failure to involve the child in the consent decision may stifle autonomy development (Kunin 1997). There is some evidence that children and parents are acutely aware of the tension between child autonomy and parental protection. Masty et al. (2006) found that a majority of both children and parents who had participated in pediatric oncology trials believed that while it was important to respect a child's decision-making abilities, parents had a responsibility to shield their children from anxiety-provoking information and to protect their children from feelings of blame or guilt if participation did not produce positive effects. HIV professionals can be sensitive to the interaction of patient disorder and parental responsibility to collaborate with parents in fitting the child's role in the research participation decision to these factors. In some family settings, the best approach to child involvement may include providing a clear description of the research for the child and encouraging active participation by asking for feedback rather than a participation choice. In this way, investigators highlight the value of the child's independent concerns while respecting the family's decision-making values. Following the child's feedback, investigators can encourage parents to take into account the child's opinion in the final health decision. Investigators can best serve the future autonomy of young study participants by facilitating the consent conversation such that the study information is conveyed clearly, the child's concerns are validated, and by promoting respectful and culturally appropriate family participation.

Confidentiality and Disclosures

Moral and Legal Frameworks

Moral and legal issues frame discussions about confidentiality and disclosure when treating or conducting research with youth with HIV. The primary questions surround who should have access to knowledge about a young person's HIV status and when should this information be disclosed? As described below, the answers to these questions are complicated by multiple factors to include age and mode of transmission.

Disclosure to young children who are perinatally infected is a well-documented issue in the area of pediatric HIV (see Wiener et al. 2007 for a comprehensive review). Parents struggle with telling their children their HIV status for a variety of reasons. Because of the nature of perinatal transmission, maternal guilt often is high and can serve as a barrier to disclosure. In cases where the biologic mother has died from AIDS, adoptive parents first must disclose the adoption to the child, which can magnify the emotional strain related to the disclosure of HIV status. In addition, biologic and adoptive parents alike often fear children's response to learning their HIV status. Understandably, parents sometimes are reluctant to disclose.

Research is mixed regarding the outcomes of disclosure with some studies revealing benefits or at least no differences in mental health outcomes pre- and postdisclosure, while other studies provide evidence of negative mental health outcomes (Wiener et al. 2007). Nonetheless, disclosure is critical. Not only do children have a right to have access to developmentally appropriate information about their health, but also ignorance of HIV status becomes a public health issue as children age into adolescence, a time marked by sexual exploration. Affirming these concerns, the American Academy of Pediatrics posits that healthcare providers who are treating children with HIV can and should disclose a child's HIV status if parents have not by the age of 13 (American Academy of Pediatrics Committee on Pediatric AIDS, 1999).

For adolescents who are behaviorally infected, the direction of the disclosure may be from minor child to parent as opposed to parent to minor child, especially given that all 50 states in the US and the District of Columbia allow most minors to be tested and treated for sexually transmitted infections, including HIV, without parental consent (The Guttmacher Institute 2015). Of note, in many states, healthcare providers may share information with parents if such disclosure is deemed to be in the best interest of the minor.

Regardless of the mode of transmission, adolescents and young adults with HIV face difficult decisions about disclosing their health status in sexual situations. Despite the importance of disclosure, some youth with HIV do not disclose their health status to sexual partners (Chenneville et al. 2014a; Dempsey et al. 2012; Marhefka et al. 2011). Among the reasons why youth with HIV are reluctant to disclose their HIV status to others, especially sexual partners, are limited communication skills and fear of rejection (Chenneville et al. 2014a). At the core of the difficulties surrounding disclosure is HIV stigma, which is the product of perceived contagion and stereotypes about the people and behavior most commonly associated with HIV (Fielden et al. 2011). Silence appears to be the means by which youth with HIV manage this stigma.

The reasons for non-disclosure notwithstanding youth with HIV may face criminal sanctions for failing to disclose their HIV status to sexual partners. As of 2011, laws had been enacted in 33 states in the US making it a crime to engage in behaviors, including sex, that pose a risk of transmission to others (Lehman et al. 2014). These laws are controversial with many HIV experts arguing that such laws serve as a barrier to HIV testing and treatment (Bernard 2006). Controversy notwithstanding, youth with HIV contend with the legal ramifications of non-disclosure although Chenneville et al. (2014a) found that moral concerns outweighed a fear of legal repercussions when contemplating the disclosure of HIV status to sexual partners.

Developmental and Family Factors

Developmental and family factors should be taken into consideration when thinking about confidentiality and disclosure among youth with HIV. Wiener et al. (2007) suggest that the abilities of both children and caregivers should be assessed when deciding when and how to disclose to a child their HIV status. Further, they recommend identifying sources of support and adequately preparing and rehearsing the actual disclosure as well as encouraging ongoing open communication.

The role of caregivers also should be considered when thinking about confidentiality and disclosure among youth with HIV. Research suggests that caregivers play an important role in adherence (Simoni et al. 2007). However, it should not be assumed that caregiver involvement will support disease management. Research suggests that caregivers sometimes hinder adherence. For example, Mellins et al. (2004) found that poor parent–child communication and high stress among caregivers were associated with poor adherence among children aged 3–13 with HIV. Gathering information about caregiver characteristics that may support or hinder adherence is important when making decisions about whether or not to disclose information to a caregiver about a minor child who has been tested or is being treated for HIV without parental consent.

Potentially, the most difficult dilemma healthcare providers face is when they are treating young people with HIV who are sexually active but are not disclosing their status to sexual partners. While medical providers and mental health providers may differ philosophically on their views about third-party disclosure, most probably agree with Rothstein and Talbott (2006) that the greatest potential threat to privacy is the compelled disclosure of health information. For physicians, enlisting the support of a local health department responsible for the oversight of partner notification programs is an acceptable option. Meanwhile, psychologists and other mental health professionals are likely to focus on helping individual clients overcome barriers to disclosure. Recognizing the factors that influence sexual health behaviors and how and why these factors may differ among different groups (e.g., sexual minority youth) is important.

Best Practices: Goodness-of-Fit Framework for Confidentiality and Disclosure Decision-Making for Children and Youth with or at Risk for HIV

Involvement of parents is often a key factor in engaging children and adolescents in psychotherapy (Dailor and Jacob 2011; Oetzel and Scherer 2003; Weisz and Hawley 2002). At the same time, establishing the boundaries of client/patient confidentiality is critical to establishing a trusting relationship among the psychologist, child client/patient, and parents. While federal and state laws grant minors limited access to medical and mental health services without guardian consent, they often permit (and sometimes require) parents to be involved in their child's treatment plan, provide parental access to treatment records (e.g., under the Health Insurance Portability and Accountability Act [HIPAA]), send all insurance billing related to a legal minor's health care directly to parents (e.g., under the Affordable Care Act Explanation of Benefits sent to policy owners), and permit the disclosure of information to protect the child or others from harm (English et al. 2010; Frerich et al. 2012; Sedlander et al. 2015; Weithorn 2006).

In making confidentiality and disclosure decisions, mental health practitioners and investigators studying treatment effectiveness should be sensitive to the influence of health disparities and medical mistrust in parents' perceptions of confidentiality as it relates to adolescent reproductive health and other health compromising behaviors (Byczkowski et al. 2010; Fisher 2003a, b, 2013; Fisher and Wallace 2000). For example, McKee et al. (2006) found that Latina and African American mothers living in impoverished neighborhoods believed that confidential reproductive care promoted risky sexual behavior and undermined mothers' efforts to protect their daughters. Practitioners must also consider practical issues such as the parent withdrawing the child from treatment for lack of access to information or children's misuse of confidentiality as a weapon in their conflict with parents. Psychologists working with children and adolescents thus need to anticipate and consistently reevaluate how they will balance confidentiality considerations with parental involvement in the child's best interests.

Establishing Confidentiality Limits at the Outset of Therapy

The nature of information that will be shared with parents should begin with a consideration of the child's cognitive and emotional maturity, presenting problem, treatment goals, and age-appropriate expectations regarding the role parents can play in facilitating treatment (Cohen and Cicchetti 2006; Morris and Mather 2007). For example, younger children's cognitive limitations and dependence on significant adults suggest that maintenance of strict confidentiality procedures may hinder treatment by failing to reflect the actual contexts in which children grow and develop. By contrast, increasing protection of private thoughts and feelings may facilitate treatment by demonstrating respect for older children's developing autonomy, comprehension of the nature and purpose of therapy, and ability to take a self-reflective perspective on their own thoughts and feelings (Hennan et al. 1997).

The Consent Conference

Engaging parents and children in discussion about the nature and rationale for confidentiality and disclosure policies is the first step in creating a trusting relationship. Empirical studies suggest that parents often respond positively to the need for adolescents to have private health consultations with practitioners and that youth are equally responsive to situations that may require disclosure to parents

(Fisher 2002, 2003b; Gilbert et al. 2014). Achieving a successful client-centered confidentiality policy begins with the consent conference during which practitioners can explain their professional ethical and legal responsibilities, provide examples of the type of information that would benefit from confidentiality versus information sharing, and obtain feedback to understand the child's and parent's concerns. This discussion should lead to an agreed-upon culturally and family sensitive confidentiality and disclosure policy that fits the child's age and treatment needs.

Parental Requests for Information

There will be times when parents request information the practitioner had not previously considered appropriate for disclosure. While parental demands should never supersede ethical, legal, and professional responsibilities, parental views should always be given respectful consideration and practitioners should be open to the possibility that the issues they raise require a reconsideration of confidentiality policies (Fisher et al. 1999; Mitchell et al. 2002; Taylor and Adelman 1989). In discussing the parent's concerns, practitioners should help the parent reframe confidentiality in terms of (a) the child's developing autonomy, (b) encouraging the child to share information with parents by choice rather than requirement, and (c) maintaining therapeutic trust. Drawing on the research indicating lack of confidentiality is a major factor in youth's failure to engage in reproductive health services can also be helpful (Frerich et al. 2012; Ringheim 2007; Thomas et al. 2006). Finally, if appropriate, suggest that the parent asks the child about the desired information or, with the parent's knowledge, explore with the child clinically indicated ways in which information might be shared.

Disclosing Confidential Information in Response to Client/Patient Risk Behavior

Practitioners working with children and adolescents often become aware of behaviors hidden from parents that place the child at some physical, psychological, or legal risk. Some of the "secret" activities that may require disclosure include when a child has or is at high risk for HIV sexual activity, alcohol and drug use, and/or self-harm. When such situations arise, it is important to consider whether parental disclosure will lead to essential protections that can only be provided outside the therapeutic context (Fisher 2013). Alternatively, sharing such information with parents may damage the therapeutic alliance or place the child at greater risk if parental reactions can be predicted to be physically violent or emotionally abusive. For example, the consequences of disclosing to parents high-risk sexual activity of sexual minority youth who have not discussed their sexual orientation with their parents are more complex and potentially more hazardous than would occur when disclosing information regarding a minor's heterosexual activities (Fisher et al. 2016; Fisher and Mustanski 2014; Gilbert et al.

2015; Mustanski 2011). Mental health providers must also consider how entering into a secrecy pact with a minor client can adversely affect the therapeutic alliance and be wary when assuming that minor clients expect and desire confidentiality when they reveal during therapy that they are engaging in high-risk behaviors (Fisher 2017; Gilbert et al. 2014).

Fisher (2017) has suggested the following steps to consider in deciding whether and how to disclose confidential information when minor clients/patients are engaging in high-risk behaviors.

Step 1: Assess and Clinically Address Risk Behaviors

The first step in any confidentiality and disclosure decision is to confirm that the child is actually engaging in the risk behavior, the level of danger to the child or others, whether it is an isolated incident or a continuing pattern, and the developmental, psychological, and situational factors that might impair the child's ability to terminate or reduce behaviors. If clinically indicated, the practitioner should then conduct and monitor the effectiveness of age and culturally appropriate intervention strategies to help the client/patient terminate or reduce risk levels of behavior.

Step 2: Consider Options if Client/Patient is Unable or Unwilling to Terminate or Reduce Behaviors

If intervention is unsuccessful, practitioners need to weigh legal, therapeutic, social, and health consequences of confidentiality and disclosure within the context of familial and cultural factors, federal and state reporting requirements, and, to the extent possible, parents' ability to appropriately respond to disclosure.

Step 3: Prepare Client/Patient for Disclosure

If disclosure is determined to be appropriate, practitioners can introduce the decision to the child in terms of the limits of confidentiality discussed during informed consent and the practitioner's responsibility to protect the welfare of the client/patient and others. Discussion should be responsive to the child's feelings and concerns without focusing on ways to avoid disclosure, explain steps that will be taken to share the information with parents, and involve the client/patient as much as possible.

Step 4: Disclosing Information to Parents

When disclosing risk information to parents, practitioners should empathize and respond to parents' feelings and concerns and focus on positive actions they can take to help their child and, whenever feasible, to place the child's actions within the context of continued treatment progress; this may include joint parent–child or more frequent goal-setting sessions and appropriate referral sources that can help parents best address their child's behaviors or their own counseling needs. Parent–child follow-up meetings should be scheduled to monitor reactions to the disclosure, to provide additional recommendations for reducing risk, and if risk increases or remains at dangerous levels, to reconsider therapeutic, community and legal options.

Addressing Heath Inequities

While HIV transmission is person to person and behavioral, the epidemic is characterized by health disparities that reflect systemic inequity resulting from the structural violence of racism and poverty, both within the US and internationally (Farmer 2004). For further information on pediatric HIV epidemiology, see Gillespie (2017). Structural racism impacts the interpersonal pathways of HIV transmission, the overall health and wellness of young people living with HIV, and access to and experience in treatment for HIV (Krieger 2012; Bassett 2015). In order to optimize ethical decision-making, clinicians must therefore consider both their own internalized biases and the impact of structural racism within the healthcare context and within their clients' lives and experiences (Griffith et al. 2007).

Within the context of structural oppression, the HIV epidemic will best be addressed through processes that support liberation, conceived of as psychological and political well-being in personal, relational, and collective domains (Prilleltensky 2003). Ethical decisions made in the context of treatment, such as interactions with children and families and decisions about clinical treatment, must take into account psychological and political context and wellness (Fisher 2014; Fisher et al. 1997, 2002). This might be especially relevant to discussions of the disclosure of HIV status. In addition, Bassett (2015) calls on physicians to engage in collective liberation efforts, specifically with regard to anti-black racism, through critical research, internal reform, and public advocacy.

Building on the frameworks of health equity and social justice described above, we present recommendations for research and practice focused on the ethics of equity in access to care (relating to institutional structures) and the ethics of people's experiences receiving care (relating to what happens once people have access and are inside institutions).

Organization and Access

The contexts of a person's life that contribute to contracting HIV may include lack of access to health care and/or occurrences of discrimination and victimization within the healthcare system. Other aspects of social, political, and economic marginalization may also cause challenges to healthcare access, such as unstable housing and food insecurity. There may also be direct barriers such as language and literacy and the burden of transportation costs. Each of these life circumstances are interconnected with structural racism and thus disproportionately burden people of color. When these factors contribute to life context that puts a person at heightened physical, emotional, and social vulnerability and the contraction of HIV, those same factors need to be addressed in order for that person to adequately and consistently access HIV treatment, be retained in care, and achieve an undetectable viral load. Thus, the distribution of resources becomes a treatment concern, particularly for adolescents, whose liminal legal status and limited developmental experience may contribute to their vulnerability within personal relationships (e.g., family relationships and sexual partners) and within healthcare institutions.

Previous experiences of discrimination and/or victimization within the healthcare system, or experiences of friends, or family members may contribute to hesitance or ambivalence around accessing HIV treatment. Such specific experiences, combined with medical distrust related to experienced or perceived discrimination based on race and ethnicity (or related to sexuality or sexual practices), can manifest in resistance to treatment, ambivalence regarding treatment, and treatment refusal (Fisher et al. 2012; Fisher and Wallace 2000).

Healthcare settings and healthcare providers can take a proactive role in addressing these effects of structural racism. Ethical obligations stem from the imperative to avoid unintentionally repeating or reinstating instances of harm and from the need to address the unjust distribution of health-enhancing resources. However, individual intentions to be "not racist" have proven to be inadequate in the face of systemic injustice. Griffith et al. (2007) propose an approach called "dismantling racism" that addresses three levels of healthcare delivery: individual, intraorganizational, and extraorganizational. Within each of these levels, the approach utilizes anti-racist community organizing methodology to uncover how racism functions through formal and informal power relationships. Anti-racist community organizing means that the voices of marginalized community members, including youth with HIV and their families, are made central, and strategies for shifting the organizational structures and individual practices in ways that address their needs and enhance their experiences are identified and enacted.

Multicultural Competence

Ethical practice entails a personal and professional commitment to examining both culture and power. Understanding the structural context of race and racism is also part of interpersonal multicultural competence (Fisher 2014). Race is a social construction rooted in systems of injustice, including social, institutional, and systemic oppression (Fisher et al. 2012). Clinical work is strengthened through understanding of the current and historical sociopolitical forces that shape individual lives and physical health and wellness (Fisher 2014). The practice of medicine in general (Bassett 2015) and, specifically, infectious disease, adolescent treatment, and HIV policy (e.g., HIV criminalization; Bernard 2006) have all been used in various ways to further oppression. That history has an impact both on the psychological experiences of people of color within the healthcare system and on the perspectives and practices that structure modern medicine. The eradication of overt and covert racism and oppressive practices from medical and pediatric practice is imperative and ongoing (Bassett 2015). Within that ongoing process, ethical responsibility of individual clinicians within medical practice includes identifying the health consequences of oppression and working within the context of their professional roles to promote psychological and political liberation (Prilleltensky 2003).

To enact these responsibilities, clinicians need to understand their own positions and roles within systems of oppression. In particular, multicultural competence involves being aware of any positions of social power and privilege and the ways it shapes personal experiences and clinical interactions (Fisher 2014). For clinicians who are white, employing practices of racial humility and cultural humility can facilitate this process of self-examination of internalized assumptions, biases, stereotypes, and default ways of treating people from marginalized social groups. This process involves humility insofar as anti-racist intentions do not guarantee that one's actions have the desired impact, and a person must accept one's involvement in oppressive systems and one's risk of perpetuating oppression in order to then take conscious steps to minimize such instances and to rectify them when they do occur (Vaught and Castagno 2008). Understanding the relational context of power and privilege needs to also involve addressing clients and families as complex, without making assumptions about their unique experiences of identity, culture, and power (Fisher et al. 2002; Fisher 2014).

Multicultural competence can be enacted throughout the implementation of GFE decision-making (Fisher 2014, 2017). Through co-learning, the clinician can exercise racial and cultural humility by learning about the perspectives and needs of the child and family (Fisher 1999, 2014). A combination of sensitivity and flexibility is needed to engage in a process of ongoing decision-making and reflection on the intended and unintended meanings and consequences of those decisions (Fisher et al. 2002; Fisher 2014).

Research Burdens and Benefits

The design and conduct of clinical research on pediatric HIV must account for the context of structural racism and health inequities. The foundational research ethics principle of justice (the National Commission for the Protection of Human Subjects of Biomedical and Behavioral Research 1979) involves equitable distribution of research burdens and research benefits. For example, youth at heightened sociopolitical vulnerability, such as youth of color, should not be burdened with being the test population for new medications. At the same time, youth have the right to participate in research to inform clinical approaches that will be better suited to their own needs. If a group of marginalized youth, for example, youth of color, or gender and sexual minority (GSM) youth, have limited access to opportunities to participate in research, then the treatment available to them may not be relevant, affirming, or effective (Fisher et al. 2016; Fisher and Mustanski 2014). In allocating research funding and planning research agendas, researchers must consider the type of research being done and the distribution of both burdens and benefits throughout the relevant populations.

As with clinical practice, cultural values and sociopolitical experiences need to be considered throughout the design and implementation of research procedures (Fisher 2014). Researchers can gather and consult with community advisory boards to elicit feedback on the appropriateness, accessibility, and acceptability of their policies, procedures, and materials for recruitment, decision-making and informed consent, confidentiality, and addressing HIV in general (Fisher et al. 2002). Researchers need to find ways to enhance both the scientific merit and the cultural competence of their research studies in tandem (Fisher et al. 1997).

Throughout the research process, and especially in the reporting and dissemination of research findings, researchers addressing pediatric HIV must be aware of how HIV stigma is differentially distributed across social groups. HIV coincides with structural racism not only in the epidemiology of the epidemic but also within interconnected layers of stigma (Fielden et al. 2011). Potentially contributing to a person's experience of stigma or to the sociopolitical stigmatization of certain groups is an ethical concern (Fisher 1999). Another area in which clinicians need to be aware of the interplay between racial stigma and HIV stigma is in the context of conversations and decision-making with regard to sexual health and the prevention of further HIV transmission.

Sexual Health

Ethical HIV treatment involves educating children and youth about the transmission of HIV, which includes sexuality education. For children who contracted HIV at birth or in childhood, this education begins with disclosure to the child of their own HIV status and how they contracted the virus. That is a good time to start communicating specifically about which fluids contain the virus and which membranes are susceptible. Before the child becomes sexually active, however, it is important to provide specific education and emotional support regarding safer sex practices and disclosure to partners. Young people who contract HIV through sexual activity also need to have conversations with their clinicians that avoid assumptions about what they may or may not have learned earlier and that also avoid blaming them for the behavior that led to their contracting the virus. The initiation of this conversation, the content of this conversation, and the outcomes of this conversation all have ethical dimensions. In particular, when addressing sexual health with all young people, it is important to use approaches that are inclusive and affirming of sexual and gender minority identities and practices (Arbeit et al. 2015).

Initiating the Conversation

In initiating a conversation about preventing further transmission of HIV, physicians need to be as proactive as possible to start a conversation prior to the onset of sexual activity, gradually building over time in order to scaffold the knowledge and skills that young people need to manage and enjoy their developing sexuality (Arbeit 2014). Different children of different ages may be responsive to different kinds of conversations at different times, depending also on pubertal status, emotional coping, social context, cultural values, and intellectual curiosity (Diamond et al. 2014). If a child or adolescent asks questions, it is important to respond with honesty and clarity, answering directly and helping them seek clarification or further information if desired (Richardson and Schuster 2004). If a child is not asking outright, the clinician can seek feedback about what might help them to feel comfortable during this conversation, or in what ways (and from whom) they would like to learn. Written materials or online resources to explore or to read privately in between conversations with a clinician may help the child feel agency and ownership over the information and its ramifications (Bay-Cheng 2005).

Depending on the treatment context, processes of informed consent or child assent may be used to allow the child and family an opportunity to affirm a decision to engage in this sexual health education process. Furthermore, for children or adolescents to feel comfortable talking to their providers about sexuality and sexual activity, clear boundaries and expectations need to be communicated around confidentiality and the involvement of parents or guardians in this conversation. To the extent possible, parents and guardians can be meaningfully involved in the process of sexual health education if they are provided with similar information and resources and with guidelines for how to continue the conversations at home, reinforcing the same messages in tandem with their family values (Grossman et al. 2014). However, in pursuing this process, the clinician needs to work within the comfort and communication style of the family. The clinician must also be attentive to sexual health values held by the parents that may contradict HIV prevention best practices and may need to address the parental resistance to supporting adolescent sexual expression, emphasizing that supporting positive sexuality development can facilitate the safety of their child and their child's sexual partners (Bay-Cheng 2013).

Young people who contract HIV through sexual activity may be reluctant to admit to their lack of knowledge about their own bodies and about sex itself. Thus, it is important to validate that many youth do not have access to information and resources about sexual health and that it is okay for them to continue learning even after sexual initiation. Starting with the basics and encouraging questions and clarifications not only has the benefit of providing information, but also can begin to build agency that can strengthen the youth's ability to engage in protection and risk reduction practices (Arbeit 2014).

The Content of the Conversation

Even though the child contracted the virus, it is imperative to have open communication about sex without inadvertently reinforcing messages of blame and shame. The virus may have been contracted as a result of their own sexual decisions, through an experience of sexual violence or coercion, or without their knowing. Feeling accepted and coping with societal stigma or with pejorative terms about HIV status may improve mental health and also provide youth with clarity and confidence in themselves that can strengthen them in communicating effectively with others and with their sexual partners (Arbeit 2014; Fielden et al. 2011). Reinforcing positive messages about the right to sexuality, love, and relationships goes along with reducing stigma (Edwards and Coleman 2004).

To have an open conversation about sexuality with a young person, and to have an effective conversation about HIV prevention, the conversation should acknowledge and address the full range of human sexual desires and behaviors (Arbeit et al. 2015). In particular, young people with same-sex desires or sexual minority identities may not readily disclose to their providers unless asked directly and assured of both confidentiality and an affirming response (Arbeit et al. 2015). In order to inform decision-making and negotiation of risk reduction with potential sexual partners, young people need open conversation about the range of sexual practices in which they can experience and share different forms of sexual pleasure, as well as the comparative transmission risks in each. Learning about a variety of barrier methods, such as gloves and dental dams, provides ways of minimizing risk even in lower-risk sexual activities. In order to have help in navigating sexual decision-making, young people will also need the opportunity to speak openly about their desires for different kinds of sexual activity and sexual access without it being stigmatized, for example, if they are using social media applications to find partners for casual sex.

To make discussions of sexual activity accessible and affirming to youth who may be gender non-conforming, questioning their gender identity, or identifying as transgender, it is imperative to talk about bodies and activities while using as few gendered terms as possible (National Center for Transgender Equality 2012). For example, instead of talking about "male condoms" and "female condoms," use more accurate and specific language, such as the "insertive condom" used for a penis, sex toy, or other phallus, and the "receptive condom," used for a vagina, anus, or other cavity. Proactively making the conversation inclusive of diverse sexual activities, sexual identities, and gender identities is an ethical issue, working to deconstruct homophobia and transphobia within healthcare systems and to avoid unintentional microaggressions or invalidations (Makadon et al. 2015; NCTE 2012). It is also an issue of effective practice, for youth may withhold information that they fear would not be received positively or disconnect from a conversation that they feel does not apply to them and their desires and experiences (Arbeit et al. 2015).

In addition to the sexual health and risk reduction information, young people need an open and honest conversation about the ethics of disclosing their HIV status to their partners. These conversations may be most effective if they acknowledge the desire for partnership and sexual connection and fear of rejection, stigma, or even violence, upon disclosure. Building upon a young person's self-confidence, and providing a young person access to counter social messages of shame and stigma regarding being HIV positive, can be emotional strengths for them to draw on when communicating with potential partners. In their communication, young people need knowledge about their own HIV status, such as viral load, and what that means for risk of transmission. They also need knowledge about the legal context, cases of HIV, and the laws and policies regulating the disclosure of HIV status to sexual partners (Bernard 2006).

The Outcomes of the Conversation

The clinician also has ethical responsibilities attending to the outcomes of these sexual health conversations. Having discussed confidentiality and parental involvement prior to beginning the conversation, those agreements will then be followed, according to the confidentiality and disclosure best practices described earlier in this chapter. It may also be that the clinician and patient together decide that there is additional information to share with parents or further conversation that the young person would like to have with their parents, for which they may want the clinicians' guidance and/or presence. The clinician and adolescent may also have made decisions about disclosure to past and present sexual partners, either directly or through partner notification programs. Access to testing for past or present partners may also be discussed.

Throughout each of these steps of the process, the emphasis needs to be on minimizing shame and stigma, both for ethical reasons and because they can psychologically interfere with the young person's ability to communicate about their HIV status and practice agency within their risk reduction practices (Arbeit 2014; Fielden et al. 2011). Talking about avoiding transmission of HIV to others may also bring up feelings about how they contracted the virus themselves, including anger at themselves, anger at other people, or reckoning with an experience of sexual coercion or trauma. Teaching safer sex practices needs to be done in a manner that is affirming to a diversity of sexual desires and identities, accurate with regard to a range of sexual activities and options, and flexible with regard to terminology about gender identities and gendered bodies (Arbeit et al. 2015).

Furthermore, many aspects of sexual feelings and values are culturally constituted. Ethical contextualism can be used as a guide for such conversations, affirming the values of the child or adolescent, parents, and family, while retaining the meaning and significance of safer sex and risk reduction practices (Fisher 2014). Clinicians can use a co-learning approach to learn about the sexual ethics of the adolescent, parent, and family while also teaching about disclosure and risk reduction through their own ethical framework (Fisher 1999).

Conclusion

Ethical care for children and adolescents with HIV requires support for their developing abilities and needs while minimizing their potential vulnerability. Learning about the family context and cultural context of the patient can inform both the process of ethical decision-making and the outcomes of those decisions. Through these approaches, clinicians can work to foster health and wellness in the lives of their patients, build groundwork for the prevention of further transmission of HIV, and address the broader health inequities of which HIV is a part.

Annotated Bibliography

Chenneville, T., Machacek, M., Tan, R., Lujan-Zilberman, J., Emmanuel, P., & Rodriguez, C. (2014). Decisional capacity among youth with HIV: Results from the MacArthur competence tool for treatment. *AIDS Patient Care and STDs*, *28*(8), 1–8. doi:10.1089/apc.2013.0374

This study assessed the decisional capacity of youth living with HIV, ages 13–24, using the MacArthur Competence Tool for Treatment. Youth demonstrated appreciation for the potential of HIV treatment to help them, but many did not demonstrate understanding of their disorder and consequential reasoning. Youth strengths and weaknesses are discussed.

Fisher, C. B., Arbeit, M. Dumont, M., Macapagal, & Mustanski, B. (2016). Self-consent for HIV prevention research involving sexual and gender minority youth: Reducing barriers through evidence-based ethics. *Journal of Research on Human Research Ethics*. doi:10.1177/1556264616633963

This study examined self-consent capacity among sexual and gender minority youth ages 14–17 for a hypothetical HIV prevention pre-exposure prophylaxis (PrEP) adherence trial. Youth highlighted guardian permission as a significant barrier to participation, and demonstrated the ability to provide informed, rational, and voluntary self-consent to age- and population-appropriate procedures.

Masty, J., & Fisher, C. B. (2008). A goodness of fit approach to parent permission and child assent pediatric intervention research. *Ethics & Behavior*, *13*, 139–160. doi:10.1080/10508420802063897

This article presents a goodness-of-fit model that frames the child's disorder-based vulnerabilities in the context of the child's cognitive and emotional maturity, the intervention approach, and the family system. Child capacity, parent understanding, history of family decision-making, and child's autonomy strivings are among factors to consider in designing consent procedures.

References

Alderson, P., Sutcliffe, K., & Curtis, K. (2006). Children's competence to consent to medical treatment. *Hasting Center Report, 36*(6), 25–34. doi:10.1353/hcr.2006.0000

American Academy of Pediatrics Committee on Pediatric AIDS. (1999). Disclosure of illness status to children and adolescents with HIV infection. *Pediatrics, 103*(1), 164–166. doi:10.1542/peds.103.1.164

Arbeit, M. R. (2014). What does healthy sex look like among youth? Towards a skills-based model for promoting adolescent sexuality development. *Human Development, 57*(5), 259–286. doi:10.1159/000367856

Arbeit, M. R., Baldi, E. A., Rubin, R. O., Harris, E. M., & Lerner, J. V. (2015). Promoting adolescent sexual health in youth programming: Implications of the 4-H study of positive youth development. In E. P. Bowers, G. J. Geldhof, S. K. Johnson, L. J. Hilliard, R. M. Hershberg, J. V. Lerner, & R. M. Lerner (Eds.). *Promoting positive youth development: Lessons from the 4-H study*. New York, NY: Springer. doi:10.1007/978-3-319-17166-1_12

Arbeit, M. R., Fisher, C. B., Macapagal, K., & Mustanski, M. (2015). They usually just assume that you're straight: LGB youth reflect on sexual health discussions with physicians. *International Academy of Sex Research*. August 10. Toronto, ON.

Barfield, R. C., & Kane, J. R. (2008). Balancing disclosure of diagnosis and assent for research in children with HIV. *Journal of the American Medical Association, 300*(5), 576–578. doi:10.1001/jama.300.5.576

Bassett, M. T. (2015). #BlackLivesMatter—A challenge to the medical and public health communities. *New England Journal of Medicine, 372*(12), 1085–1087. doi:10.1056/NEJMp1500529

Bay-Cheng, L. Y. (2005). Left to their own devices: Disciplining youth discourse on sexuality education electronic bulletin boards. *Sexuality Research and Social Policy, 2*, 37–50. doi:10.1525/srsp.2005.2.1.37

Bay-Cheng, L. Y. (2013). Ethical parenting of sexually active youth: Ensuring safety while enabling development. *Sex Education, 13*, 133–145. doi:10.1080/14681811.2012.700280

Bernard, E. (2006). US criminal HIV disclosure laws may do more harm than good. NAM AIDSmap: HIV & AIDS, sharing knowledge and changing lives. Retrieved from http://www.aidsmap.com/US-criminal-HIV-disclosurelaws-may-do-more-harm-than-good/page/1424402/

Broome, M. E., Richards, D., & Hall, J. (2001). Children in research: The experience of ill children and adolescents. *Journal of Family Nursing, 7*(1), 32–49. doi:10.1177/107484070100700103

Byczkowski, T. L., Kollar, L. M., & Britto, M. T. (2010). Family experiences with outpatient care: Do adolescents and parents have the same perceptions? *Journal of Adolescent Health, 47*(1), 92–98. doi:10.1016/j.jadohealth.2009.12.005

Chenneville, T., Clutter, M., Hintz, S., Walsh, A., Emmanuel, P., Lujan-Zilberman, J., et al. (2015). Decisional capacity and medication adherence among youth with HIV. *AIDS Care, 27*(3), 338–341. doi:10.1080/09540121.2014.993582

Chenneville, T., Lynn, V., Peacock, B., Turner, D., & Marhefka, S. (2014a). Disclosure of HIV status among female youth with HIV. *Ethics and Behavior, 25*(4), 314–331. doi:10.1080/10508422.2014.934371

Chenneville, T., Machacek, M., Tan, R., Lujan-Zilberman, J., Emmanuel, P., & Rodriguez, C. (2014b). Decisional capacity among youth with HIV: Results from the MacArthur competence tool for treatment. *AIDS Patient Care and STDs, 28*(8), 1–8. doi:10.1089/apc.2013.0374

Chenneville, T., Sibille, K., & Bendell-Estroff, D. (2010). Decisional capacity among minors with HIV: A model for balancing autonomy rights with the need for protection. *Ethics and Behavior, 20*(2), 83–94. doi:10.1080/10508421003595901

Childress, J. F. (1990). The place of autonomy in bioethics. *Hastings Center Report, 20*, 12–17. doi:10.2307/3562967

Cohen, D. J., & Cicchetti, D. (2006). *Developmental psychopathology*. New York, NY: John Wiley.

Committee on Bioethics. (2013). Conflicts between religious or spiritual beliefs and pediatric care: Informed refusal, exemptions, and public funding. *Pediatrics, 132*, 962–965. doi:10.1542/peds.2013-2716

Crisp, J., Ungerer, J. A., & Goodnow, J. J. (1996). The impact of experience on children's understanding of illness. *Journal of Pediatric Psychology, 21*, 57–72. doi:10.1093/jpepsy/21.1.57

Dailor, A. N., & Jacob, S. (2011). Ethically challenging situations reported by school psychologists: implications for training. *Psychology in the Schools, 48*(6), 619–631. doi:10.1002/pits.20574

Dempsey, A. G., MacDonell, K. E., Naar-King, S., Lau, C. Y., & Adolescent Medicine Trials Network for HIV/AIDS Interventions. (2012). Patterns of disclosure among youth who are HIV-positive: A multisite study. *Journal of Adolescent Health, 50*, 315–317. doi:10.1016/j.jadohealth.2011.06.003

Department of Health and Human Services (1990). *Title 45 public welfare, part 1340, code of federal regulations, child abuse and neglect prevention and treatment.* Washington, DC: Government Printing Office. Retrieved from https://www.gpo.gov/fdsys/pkg/CFR-2013-title45-vol4/pdf/CFR-2013-title45-vol4-subtitleB-chapXIII-subchapE.pdf

Diamond, L. M., Bonner, S. B., & Dickenson, J. (2014). The development of sexuality. In M. E. Lamb, A. M. Freud, & R. M. Lerner (Eds.), *Social and emotional development* (The handbook of child psychology and developmental science, 7th ed., Vol. 3). Hoboken, NJ: Wiley.

Dunn, L. B., Nowrangi, M. A., Palmer, B. W., Jeste, D. V., & Saks, E. R. (2006). Assessing decisional capacity for clinical research or treatment: A review of instruments. *American Journal of Psychiatry, 163*(8), 1323–1334. doi:10.1176/ajp.2006.163.8.1323

Edwards, W. M., & Coleman, E. (2004). Defining sexual health: A descriptive overview. *Archives of Sexual Behavior, 33*(3), 189–195. doi:10.1023/B:ASEB.0000026619.95734.d5

Eiser, C., Davies, H., Jenney, M., & Glaser, A. (2005). Mother's attitudes to the randomized controlled trial (RCT): The case of acute lymphoblastic leukemia (ALL) in children. *Child: Care, Health and Development, 31*, 517–523. doi:10.1111/j.1365-2214.2005.00538.x

English, A., Bass, L., Boyle, A. D., & Eshragh, F. (2010). *State minor consent laws: A summary* (3rd ed.). Chapel Hill, North Carolina: Center for Adolescent Health & the Law. doi:10.1016/j.clinthera.2013.11.001

Farmer, P. (2004). *Pathologies of power: Health, human rights, and the new war on the poor.* Los Angeles, CA: University of California Press.

Field, M. J., & Behrman, R. E. (2004). *Ethical conduct of clinical research involving children.* Washington DC: Institute of Medicine.

Fielden, S. J., Chapman, G. E., & Cadell, S. (2011). Managing stigma in adolescent HIV: Silence, secrets and sanctioned spaces. *Culture, Health & Sexuality, 13*(3), 267–281. doi:10.1080/13691058.2010.525665

Fisher, C. B. (1999). *Relational ethics and research with vulnerable populations.* In *Reports on research involving persons with mental disorders that may affect decision-making capacity* (Vol. 2, pp. 29–49). Commissioned Papers by the National Bioethics Advisory Commission. Rockville, MD: National Bioethics Advisory Commission. Retrieved August 1, 2015, from http://www.bioethics.gov/reports/past_commissions/nbac_mental2.pdf

Fisher, C. B. (2000). Relational ethics in psychological research: One feminist's journey. In M. M. Brabeck (Ed), *Practicing feminist ethics in psychology*: *Psychology of women book series* (pp. 125–142). Washington, DC, US: American Psychological Association. doi:10.1037/10343-006

Fisher, C. B. (2002). Participant consultation: Ethical insights into parental permission and confidentiality procedures for policy relevant research with youth. In R. M. Lerner, F. Jacobs, & D. Wertlieb (Eds.), *Handbook of applied developmental science* (Vol. 4, pp. 371–396). Thousand Oaks, CA: Sage. Also in R. M. Lerner, F. Jacobs, & D. Wertlieb (Eds.) (2005), *Applied developmental science*: *An advanced textbook* (pp. 113–138). Thousand Oaks, CA: Sage.

Fisher, C. B. (2003a). A goodness-of-fit ethic for informed consent to research involving persons with mental retardation and developmental disabilities. *Mental retardation and developmental disabilities research reviews, 9*, 27–31. PMID: 12587135. doi:10.1002/mrdd.10052

Fisher, C. B. (2003b). Adolescent and parent perspectives on ethical issues in youth drug use and suicide survey research. *Ethics & Behavior, 13*(4), 303–332. PMID: 15000093. doi:10.1207/S15327019EB1304_1

Fisher, C. B. (2005). Commentary: SES, ethnicity and goodness-of-fit in Clinician–parent communication during pediatric cancer trials. *Journal of Pediatric Psychology, 30*, 232–234. doi:10.1093/jpepsy/jsi033

Fisher, C. B. (2013). Confidentiality and disclosure in non-intervention adolescent risk research. *Applied Developmental Science, 17*(2), 88–93. doi:10.1080/10888691.2013.775915

Fisher, C. B. (2014). Multicultural ethics in professional psychology practice, consulting, and training. In F. T. Leong (Ed.), *APA handbook of multicultural psychology, Vol. 2: Applications and training* (pp. 35–57). American Psychological Association: Washington, DC. doi:10.1037/14187-003

Fisher, C. B. (2015). Enhancing the responsible conduct of sexual health prevention research across global and local contexts: Training for evidence-based research ethics. *Ethics and Behavior, 25*(2), 87–96. doi:10.1080/10508422.2014.948956

Fisher, C. B. (2017). *Decoding the ethics code: A practical guide for psychologists* (4th ed.). Los Angeles, CA: Sage Publications.

Fisher, C. B., Arbeit, M. R., Dumont, M. S., Macapagal, K., & Mustanski, B. (2016). Self-consent for HIV prevention research involving sexual and gender minority youth reducing barriers through evidence-based ethics. *Journal of Empirical Research on Human Research Ethics, 11* (1), 3–14. doi:10.1177/1556264616633963

Fisher, C. B., Busch-Rossnagel, N. B., Jopp, D. S., & Brown, J. L. (2012). Applied developmental science, social justice and socio-political well-being. *Applied Developmental Science, 16*, 54–64. doi:10.1080/10888691.2012.642786

Fisher, C. B., & Goodman, S. J. (2009). Goodness-of-fit ethics for non-intervention research involving dangerous and illegal behaviors. In D. Buchanan, C. B. Fisher, & L. Gable (Eds.), *Research with high-risk populations: Balancing science, ethics, and law* (pp. 25–46). Washington, DC: APA Books.

Fisher, C. B., Hatashita-Wong, M., & Isman, L. (1999). Ethical and legal issues. *Developmental issues in the clinical treatment of children*, 470–486.

Fisher, C. B., Hoagwood, K., Boyce, C., Duster, T., Frank, D. A., Grisso, T., … & Zayas, L. H. (2002). Research ethics for mental health science involving ethnic minority children and youths. *American Psychologist, 57*(12), 1024. doi:10.1037/0003 066X.57.12.1024

Fisher, C. B., Jackson, J. J., & Villarruel, F. A. (1997). The study of ethnic minority children and youth in the United States. *Theoretical Models of Human Development, 1*.

Fisher, C. B., & Masty, J. K. (2006). A goodness-of-fit ethic for informed consent to pediatric cancer research. In R. T. Brown (Ed.), *Comprehensive handbook of childhood cancer and sickle cell disease* (pp. 205–217). New York: Oxford University Press.

Fisher, C. B., & Mustanski, B. (2014). Reducing health disparities and enhancing the responsible conduct of research involving LGBT youth. *Hastings Center Report, 44*(Suppl. 4), S28–S31. doi:10.1002/hast.367

Fisher, C. B., & Ragsdale, K. (2006). A goodness-of-fit ethics for multicultural research. In J. Trimble and C. B. Fisher (Eds.), *The handbook of ethical research with ethnocultural populations and communities* (pp. 3–26). Thousand Oaks, CA: Sage. doi:10.4135/9781412986168.n1

Fisher, C. B., & Wallace, S. A. (2000). Through the community looking glass: Re-evaluating the ethical and policy implications of research on adolescent risk and psychopathology. *Ethics and Behavior, 33*(4), 470–487. doi:10.1207/s15327019eb1002_01

Frerich, E. A., Garcia, C. M., Long, S. K., Lechner, K. E., Lust, K., & Eisenberg, M. E. (2012). Health care reform and young adults' access to sexual health care: an exploration of potential confidentiality implications of the affordable care act. *American Journal of Public Health, 102* (2), 1818–1821. doi:10.2105/AJPH.2012.300857

Geller, G., Tambor, E. S., & Bernhardt, B. A. (2003). Informed consent for enrolling minors in genetic susceptibility research: A qualitative study of at-risk children's and parents' views about children's role in decision-making. *Journal of Adolescent Health, 32*, 260–271. doi:10.1016/S1054-139X(02)00459-7

Gilbert, A. L., Knopf, A. S., Fortenberry, J. D., Hosek, S. G., Kapogiannis, B. G., & Zimet, G. D. (2015). Adolescent self-consent for biomedical human immunodeficiency virus prevention research. *Journal of Adolescent Health, 57*(1), 113–119. doi:10.1016/j.jadohealth.2015.03.017

Gilbert, A. L., Rickert, V. I., & Aalsma, M. C. (2014). Clinical conversations about health: the impact of confidentiality in preventive adolescent care. *Journal of Adolescent Health, 55*(5), 672–677. doi:10.1016/j.jadohealth.2014.05.016

Gillespie, S. (2017). Epidemiology of Pediatric HIV Infection. In T. Chenneville (Ed), *A Clinical Guide to Pediatric HIV*, 1–14. Dordrecht: Springer.

Gilligan, C. (1982). *In a different voice*. Cambridge, MA: Harvard University Press.

Griffith, D. M., Mason, M., Yonas, M., Eng, E., Jeffries, V., Plihcik, S., et al. (2007). Dismantling institutional racism: Theory and action. *American Journal of Community Psychology, 39*(3–4), 381–392. doi:10.1007/s10464-007-9117-0

Grisso, T., & Appelbaum, P. S. (1998). *Assessing competence to consent to treatment*. New York: Oxford University Press.

Grisso, T., Appelbaum, P. S., & Hill-Fotouhi, C. (1997). The MacCAT–T: A clinical tool to assess patients' capacities to make treatment decisions. *Psychiatric Services, 48*, 1415–1419. doi:10.1176/ps.48.11.1415

Grodin, M. A., & Burton, L. A. (1988). Context and process in medical ethics: The contribution of family-systems theory. *Family Systems Medicine, 6*(4), 421–438. doi:10.1037/h0089755

Grossman, J. M., Tracy, A. J., Charmaraman, L., Ceder, I., & Erkut, S. (2014). Protective effects of middle school comprehensive sex education with family involvement. *Journal of School Health, 84*, 739–747. doi:10.1111/josh.12199

Guttmacher Institute. (2015). State policies in brief as of June 1, 2015: Minors access to STI services. Accessed from http://www.guttmacher.org/statecenter/spibs/spib_MASS.pdf

Hall, D. E., Prochazka, A. V., & Fink, A. S. (2012). Informed consent for clinical treatment. *Canadian Medical Association Journal, 184*(5), 533–540. doi:10.1017/S0009840X00087515

Hein, I. M., De Vries, M. C., Troost, P. W., Meynen, G., Van Goudoever, J. B., & Lindauer, R. J. L. (2015). Informed consent instead of assent is appropriate in children from the age of twelve: Policy implications of new findings on children's competence to consent to clinical research. *BMC Medical Ethics, 16*(1), 76. doi:10.1186/s12910-015-0067-z

Hennan, M. R., Dornbusch, S. M., Herron, M. C., & Herting, J. R. (1997). The influence of family regulation, connection, and psychological autonomy on six measures of adolescent functioning. *Journal of Adolescent Research, 12*, 34–67. doi:10.1177/0743554897121004

Kodish, E., Eder, M., Noll, R. B., Ruccione, K., Lange, B., Angiolillo, A., … & Drotar, D. (2004). Communication of randomization in childhood leukemia trials. *JAMA, 291*(4), 470–475. doi:10.1001/jama.291.4.470

Kohlberg, L. (1984). *The psychology of moral development: The nature and validity of moral stages. Essays on moral development* (Vol. 2). New York: Harper & Row.

Krieger, N. (2012). Methods for the scientific study of discrimination and health: An ecosocial approach. *American Journal of Public Health, 102*(5), 936–944. doi:10.2105/AJPH.2011.300544

Kunin, H. (1997). Ethical issues in pediatric life-threatening illness: Dilemmas of consent, assent, and communication. *Ethics and Behavior, 7*, 43–57. doi:10.1207/s15327019eb0701_4

Kupst, M. J., Patenaude, A. F., Walco, G. A., & Sterling, C. (2003). Clinical trials in pediatric cancer: Parental perspectives on informed consent. *Journal of Pediatric Hematology and Oncology, 25*, 787–790. doi:10.1097/00043426-200310000-00009

Lehman, J. S., Carr, M. H., Nichol, A. J., Ruisanchez, A., Knight, D. W., Langford, A. E., … & Mermin, J. H. (2014). Prevalence and public health implications of state laws that criminalize potential HIV exposure in the United States. *AIDS and Behavior, 18*, 997–1006. doi:10.1007/s10461-014-0724-0

Makadon, H. J., Mayer, K. H., Potter, J., & Goldhammer, H. (2015). *The Fenway guide to Lesbian, gay, bisexual, and transgender health* (2nd ed.). ACP Press.

Marhefka, S. L., Valentin, C. R., Pinto, R. M., Demetriou, N., Wiznia, A., & Mellins, C. (2011). "I feel like I'm carrying a weapon". Information and motivations related to sexual risk among girls with perinatally acquired HIV. *AIDS Care, 23*, 1321–1328. doi:10.1080/09540121.2010.532536

Marshall, P. A., Magtanong, R. V., Leek, A. C., Hizlan, S., Yamokoshi, A. D., & Kodish, E. D. (2012). Negotiating decisions during informed consent for pediatric phase I oncology trials. *Journal of Empirical Research on Human Resource Ethics., 7*(2), 51–59. doi:10.1525/jer.2012.7.2.51

Masty, J., & Fisher, C. B. (2008). A goodness of fit approach to parent permission and child assent pediatric intervention research. *Ethics and Behavior, 13*, 139–160. doi:10.1080/10508420802063897

Masty, J. K., Fisher, C. B., Cruz-Arrieta, E., & Reisman, J. (2006). Adolescent involvement in cancer research decisions: A pilot study. Poster session presented at the 2006 American Psychological Association convention, New Orleans, LA.

McCabe, M. A. (1996). Involving children and adolescents in medical decision making: Developmental and clinical considerations. *Journal of Pediatric Psychology, 21*(4), 505–516. doi:10.1093/jpepsy/21.4.505

McKee, M. D., O'Sullivan, L. F., & Weber, C. M. (2006). Perspectives on confidential care for adolescent girls. *The Annals of Family Medicine, 4*(6), 519–526. doi:10.1370/afm.601

Meaux, J. B., & Bell, P. L. (2001). Balancing recruitment and protection: Children as research subjects. *Issues in comprehensive pediatric nursing, 24*(4), 241–251. doi:10.1080/014608601753260335

Mellins, C. A., Brackis-Cott, E., Dolezal, C., & Abrams, E. (2004). The role of psychosocial and family factors in adherence to antiretroviral treatment in human immunodeficiency-infected children. *Pediatric Infectious Disease Journal, 23*(11), 1035–1041. doi:10.1097/01.inf.0000143646.15240.ac

Melton, G. B. (1999). Parents and children: Legal reform to facilitate children's participation. *American Psychologist, 54*, 935–944. doi:10.1037/h0088201

Miller, V. A., Drotar, D., Burant, C., & Kodish, E. (2005). Clinician–parent communication during informed consent for pediatric leukemia trials. *Journal of Pediatric Psychology, 30*, 219–229. doi:10.1093/jpepsy/jsi032

Mitchell, C. W., Disque, J. G., & Robertson, P. (2002). When parents want to know: responding to parental demands for confidential information. *Professional School Counseling, 6*(2), 156–161.

Morris, R. J., & Mather, N. (Eds.). (2007). *Evidence-based interventions for students with learning and behavioral challenges*. Oxford, UK: Taylor & Francis.

Mustanski, B. (2011). Ethical and regulatory issues with conducting sexuality research with LGBT adolescents: A call to action for a scientifically informed approach. *Archives of Sexual Behavior, 40*(4), 673–686. doi:10.1007/s10508-011-9745-1

Mustanski, B., & Fisher, C. B. (2016). HIV rates are increasing in gay/bisexual teens: IRB barriers to research must be resolved to bend the curve. *American Journal of Preventive Medicine,*. doi:10.1016/j.amepre.2016.02.026

National Center for Transgender Equality. (2012). *Transgender sexual and reproductive health: Unmet needs and barriers to care*. Washington, DC: TransEquality.org.

National Commission for the Protection of Human Subjects of Biomedical and Behavioral Research. (1979). *The belmont report: Ethical principles and guidelines for the protection of human subjects of research*. Washington, DC: Department of Health, Education, and Welfare.

Oetzel, K. B., & Scherer, D. G. (2003). Therapeutic engagement with adolescents in psychotherapy. *Psychotherapy: Theory, Research, Practice, Training, 40*(3), 215–225. doi:10.1037/0033-3204.40.3.215

Prilleltensky, I. (2003). Understanding, resisting, and overcoming oppression: Toward psychopolitical validity. *American Journal of Community Psychology, 31*(1–2), 195–201. doi:10.1023/A:1023043108210

Pustilnik, A. C., & Henry, L. M. (2012). Adolescent medical decision making and the law of the horse. *Journal of Health Care Law & Policy, 15*(1), 1–14.

Richardson, J., & Schuster, M. A. (2004). *Everything you never wanted your kids to know about sex (but were afraid they'd ask): The secrets to surviving your child's sexual development from birth to the teens*. Harmony Books.

Ringheim, K. (2007). Ethical and human rights perspectives on providers' obligation to ensure adolescents' rights to privacy. *Studies in Family Planning, 38*(4), 245–252. doi:10.1111/j.1728-4465.2007.00137.x

Ross, L. F. (1997). Health care decision-making by children: Is it in their best interest? *Hastings Center Report, 27*(6), 41–46. doi:10.2307/3527717

Rothstein, M. A., & Talbott, M. K. (2006). Compelled disclosure of health information: Protecting against the greatest potential threat to privacy. *The Journal of the American Medical Association, 295*(24), 2882–2885. doi:10.1001/jama.295.24.2882

Ruggeri, A., Gummerum, M., & Hanoch, Y. (2014). Braving difficult choices alone: Children's and adolescents' medical decision making. *PLoS One, 9*(8), e103287. doi:10.1371/journal.pone.0103287

Sedlander, E., Brindis, C. D., Bausch, S. H., & Tebb, K. P. (2015). Options for assuring access to confidential care for adolescents and young adults in an explanation of benefits environment. *Journal of Adolescent Health, 56*, 7–9. doi:10.1016/j.jadohealth.2014.10.262

Simoni, J. M., Montgomery, A., Martin, E., New, M., Demas, P. A., & Rana, S. (2007). Adherence to antiretroviral therapy for HIV infection: A qualitative systematic review with recommendations for research and clinical management. *Pediatrics, 119*(6), 1371–1383. doi:10.1542/peds.2006-1232

Taylor, L., & Adelman, H. S. (1989). Reframing the confidentiality dilemma to work in children's best interest. *Professional Psychology: Research and Practice, 20*, 79–83. doi:10.1037/0735-7028.20.2.79

Thomas, N., Murray, E., & Rogstad, K. E. (2006). Confidentiality is essential if young people are to access sexual health services. *International Journal of STD and AIDS, 17*(8), 525–529. doi:10.1258/095646206778145686

Varni, J. W., Katz, E. R., Colgrove, R., & Dolgin, M. (1996). Family functioning predictors of adjustment in children with newly diagnosed cancer: A prospective analysis. *Journal of Child Psychology and Psychiatry and Allied Disciplines, 37*, 321–328. doi:10.1111/j.1469-7610.1996.tb01409.x

Vaught, S. E., & Castagno, A. E. (2008). "I don't think I'm a racist": Critical race theory, teacher attitudes, and structural racism. *Race Ethnicity and Education, 11*(2), 95–113. doi:10.1080/13613320802110217

Walker, N. E. (2002). Meaningful participation of minors with HIV/AIDS in decisions regarding medical treatment: Balancing the rights of children, parents, and the state. *International Journal of Law and Psychiatry, 25*(3), 271–297. doi:10.1016/S0160-2527(02)00106-1

Weisz, J. R., & Hawley, K. M. (2002). Developmental factors in the treatment of adolescents. *Journal of Consulting and Clinical Psychology, 70*, 21–43. doi:10.1037/0022-006X.70.1.21

Weithorn, L. A. (2006). The legal contexts of forensic assessment of children and families. In Sparta, S. N., & Koocher, G. P. (Eds.) *Forensic mental health assessment of children and adolescents*. Oxford, New York. doi:10.1093/med:psych/9780195145847.003.0002

Wiener, L., Mellins, C. A., Marhefka, S., & Battles, H. B. (2007). Disclosure of an HIV diagnosis to children: History, current research, and future directions. *Journal of Developmental and Behavioral Pediatrics, 28*(2), 155–166. doi:10.1097/01.DBP.0000267570.87564.cd

Young, A. J., Kim, L., Li, S., Baker, J. N., Schmidt, M., Camp, J. W., et al. (2010). Agency and communication challenges in discussions of informed consent in pediatric cancer research. *Qualitative Health Research, 20*(5), 623–643. doi:10.1177/1049732310361467

Chapter 10
Cultural Considerations for Pediatric HIV Research and Practice

Guitele J. Rahill, Manisha Joshi and Celia M. Lescano

Introduction

While there has been a global decline in new cases of the human immunodeficiency virus (HIV) and of the acquired immune deficiency syndrome (AIDS), HIV and AIDS have had a devastating impact on the physical and mental health of individuals regardless of race, nationality, gender or chronological age. Since we first became aware of HIV/AIDS, more than 34 million people have died from complications related to the virus, both as a consequence of its effect on the body and as a consequence of disparate access to HIV knowledge, testing, and treatment (UNAIDS 2010; World Health Organization [WHO] 2011). A tenth of these were children younger than 15 years. In the United States (US), approximately 21% of persons who acquired the virus were between the ages of 13 and 24, and the preponderance of these was cultural minorities (i.e., sexual minorities such as gay and bisexual males and racial minorities such as males of African descent). Culture is among the factors that either facilitate or hinder access to interventions ranging from education about the virus and its consequences, to treatment and a reduced level of the virus in the blood. Although we emphasize race, ethnicity, chronological age and HIV status in the present work, we recognize that culture is not always observable or subject to a biological or mental health diagnosis. In fact, culture is elusive, often presenting as minimally discernible cues that inform

G.J. Rahill (✉) · M. Joshi · C.M. Lescano
University of South Florida, Tampa, FL, USA
e-mail: gjrahill@usf.edu

M. Joshi
e-mail: manishaj@usf.edu

C.M. Lescano
e-mail: lescano@usf.edu

T. Chenneville (ed.), *A Clinical Guide to Pediatric HIV*,
DOI 10.1007/978-3-319-49704-4_10

whether or not the client or targeted population is operating from a base of power or marginality.

In the present work, we highlight youth as a minority culture and consider the mental health aspects of youth who are members of racial and ethnic minority groups and who also receive a diagnosis of HIV/AIDS. We do so because racial and cultural/ethnic minority youth in the US, youth who reside in resource-limited settings and youth from the latter nations who immigrate to the US have disparate access to treatment for HIV/AIDS and to evidence-based mental health interventions compared to youth in developed countries (Grelotti 2013). We include a discussion of culture, including the culture of youth, and review the differential impact of HIV among cultural groups in the US (e.g., African-Americans and subgroups, and Hispanics and subgroups), as well as the culture of living with HIV. Within that discussion, we emphasize cultural and ethnic minority youth in the US and youth who live in developing countries, (i.e., the differential impact of HIV among youth in the US compared to youth who live in developing countries). Since even a diagnosis of HIV can be traumatic and stigmatizing to the patient and to significant others and can evoke bullying behaviors as well as stigmatizing and discriminatory attitudes, we discuss mental health concerns among populations of youth with HIV, highlighting issues of global relevance for youth with HIV who are also in need of mental health services—for example, the disparate access to mental health services in the US and around the globe. Following, we review the latest research in the aforementioned areas and offer recommendations for working with cultural groups in the context of cultural competence, cultural humility and ethical practice as clinicians and researchers.

Culture

Culture includes how persons act, how they react and how they interact in the various contexts in which they live and with the various systems of which they are a part. Culture includes not only race, age and ethnicity or disease status, but also geographical context or place, religion and spirituality, sexuality, gender identification, physical and mental ability versus disability, poverty versus financial power, mental health status, and cultural taboos. Purnell and Palaunka (2003) include in their definition of culture:

> … The totality of socially transmitted behavioral patterns, arts, beliefs, values, customs, lifeways … and thought characteristics … that guide worldview and decision making … explicit or implicit–primarily learned and transmitted within the family … shared by most members of the culture–emergent phenomena that change in response to global phenomena … (p. 3).

Purnell and Palaunka's definition of culture acknowledges internal (e.g., beliefs, values), external (e.g., contexts and observable customs) and intersecting (e.g., shared values, artifacts) aspects of culture.

Geographical context and place are aspects of cultures that affect coexisting experiences of race, ethnicity, sexual or gender identity, religious or spiritual affiliation and age as well as mental health or mental disorder. The geographical context or cultural enclave in which a person lives can shape the physical, affective and financial experiences of being diagnosed with HIV/AIDS, and can evoke tremendous financial, personal, interpersonal, biological and mental consequences on the person diagnosed, on caregivers, and on those who share the context. For example, in recent years, the National Institute on Minority Health and Health Disparities of the National Institutes of Health (NIMHD/NIH) included residents of rural regions of America as cultural minorities by virtue of the geographical, socioeconomic and cultural barriers they experience to positive health outcomes, and in light of the health disparities they experience in relation to urban residents, e.g., health infrastructure (NIMHD/NIH 2011).

Adding to the influence of geographical place or cultural enclave in which one resides, values, beliefs and norms that dictate what constitutes normal as opposed to abnormal behaviors can result in the association of HIV/AIDS with certain sexual taboos and thus with members of sexual or racial minority groups; for example, in rural areas of the southern US, as in India, HIV/AIDS still evokes the perception that the person may have been sexually promiscuous or may have engaged in homosexual behavior, both of which are cultural taboos. Such cultural taboos also affect whether or not clients seek testing and treatment.

Being a member of a racial or cultural minority culture can also determine whether an individual has access to good health or to the treatment of diseases, since culture is linked to socioeconomic status and socioeconomic status contributes to health disparities for racial and cultural minorities in relation to non-minorities, but the region of the globe in which a person lives, a person's age, and whether or not a person is male or female can also contribute to health disparities. As an example, between 2009 and 2011, there was a 32% decline in the number of children acquiring HIV in the Caribbean, and a 24% decline in new HIV infections among children in Latin America; despite the fact that Latin America enjoys the highest access to antiretroviral therapies of any low- and middle-income areas around the world, that region's women and children have disparate access to treatment compared to men. Youth in non-Spanish speaking countries of Latin America and the Caribbean (e.g., Haiti) have the least access to care (Garcia et al. 2014).

In addition to the association of racial or cultural minority status with health access, cultural minority status and disease status (in contrast to cultural majority status or the experience of positive health) can contribute to how clients view themselves. And, the manner in which clients view themselves results, in part, from how we label clients and from how we as clinicians and researchers interact with them. The way in which we view and treat clients ultimately influences how they experience the disease and their health outcomes. In addition, the place or environment which shapes the experiences of cultural minorities as they observe, interact and speak with those who share their geographical and neighborhood milieus can either contribute to positive health outcomes or result in morbidity.

Culture of Youth

The National Institutes of Health (NIH) classifies children or youth as individuals under the age of 18. Individuals within the 10–24 age range contend with developing intimate relationships and gaining close friends and avoiding isolation from peers and alienation from society (NIH 2015). The NIH includes a subcategory of youth who are either at risk for or who use drugs, who are at risk for HIV/AIDS, who are living with HIV/AIDS regardless of how they became infected with the virus (i.e., perinatally or behaviorally acquired) and who have lost a loved one or both parents to AIDS-related complications.

Pediatric HIV/AIDS and the mental health of culturally diverse youth are interrelated issues that are significant for several reasons. First, the varied developmental rates and capacities of persons classified as youth can cause them to experience difficulties making good health promoting decisions and engaging in safer sex behaviors. Second, conflicts emerge during this developmental time frame as youth strive to take social norms into account on the one hand, and on the other hand, to conform to normative roles and behaviors adopted by their peers. Thus, these individuals are vulnerable as they attempt to develop a stable identity and to manage confusion about their niche in their social environment. For youth, then, HIV/AIDS is both a risk factor and a condition which has both medical and psychological consequences, especially for those who live in social environments where they are exposed to psychological or behavioral risk factors for HIV/AIDS (i.e., absence of stable and consistent caregivers/homes, exposure to drugs and or violence). Pediatric HIV/AIDS and the mental health of culturally diverse youth are also important because engagement in the whole spectrum of HIV care is often context dependent and dependent on race, ethnicity and other minority classes.

Differential Impact of HIV/AIDS Among Youth Globally

In 2012, the Centers for Disease Control and Prevention (CDC) reported that only about one quarter of the 1.1 million people living with HIV/AIDS (PLWHA) in the US "have their virus under control—and that African-Americans and young people are least likely to receive ongoing care and effective treatment". (CDC 2012b, p. 1). In that same report, the CDC identified five central phases of HIV care: (1) testing/diagnosis, (2) linkage to care for seropositive persons, (3) long-term retention in care, (4) access and use of antiretroviral medications and (5) achievement of viral suppression (i.e., the seropositive individual is healthy and the risk of transmitting the virus is significantly reduced) (CDC 2012b). Significantly, Flores (2010) had noted prior to the 2012 report from the CDC that there were inconsistencies and errors even in the methods used to assess HIV and mental health disparities for racial and ethnic minority youth, and in methods applied to the evaluation of health disparities across the cascade of health and health care, regardless of the type of disease or the nature of the ailment (i.e., chronicity and the extent to which the disease is life threatening). Gardner and colleagues (2013) also underscored the need for fully engaging PLWHA in care, because partial or non-engagement is a critical risk for HIV transmission.

More recently, the Agency for Healthcare Research and Quality Report (AHRQ) on National Health Disparities (United States Department of Health and Human Services 2013, 2015a) confirmed that racial and ethnic minority youth and their families who reside in the US receive poorer care than majority peers and highlighted the increased needs of persons who have physical or mental disabilities, especially youth with special health care needs. However, these disparities in access to care are not restricted to the US.

Recent years have shown a decrease in maternal-to-child transmission of HIV (United States Department of Health and Human Services [DHHS] 2015). In resource-poor settings, there remain disparities in access to HIV treatment for youth in developing countries compared to those in low- to middle-income countries. One example is Haiti, which still has the highest prevalence of HIV in the western hemisphere (United Nations Children's Fund [UNICEF] 2010) although it has seen a decline from 12 to 2.2% in the past decade. There has also been a decline in mother-to-child transmission of the virus in Haiti as a consequence of availing pregnant women who are HIV seropositive with HIV medicines during labor and delivery and providing a pre-planned cesarean section approximately two weeks before a woman's scheduled delivery date (Theodore et al. 2011); however, poverty and hunger continue to impact the general health of women of child-bearing age and of children in Haiti, such that inadequate nutrition can reduce the benefits of ARVs. Indeed, Martinez and Chakraborty (2014) submit that socioeconomic factors in disadvantaged communities are key factors which prevent racial and ethnic minorities to benefit from the more modern and potent antiretrovirals (ARVs); they maintained that socioeconomic factors in disadvantaged and underserved communities contribute to the propagation of the virus, to the physical and mental health status of those who are seropositive and to the progression of the virus to AIDS and even death. As a remedy, they urged a holistic approach that takes into account the whole person and not just the virus and its attending consequences. Culture is a factor which must be taken into account if we are to take a holistic approach, as culture can be a protective factor or an obstacle to successful negotiation of all the phases of care.

Cultural Barriers to Mental Health and HIV Testing

For Latino, African-American and Haitian youth in the US, cultural differences can serve as protective as well as risk factors for HIV/AIDS and mental health or disorder (Lescano et al. 2009). Nevertheless, for youth who are cultural minorities, in the US or abroad, non-adherence to treatment and resistance to treatment are compounded barriers that pose significant challenges throughout the spectrum of care. For cultural minority youth, the obstacles often begin with energy invested in striving to survive culturally and psychologically from assaults targeting their differences. When in the US, youth who are born of racially and ethnically diverse immigrants can experience acculturation stressors, stigma associated with being from another country or from experiencing language barriers along with discrimination that can stem from having multiple minority statuses associated with race, ethnicity, language, sexual and gender identity and even having their entire nationality associated with being HIV carriers (Portes and Rumbaut 2001; Antoine et al. 1990; Farmer 2006; Rumbaut and Portes 2001). In addition, racial and ethnic minority youth are often not seen at local mental health venues due to a metaphor of mental health problems within a family as "dirty laundry" that should neither be aired (i.e., disclosed to others outside the family) nor washed in public (i.e., handled or resolved with non-family members). Furthermore, non-ethnic and even co-ethnic clinicians may at times confound the ability to speak a client's native language with cultural or clinical competence, obfuscating the salient within-cultural values and beliefs that may translate into health decisions and practices which in turn can inform risk and treatment.

Cultural Beliefs and Health Practices in Relation to HIV Risk

Cultural beliefs can shape health practices, which may increase risk for HIV. An important example of the impact of cultural health beliefs and practices on HIV and mental health outcomes is from the 2014 HIV outbreak in a rural Cambodian village, in which hundreds of people were infected via non-medical injections by a respected village injectionist. That situation also underscores the threat of unsafe injections in developing countries, where ethnic immigrants sometimes seek out traditional healers to overcome cultural and financial barriers to health care (Rahill and Rice 2010). Naturally, there was a great deal of distress among directly and indirectly impacted persons in that Cambodian town, including children and adolescents who were brought to the injectionist for treatment by well-meaning caregivers (Fuller 2015). Thus, we see the potential impact of cultural beliefs and traditional health practices on HIV risk, and unanticipated risks and the accompanying stressors can in turn impact mental health and mental disorders.

Mental Disorder and Mental Health

When a diagnosis of disease such as HIV/AIDS is introduced in pediatric populations, whatever the residential or global enclave and whatever the racial or ethnic classification, stigma (negative beliefs and attitudes about the condition) and associated emotional distress or mental disorders can occur. The fifth edition of the Diagnostic and Statistical Manual of Mental Disorders defines mental disorders as:

> A syndrome characterized by clinically significant disturbance in an individual's cognition, emotion regulation, or behavior that reflects a dysfunction in the psychological, biological, or developmental processes underlying mental functioning ... usually associated with significant distress in social, occupational, or other important activities (American Psychiatric Association [APA], 2013, p. 20).

Pertinent to pediatric clients who are members of racial and ethnic minority cultural groups, culturally consonant social, religious and sexual responses are not classified as mental disorders, except in cases where the dysfunction stems from the individual. Nevertheless, when working with pediatric populations who are members of racial and ethnic minority groups, clinicians need to be aware that caregivers' culturally embedded beliefs about the nature and origin of HIV/AIDS, mental illness and the hierarchy of resort they proceed through when they are engaged in health seeking can differ from that of the youth; the child or adolescent's ascribed roles based on notions of gender and/or power within the particular culture or subculture can translate into health or disease and can exacerbate distress associated with the diagnosis and prevent treatment seeking and/or adherence to treatment (Rahill and Rice 2010). This is particularly important as roles and notions of power versus disenfranchisement convey strong messages regarding the ability or inability of children to contribute to decisions about their health and mental health care.

Additional factors that impact the mental health of cultural minority youth include HIV stigma, the stigma of having mental health issues and the subjective experience of having or not having access to care across the different stages of development. These all can impact the ability of racial, ethnic and age minority youth to access and benefit from HIV care and prevention and from the associated mental health struggles. That is, ethnic or racial minority youth who are already stigmatized by virtue of their being members of minority groups may resist identifying with an additional stigmatized group (i.e., PLWHA). Consequently, these youth may not risk disclosure to family members or friends who might influence them to engage fully in the cascade of care. Internalized stigma surrounding other minority statuses in addition to taking on an additional HIV diagnosis/classification can compound mental distress and contribute to suicidal ideation or behaviors, particularly among youth such as Haitians who were previously classified as HIV carriers (Antoine et al. 1990).

Culturally Relevant Issues for Clinicians

The aforementioned discussion underscores several issues that are of relevance for clinicians who engage and treat pediatric populations who are HIV positive and also experience mental health issues. First, even hearing about the global decline in new cases of HIV/AIDS can lead to HIV complacency, especially among youth who often erroneously feel as if they are immune from certain conditions. Second, the fear of disclosing HIV status to relatives and peers in order to avoid bullying and discrimination can lead to HIV transmission on the one hand or to a barrier in developing age-appropriate emotional and sexual intimacy on the other. Third, family dynamics can hinder treatment seeking and disclosure—for example, when protective parents attempting to shelter their children from societal stigma and shame encourage them not to disclose. Fourth, clinicians' assumptions that confound speaking the language of the co-ethnic or co-racial client group with cultural competence can result in more harm than good for the pediatric HIV client. This can be the case in second-generation clinicians, i.e., children of first-generation immigrants who may speak their clients' language semantically, but for whom their clients' subtle cultural, affective, linguistic and behavioral nuances are not always evident. Moreover, second-generation clinicians who are acculturated to the host American culture and who hold perceptions that culturally non-normative health beliefs and practices of their co-ethnic group members are deviant can hinder the process of developing rapport and of ethical and effective care. Thus, it is important for clinicians, whatever their original language or their racial or ethnic backgrounds, to be aware of as well as manage their personal biases. In so doing, the focus of service and treatment will be to harness clients' personal and cultural strengths and to disentangle cultural myths and stereotypes from different beliefs and practices that might indeed serve the client as protective factors.

Future Directions for Research and Practice

Prior to offering recommendations for future directions, we remind the reader that the context for the present work is that over the past three decades, minority populations have shown a 15% increase (from 25% to almost 40% of the US population), with Asian and Latino immigrants in the US being expected to experience increases due to new immigrants and high birth rates (Lum 2011). However, there remains the need to understand diversity in all its forms, not just racial and ethnic diversity. There is also the need to increase cultural competence if we are to achieve gains in delivering effective interventions and in conducting high-impact research.

Clearly, the culturally relevant challenges for clinicians and researchers underscore the need for cultural competence. Lum (2011) defines cultural competence as a process which involves the informed and mutual consent of both the clinician and the client in a conscious collaboration to explore, learn and share each others' experiences as impacted by race, ethnicity, sexual or religious identity as well as other minority or majority status. As applied to this work, cultural competence pertains to the clinician's viewing an HIV diagnosis through the cultural lenses of the client, to view him or herself as a helper or facilitator whose roles include the management of personal biases and the development of interventions and policies which benefit youth who are culturally and ethnically diverse.

Moving beyond efforts to achieve the elusive cultural competence to practicing cultural humility through critical consciousness is essential for clinicians and researchers who work in all facets of pediatric HIV and pediatric psychology. Cultural humility involves acquiring knowledge of clients' diversity and allowing that knowledge to impact the clinician's or researcher's personal awareness in such a manner that the client is empowered and that there is a positive change or outcome that benefits the client in a way that is appropriate for the client's cultural context. That is when therapeutic gain occurs and that is when we can be assured that our research is ethical and safely protects our clients. As important, we must not only incorporate culture as a vehicle for testing the applicability of psychological processes or for facilitating uptake of scientifically proven interventions, but we must emphasize how internalized beliefs and attitudes and cultural practices shape HIV risk behaviors as well as psychological processes. That would optimally result in shared meanings between the client/ research participant and the clinician/ researcher.

One useful approach to address pediatric HIV and mental health disparities is to adapt, disseminate and implement evidence-based interventions for diverse cultural groups (e.g., the CDC's Compendium of Evidence-based Interventions) (CDC 2012a). In fact, there is a very useful model to accomplish this process, ADAPT-ITT (Wingood and DiClemente 2008). The ADAPT-ITT model reflects cultural humility in that it incorporates clients, their families and significant others as well as cultural experts and community gatekeepers in all phases of the intervention adaptation. Cultural humility is essential to meeting our ethical responsibilities to our clients, to ourselves, to our colleagues who engage the same populations and to our profession.

Professional and cultural training is needed to help foster clinician/ researcher recognition of the manner in which personal values can impact and may conflict with or accommodate the needs of diverse clients such as a youth living with HIV. Education and training can also help clinicians/researchers develop a clearer understanding of their own cultural beliefs and values in relation to the multiple identities that a racial, religious, ethnic, disabled or sexual minority youth who is also HIV positive may be experiencing. Continuing education can foster the development of more detailed knowledge and understanding of clients' targeted populations' beliefs, traditions and values concerning treatment or participation in research. This, in turn, would help clinicians and researchers to develop useful techniques and appropriate research designs and measures which reflect understanding of the role of culture in the helping or research process (Rahill et al. 2011).

There also is a need to increase clinicians' knowledge of HIV and mental health resources that are available around the globe, even going so far as to share resources in a global network to address pediatric HIV and mental health in the most impacted settings. That involves remaining vigilant for opportunities to intentionally engage and empower researchers from low- to middle-income countries in global partnerships for social science research. Indeed, the National Institute for Child Health and Human Development has funded several such initiatives in the past decade.

Cultural humility underscores involvement of community leaders, gatekeepers and stakeholders as leaders and partners in collaborations. This engagement includes involving HIV-impacted youth, including those who are effectively managing and living with a mental health or HIV diagnosis. It also includes involving families and community gatekeepers in research that examines the interaction among culture, HIV status, mental health status, neighborhood conditions, policies and biological health status (Singer 2012). Finally, clinicians and researchers can acknowledge that HIV and mental health disparities for children are social justice issues that require collaboration between them and families as well as advocacy to combat the oppressive conditions that impede the well-being of diverse populations and communities; we can strive to influence policies which are conducive to positive health outcomes for all youth, regardless of minority or health status (American Academy of Pediatrics 2009).

Conclusion

In summary, as disparities remain with regard to the burden of HIV/AIDS and cultural minority youth around the globe, biological and psychological, as well as cultural, factors often interact to exacerbate negative health outcomes. The takeaway message from the CDC, from the AHRQ and from our own ethical mandates as clinicians, is that individuals must be engaged throughout all the phases of HIV care if we are to significantly diminish the impact of HIV/AIDS nationally and internationally (CDC 2012b). No longer are test-and-treat, non-adherence to antiretroviral therapy and antiretroviral medication resistance the primary barriers to controlling the HIV epidemic among racial and ethnic minority youth in the US or around the world. Indeed, the CDC suggests that reducing the impact of HIV/AIDS disparities in the US necessitates progress in serving individuals throughout the spectrum or cascade of care, with emphasis on racial and age minorities such as youth and the elderly. Moreover, Foy and Perrin (2010) suggested the need for partnerships with professionals from other disciplines (e.g., social workers, psychiatrists, nurses, school personnel, public health professionals, and the criminal justice system). We add that religious leaders, however far outside our cultural norms they may be, should also be engaged, insofar as they are relevant to the particular youth and his or her family. Such an approach, combined with cultural humility, would appear optimal to bring multilevel and multifaceted mental health interventions to cultural minority pediatric populations who bear a diagnosis of HIV.

Annotated Bibliography

American Academy of Pediatrics. (2009). Principles to reduce disparities and promote equity in children's health care. Retrieved from http://www.aap.org/en-us/about-the-aap/Committees-Councils-Sections/Council-on-Community-Pediatrics/Documents/Health_Equity_Principles.pdf

This is a one-page list/summary of principles reflecting the American Academy of Pediatrics' commitment to mitigate health disparities and to enhance health equity for young persons.

Centers for Disease Control and Prevention. (2012). HIV in the United States: The stages of care. Retrieved from http://www.cdc.gov/hiv/pdf/research_mmp_stagesofcare.pdf

This fact sheet from the CDC provides crucial information regarding the more than one million persons living with HIV/AIDS in the United States and highlights that African Americans and youth remain underserved in HIV testing/ diagnosis, care and receipt of treatment and ultimately in suppression of the virus load/ better health.

Fuller, T. (2015). Shock and anger in cambodian village struck with HIV. Retrieved from http://www.nytimes.com/2015/01/20/world/asia/farming-village-in-cambodia-grieves-as-hundreds-learn-they-have-hiv.html?_r=0

Fuller details that injections administered by a cultural healer in Cambodia resulted in adults and youth acquiring HIV/AIDS. It underscores that, like intravenous drug use, unsafe injections that are not self-administered can be HIV vectors. Rahill and colleagues (2010, 2011) introduced this risk based on research with Florida Haitian immigrants.

United States Department of Health and Human Services (DHHS). (2015). HIV and women: Preventing mother-to-child transmission of HIV during childbirth. Retrieved from https://aidsinfo.nih.gov/education-materials/fact-sheets/24/70/preventing-mother-to-child-transmission-of-hiv-during-childbirth

This page summarizes how to minimize the risk of HIV transmission from pregnant women to their offspring, from pregnancy through childbirth. It includes specific prophylactics that are used with prepartum women whose HIV viral loads are high or unknown and optimal delivery methods for seropositive mothers.

World Health Organization (WHO). (2011). Global health sector strategy on HIV AIDS 2011–2015. Retrieved from http://whqlibdoc.who.int/publications/2011/9789241501651_eng.pdf?ua=1

This article summarizes the WHO's plan for combatting HIV/AIDS, so as to "achieve universal access" (WHO, 2011, p. 3) to HIV prevention, diagnosis, treatment, care and support.

References

American Academy of Pediatrics. (2009). Principles to reduce disparities and promote equity in children's health care. Retrieved from http://www.aap.org/en-us/about-the-aap/Committees-Councils-Sections/Council-on-Community-Pediatrics/Documents/Health_Equity_Principles.pdf

American Psychiatric Association. (2013). *Diagnostic and statistical manual of mental disorders* (5th ed.). Washington, DC: Author.

Antoine, L. B., Pierre, L., & Page, J. B. (1990). Exclusion of blood donors by country of origin and discrimination against Black foreigners in the USA. *AIDS, 4*, 818. doi:10.1097/00002030-199008000-00018

CDC. (2012a). Compendium of evidence-based HIV behavioral interventions. Retrieved from http://www.cdc.gov/hiv/prevention/research/compendium/index.html

CDC. (2012b). HIV in the United States: the stages of care. Retrieved from http://www.cdc.gov/hiv/pdf/research_mmp_stagesofcare.pdf

Farmer, P. (2006). *AIDS and accusation: Haiti and the geography of blame*. Berkeley, CA: University of California Press.

Flores, G. & The Committee on Pediatric Research. (2010). Racial and ethnic disparities in the health and health care of children. *Pediatrics, 125*(4), e979–1020.

Foy, J. M., & Perrin, J. (2010). Enhancing pediatric mental health care: Strategies for preparing a community. *Pediatrics, 125*(S3), S75–S86. doi:10.1542/peds.2010-0788D

Fuller, T. (2015). Shock and anger in Cambodian village struck with HIV. Retrieved from http://www.nytimes.com/2015/01/20/world/asia/farming-village-in-cambodia-grieves-as-hundreds-learn-they-have-hiv.html?_r=0

Garcia, P. J., Bayer, A., & Carcamo, C. P. (2014). The changing face of HIV in Latin America and the Caribbean. *Current HIV/AIDS Reports, 11*(2), 146–157. doi:10.1007/s11904-014-0204-1

Gardner, E. (2013). Retention in HIV care and treatment adherence. Retrieved from http://www.acthiv.org/2013_presentations/3-ACTHIV2013-SessionI-Gardner-03-15-13-approved.pdf
Grelotti, D. V. (2013). Even more mountains: Challenges to implementing mental health services in resource-limited settings, *Journal of the American Academy of Child & Adolescent Psychiatry*, 52(4), 339–343. Retrieved from http://www.sciencedirect.com/science/article/pii/S0890856712009999. doi:10.1016/j.jaac.2012.12.013
Lescano, C. M., Brown, L. K., Raffaelli, M., & Lima, U. (2009). Cultural factors and family–based HIV prevention for Latino youth. *Journal of Pediatric Psychology, 34*(10), 1041–1052. doi:10.1093/jpepsy/jsn146
Lum, D. (2011). *Culturally competent practice: A framework for understanding diverse group and justice issues*. Belmont, CA: Brooks/Cole.
Martinez, J., & Chakraborty, R. (2014). Psychosocial support for youth living with HIV. *Pediatrics, 133*(3), 558–562. doi:10.1542/peds.2013-4061
National Institute on Minority Health and Health Disparities of the National Institutes of Health (NIMHD/NIH). (2011). Retrieved from http://www.nimhd.nih.gov/programs/extra/rrr.html
National Institutes of Health. (2015). Inclusion of children in clinical research: Change in NIH definition. Notice number: NOT-OD-16-010. Retrieved from http://grants.nih.gov/grants/guide/notice-files/NOT-OD-16-010.html
Portes, A., & Rumbaut, R. G. (2001). *Legacies: The story of the immigrant second generation*. Berkeley, CA: University of California Press.
Purnell, L. D., & Paulanka, B. J. (Eds.). (2003). *Transcultural health care: A culturally competent approach* (2nd ed.). Philadelphia, PA: F.A. Davis.
Rahill, G. J., Jean-Gilles, M., Thomlison, B., & Pinto, E. (2011). Metaphors as contextual evidence for engaging Haitian clients in practice: A case study. *American Journal of Psychotherapy, 65* (2), 133–149.
Rahill, G. J., & Rice, C. (2010). Correlates of picuriste use in a sample of health-seeking Haitian immigrants and adult children of immigrants in Miami-Dade County, Florida. *American Journal of Public Health: Special Issue: The Science of Eliminating Health Disparities, 100*(1), S140–S145. doi:10.2105/AJPH.2009.162479
Rumbaut, R. G., & Portes, A. (2001). *Ethnicities: Children of immigrants in America*. Berkeley, CA: University of California Press.
Singer, K. M. (2012). Applying the concept of culture to reduce health disparities through health behavior research. *Preventive Medicine, 55*(5), 356–361. doi:10.1016/j.ypmed.2012.02.011
Theodore, H., Christophe, M. I., Morantus, S., Anglade, S. B., Deschamps, M. M., & Pape, J. W. (2011, November). Gender-based violence in emergencies. Paper presented at the 2011 Caribbean HIV Conference: Strengthening Evidence to Achieve Sustainable Action, The Bahamas. Abstract retrieved from https://www.2011caribbeanhivconference.org/abstract/gender-based-violence-emergencies
UNAIDS. (2010). Joint United Nations Programme on HIV/AIDS (UNAIDS). Global report: UNAIDS report on the global AIDS epidemic 2010. Retrieved from http://www.unaids.org/documents/20101123_globalreport_em.pdf
United Nations Children's Fund (UNICEF). (2010). The Americans and the Caribbean: Haiti. Humanitarian Action Report. Retrieved from http://www.unicef.org/har2010/index_haiti.php
United States Department of Health and Human Services (DHHS). (2015). HIV and women: Preventing mother-to-child transmission of HIV during childbirth. Retrieved from https://aidsinfo.nih.gov/education-materials/fact-sheets/24/70/preventing-mother-to-child-transmission-of-hiv-during-childbirth
United States Department of Health and Human Services, Agency for Healthcare Research and Quality. (2013). Highlights: 2013 national healthcare quality and disparities reports. Retrieved from http://www.ahrq.gov/research/findings/nhqrdr/nhqr13/2013highlights.pdf

Wingood, G. M., & DiClemente, R. J. (2008). The ADAPT-ITT model: A novel method of adapting evidence-based HIV Interventions. *Journal of Acquired Immune Deficiency Syndrome, 47*(S1), S40–S46. doi:10.1097/QAI.0b013e3181605df1

World Health Organization (WHO). (2011). Global health sector strategy on HIV AIDS 2011–2015. Retrieved from http://whqlibdoc.who.int/publications/2011/9789241501651_eng.pdf?ua=1

Chapter 11
HIV Prevention Among Youth: Designing Effective Evidence-Based HIV Risk-Reduction Programs for Adolescents

Ralph J. DiClemente and Nihari Patel

Introduction

In response to the human immunodeficiency virus (HIV) epidemic among adolescents, there is an overriding urgency to develop and implement prevention interventions designed to motivate adolescents' adoption and maintenance of HIV-preventative practices. Surveillance data suggest that about 16% of all reported AIDS cases resulted from HIV acquisition during the second decade of life (10–19 years of age) (Centers for Disease Control and Prevention [CDC] 2005). At the end of 2014, 36.9 million persons were living with HIV worldwide. Of these, four million were aged 15–24; 29% of whom were adolescents aged 15–19 years. Furthermore, approximately 3.2 million children younger than 15 years were living with HIV. This finding is especially alarming because adolescents, as a population, are less likely to be sexually active than their adult counterparts. The majority of HIV transmission among adolescents is attributed to sexual contact as opposed to other methods, for instance, injection drug use with shared needles and syringes (Rosenberg and Biggar 1998; CDC 1998). Because of these high rates coupled with the associated mortality and morbidity, both physical and psychological, the risk of acquiring HIV is one of the most substantial and immediate threats to the health and well-being of adolescents. In the past decade, numerous HIV prevention programs have been designed, implemented, and evaluated. While modifying adolescents' HIV risk behavior has been a formidable challenge, accumulating empirical evidence suggests that, in general, some of these programs are effective (DiClemente and Crosby 2003).

R.J. DiClemente (✉) · N. Patel
Emory University, Druid Hills, GA, USA
e-mail: rdiclem@emory.edu

N. Patel
e-mail: nihari.patel@emory.edu

T. Chenneville (ed.), *A Clinical Guide to Pediatric HIV*,
DOI 10.1007/978-3-319-49704-4_11

Although the risk behaviors for STI infection have been articulated in the previous literature (DiClemente and Crosby 2003), understanding the antecedents of these behaviors has been a complex and formidable challenge among prevention scientists. The task is particularly daunting because empirical investigation of such a personal and often nonpublic, nondisclosed behavior is logistically complicated. Historically, the STI/HIV epidemic has been viewed largely as an individual-level phenomenon where much effort has been focused on understanding intrapsychic influences that affect adolescents' decision making. Consequently, many intervention efforts that target adolescents with the goal of eliminating or reducing specific STI/HIV-associated risk behavior fail to address pervasive contextual influences that directly and indirectly affect disease acquisition.

Within the last decade, health researchers have begun to recognize the value of adopting a socioecological approach to examine the individual risk behavior (DiClemente et al. 2005). A socioecological approach involves examining individuals' behavior within the context of their social and physical environment, inclusive of familial, relational, peer, and societal influences (DiClemente et al. 2005; Bronfenbrenner 1979). The integration of these psychosocial influences reciprocally shapes one another and collectively affects the balance of risk for STI/HIV infection.

In this chapter, we highlight research assessing adolescents' sexual risk behavior and place the findings in the context of the diverse array of factors that influence adolescents' behavior. This synthesis provides an opportunity to examine why adolescents engage in risky sexual behavior and to review the effectiveness of the prevention programs. Next, we discuss the previous prevention approaches and highlight the strengths and weaknesses in these approaches. Subsequently, we articulate directions for future research to address gaps in the literature, while proposing an integrated strategy that targets the social ecology of the HIV epidemic among adolescents.

Predictors of Risk Behavior

Individual

Although adolescents typically perceive STI/HIV as a severe disease, a great deal of variability exists regarding individual perception of susceptibility. Studies have suggested that adolescents who perceive that they are at risk of STI/HIV tend to engage in less risky sexual behavior than those who do not have these perceptions (Boyer et al. 2000; Sieving et al. 1997; Zimet et al. 1992). Furthermore, adolescents who feel confident in using condoms (Bandura 1994; Jemmott et al. 1992; Rosenthal et al. 1991), in their ability to negotiate condom use with their partners (DiClemente et al. 2001a), in their ability to refuse sexual intercourse without condom use (Sionéan et al. 2002), and in their ability to discuss sexual matters

(DiClemente et al. 2001a; Crosby et al. 2002a) tend to use condoms more often and have lower rates of STIs (Crosby et al. 2001a). Additional individual characteristics, such as low self-esteem, psychological distress, sexual abuse, and depression, may also contribute to adolescents' risk for engaging in STI/HIV-associated sexual behaviors (DiClemente et al. 2001b; Shrier et al. 2001, 2002; Spencer et al. 2002; Parillo et al. 2001).

Adolescents' STI/HIV risk behavior appears to cluster with other risk behaviors such as alcohol or drug use (Doljanac and Zimmerman 1998; Millstein and Moscicki 1995; Shafer and Boyer 1991), antisocial behavior and delinquency (Doljanac and Zimmerman 1998), and pregnancy (Crosby et al. 2002b). Moreover, adolescents with high levels of impulsivity or who are prone toward sensation-seeking behaviors may place themselves at greater risk for contracting an STI/HIV (Donohew et al. 2000; Kahn et al. 2002; Stanton et al. 2000).

Family

Adolescents' sexual risk behavior has also been associated with their family structure. Perceived family support, family cohesiveness, parental monitoring, and parent–adolescent communication about sex have each been shown to help prevent adolescents from engaging in risky sexual behavior (Crosby et al. 2001b; DiClemente et al. 2001c; DiIorio et al. 1999; Resnick et al. 1997; Romer et al. 1999). Parental monitoring is a particularly important familial factor. Evidence suggests that adolescents who perceive that their parents (or parental figure) know where they are and who they are with outside of the home are substantially less likely to engage in STI/HIV sexual risk behaviors (Crosby et al. 2003; Li et al. 2000). In addition, positive parental influence can buffer adolescents against the influence of negative peer norms that could lead to risky sexual behavior (Whitaker and Miller 2000).

Relationships

Relationship characteristics also play an important role in influencing adolescents' risk behavior and the likelihood of contracting an STI/HIV. Although commonalities exist across gender, some differences are evident in the role that social and intimate relationships play on risky behavior. Key issues that affect females include their lack of relationship control (Crosby et al. 2000), engagement in longer relationships (Fortenberry et al. 2002; Plichta et al. 1992), fear of condom negotiation with their male partner (Sionéan et al. 2002), communicating less frequently with their partner about sex (DiClemente et al. 2001a), and having older sexual partners (Catania et al. 1989; Begley et al. 2003; DiClemente et al. 2002c; Miller et al. 1997); all of these issues have been associated with greater likelihood of engaging in STI/HIV sexual risk behavior.

Emerging research on male partner influences (Rosenthal et al. 1999) and perceived male partner support (Weisman et al. 1991) as relational risk factors have likewise been documented. For males, partner communication about sex (Lindberg et al. 1998; Wilson et al. 1994), belief in contraception responsibility (Pendergrast et al. 1992), being in the early stages of a relationship (Ku et al. 1994), and perceptions of partners' sexual inexperience have been associated with increased condom use (Brown et al. 1986), thus acting more as protective factors against risky sexual behavior. Among both males and females, perceived partners' negative attitude toward condom use has been related to unprotected intercourse and an increased number of sexual partners (Brown et al. 1986).

Peers

Perhaps one of the most powerful psychosocial influences on adolescents' sexual risk behavior is the perception about the behavior of their peers. Although parents have considerable influence on adolescents' decisions to engage in risk behaviors relative to adolescents' peers (Tremblay et al. 1995), perceived peer norms surrounding sexual behavior and condom use have been shown to also be key influencers of risky sexual behavior. If adolescents and young adults perceive that their friends are having unprotected sex or engaging in risky sex, they may be more likely to adopt their friends' behaviors (Boyer et al. 2000; Doljanac and Zimmerman 1998; Crosby et al. 2000; Bachanas et al. Bachanas et al. 2002). Similarly, general perceptions of low levels of social support among peers have also been associated with the likelihood of participating in risky sexual behavior (Lawrence et al. 1994). In contrast, perceived peer norms supportive of STI/HIV-protective behaviors can have a significant influence on the adoption and maintenance of protective behaviors (Doljanac and Zimmerman 1998; Millstein and Moscicki 1995).

Society

Societal factors play distinct roles in shaping cultural norms and influencing behavior. Surveillance data indicate that African American adolescent females are disproportionately affected by STI/HIV relative to other racial/ethnic groups and males (DiClemente and Crosby 2003). The apparent influence of race/ethnicity may be confounded by a variety of environmental factors (Fullilove 1998). Societal influences, such as neighborhoods devoid of adequate community resources (Small and Luster 1994), poor community supervision, and extreme poverty (Aral and Wasserheit 1995), are each likely to be key social determinants of STI/HIV risk behavior. Among poverty-stricken populations, in particular, incidence of sexual abuse is often high and may play a role in individual risk-taking behavior. Adolescents living in stressful environments are generally more likely to take sexual risks (Ennett et al. 1999; Lown et al. 1993). More recently, a dominant influence on the sexual health of adolescents is the media. Implicit and explicit sexual imagery coupled with situations depicting unprotected sexual intercourse, violence, and aggression toward females is ubiquitous (Peter and Valkenburg 2006). There is evidence of an association between exposures to both rap music (Wingood et al. 2003) and pornographic movies (Wingood et al. 2001) with greater levels of problem behavior and more sexual risk taking. Unfortunately, little is known about the psychosocial mechanism that might explain the observed associations between the media and adolescent risk behavior. Recent studies suggested that one potentially important community-level predictor of adolescents' sexual risk behavior may be their affiliation with organized social groups (Crosby et al. 2002c, d; Ramirez-Valles et al. 1998; Schinke et al. 1992). Future research in this area is warranted.

The Importance of an Ecological Approach for HIV Prevention

Primary prevention to reduce the incidence of STI/HIV is essential. The following strategies reduce STI/HIV transmission (Centers for Disease Control and Prevention 2015):

- Abstaining from oral, anal, or vaginal sex;
- Engaging in less risky sexual behaviors;
- Using condoms correctly and consistently during oral, anal, or vaginal sex;
- Limiting the number of sex partners;
- Getting tested for HIV and other STIs and have sex partners engage in routine testing; the CDC recommends annual testing for sexually active individuals; and
- Preventing mother-to-child transmission.

Primary prevention reduces transmission of STI/HIV, ensuring fewer people become infected from individuals who are STI/HIV positive. Secondary prevention is a key factor to prevent being infected with a new strain of HIV or infecting another person. Secondary prevention also reduces the severity of HIV by early identification of cases through testing and rapid intervention (Groseclose et al. 1995).

Many interventions efforts, as seen above, have targeted individual-level factors as a means of achieving significant behavioral change. In the past two decades, there have been scores of programs designed to enhance adolescents' STI/HIV-preventive knowledge, foster positive attitudes toward condom use, develop norms supportive of abstinence and condom use, teach skills to foster self-efficacy, and motivate adolescents to adopt preventive behaviors and to decrease risk behaviors. Typically, these programs have used small-group educational formats and recruited participants through clinics, schools, and communities. In general, the weight of empirical evidence indicates that small-group interventions emphasizing cognitive decision making and behavioral skills were effective in reducing sexual risk behaviors (Centers for Disease Control and Prevention 1999; Robin et al. 2004). One review, for example, examined 23 randomized clinical trials (RCTs) conducted with adolescents and that used sexual behavior change as an outcome. Of these interventions, 13(57%) achieved significant risk-reduction effects. No studies found the reverse effect; that is, in no case, did the experimental intervention do worse than the control intervention. Across studies, frequency of unprotected sex was reduced in 75% of studies that measured this outcome, condom use improved in 53% of studies, and number of sex partners was reduced in 27%. The lowest rates of behavior change were found for abstinence, which was improved in only 14% of studies that measured it (Pedlow and Carey 2004). These findings have been confirmed by another meta-analysis of HIV-reduction interventions for youth (Jemmott and Jemmott, 2000).

Although there is ample evidence to support the efficacy of individual-level approaches; there is also substantial evidence indicating that intervention effects tend to diminish over time (DiClemente et al. 2013). Thus, while efficacious in promoting the adoption of STI/HIV-preventive behaviors in the near-term, individual-level interventions appear to be insufficient in sustaining newly adopted preventive behavior changes over protracted periods of time. In fact, a recent meta-analysis of randomized HIV prevention trials indicated that the effects of interventions diminish substantially, often back to baseline levels as a direct function of time from intervention-to-follow-up (Pedlow and Carey 2004). Unfortunately, for behavior change to be meaningful, it must be enduring. Thus, as individual-level interventions lack sufficient impact to sustain behavioral change, there is a critical need to modify the current STI/HIV prevention paradigm for adolescents.

The development of an intervention approach that promotes consistent, sustained behavior change represents an important challenge to STI/HIV prevention science (DiClemente et al. 2003). Researchers and practitioners have recognized the importance of a perspective that expands investigational and intervention efforts beyond the individual level. A diverse array of factors that represent a web of causality influencing adolescents' risk taking exists. Thus, we cannot hope to optimize changes in adolescents' sexual behavior without addressing both the proximal and distal environmental influences that affect adolescents' decision making and, in turn, their likelihood of engaging in risky sexual behavior (Maton 2000).

Emerging evidence suggests that some environmental factors may also have an equal if not greater effect than individual-level factors on adolescents' sexual risk behaviors and, ultimately, on STI and HIV transmission (Rotheram-Borus 2000). Discrete individual, interpersonal, social, and economic influences are embedded within a cultural context superimposed over traditions, values, and patterns of social organization. Figure 11.1 illustrates the individual embedded within the proximal context of an environment defined by peers, community, family, and sexual and dating relationships. Further, the figure illustrates that these proximal influences are embedded within the broader, distal influences of society such as economics, tradition, norms, laws, and mores. In essence, the distal elements influence the proximal elements, which mutually influence each other as well as the adolescent,

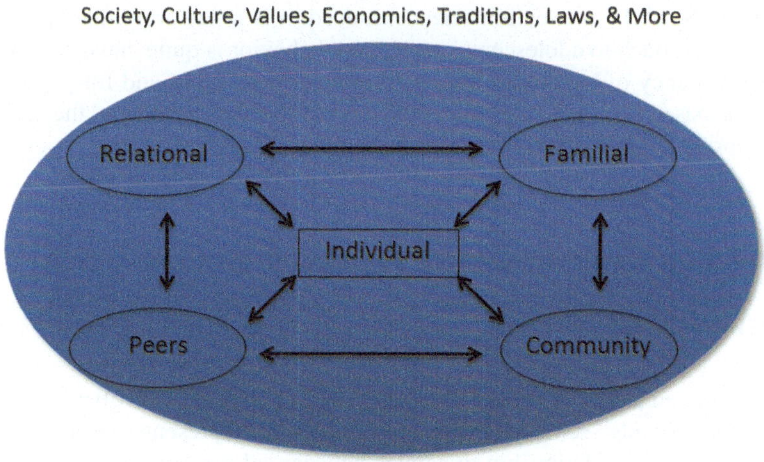

Fig. 11.1 Multiple influences underlying adolescent sexual risk behavior

thereby making the adolescent the victim or the benefactor of these larger influences. Not surprising, few studies have attempted to understand wholly the complexity of these interactions let alone conceptualize interventions to modify them. What is needed is a complementary approach that addresses these multiple spheres of influence as well as the interaction among spheres.

As a useful and familiar heuristic framework for understanding these proximal and distal influences, Bronfenbrenner (1979) defined this social ecology of human development as involving the study of mutual transactions between human beings and the properties of the environmental systems in which they interact. The goodness of fit between the person and the environment influences whether outcomes are successful or strained. He identified four system levels: (a) the microsystem—the roles and characteristics of the developing individual; (b) the mesosystem—the settings with which the developing person interacts, (c) the exosystem—settings with which the individual does not interact but nevertheless have an effect on the person's development; and the (d) the macrosystem—cultural values and larger societal factors that influence the individual. Because adolescents interact simultaneously in several social spheres—family, peer, neighborhood systems—that can either serve to inhibit or promote behavior.

Applying an ecological approach to adolescent sexual risk behavior would entail first examining their sexual behaviors within the context of their social and physical environments, and then designing concurrent interventions aimed at multiple relevant, modifiable levels. The use of an ecological approach may provide a more efficacious strategy for influencing numerous leverage points of long-term behavior change and address the issue of the limited sustainability of intervention effects observed in STI/HIV prevention science. Indeed, it is noteworthy that applying an ecological approach to adolescents' sexual risk behavior is quite consistent with the growing tendency of health promotion programs (of all types and for people of all ages) to be based on expansive theoretical models that extend beyond the constructs that comprise the individual level (DiClemente et al. 2002a).

Intervention Approaches that Transcend Multiple Levels

Mesosystems Approaches

By definition, engaging in sexual risk and protective behaviors involve, at least, two people. Adolescents' sexual relationships, therefore, represent one aspect of the mesosystem, as the relationship dynamics between adolescents and their sex partners may be an important point for intervention. Activities designed to enhance the quality and frequency of communication between partners, help adolescents select partners similar in age, teach condom negotiation skills as well as sexual refusal skills, and reduce dating violence and date rape perpetration may be effective in achieving behavioral change. Although some of these factors have been addressed previously with activities in small-group interventions, these efforts have traditionally focused entirely on one of the partners rather than the dyad. A dyadic intervention would address these salient relational influences associated with STI/HIV risk and protective behaviors, while also transferring the burden to initiate STI/HIV-protective behaviors from one person to the dyad. This is particularly important for adolescent females who are often in power imbalanced relationships with their male partners (Begley et al. 2003; DiClemente et al. 2002b; Gollub 1995; Wingood et al. 2002). Additionally, this type of intervention holds great promise for enhancing not only the adoption of STI/HIV-preventive behaviors by the dyad, but also, in the event of dissolution, not unexpected among adolescents, there may be a generalization of recently adopted STI/HIV-preventive behaviors to new relationships. Unfortunately, a review of the literature indicated only one dyadic STI/HIV-preventive intervention, which was designed for inner-city Latino teen parenting couples. Its efficacy has not been reported as of yet (Lesser et al. 2005).

Another aspect of adolescents' mesosystem and one related to their engaging in STI/HIV risk and protective behaviors is the family since familial factors are critical in keeping adolescents safe. Particularly important is parental monitoring. Emerging evidence suggests that adolescents who perceive that their parents or parent figure know where they are and who they are with outside of school or work are substantially less likely to engage in sexual risk behaviors or to have an STI (Crosby et al. 2003; DiClemente et al. 2001c; Doljanac and Zimmerman 1998; Li et al. 2000; McNeely et al. 2002; Rodgers 1999; Romer et al. 1999; Voisin et al. 2006; Williams et al. 2002). Furthermore, parents' influence can also buffer adolescents' against the influence of peer norms that encourage risky sexual behaviors

—one example of the interaction of multiple influences (Fisher and Feldman 1998). Acknowledging the importance of family-level interventions, the National Institute of Mental Health has established a consortium of family grants specifically designed to enhance parent–adolescent interactions surrounding STI/HIV prevention (Pequegnat et al. 2001).

Family-level interventions typically promote increased communication between adolescents and parents about STI/HIV prevention (Stanton et al. 2001). These interventions may also attempt to increase parental monitoring of adolescents and adolescents' perceptions of enhanced parental monitoring, as well as foster a sense of increased family support. Although promising in that family-level interventions go beyond the individual-level only, the preliminary evidence suggests that intervention effectiveness has been modest (DiIorio et al. 2000; Hawkins et al. 1999; Jemmott et al. 2000; Stanton et al. 2000).

Moving beyond the relationship and the family levels, most adolescents also interact with their schools and community through myriad social activities, programs, sports, or exposure to other institutions such as their church. Not surprising, research has identified several community-level influences on adolescents' risk and protective behaviors. One important community-level influence is adolescents' perception of social norms. Social norms theory (Perkins and Berkowitz 1986) posits that behavior is influenced by the pervasive and underlying social norms surrounding a behavior. Moreover, the influence exerted by social norms is based on people's perception of those norms, and perceptions may not accurately reflect actual norms. The influence of perceived peer norms on behavior is also emphasized by the theory of reasoned action (Fishbein 2000). Peer norms surrounding sexual behaviors and condom use have been shown to be robust influences on both risky and protective sexual behavior. When adolescents perceive that friends and similar-aged teens engage in risky sexual behavior, even if their perception is skewed, then they are more likely to adopt those same behaviors. In contrast, perceiving that friends and other teens abstain from sex or practice safer sex would influence youth to adopt those protective behaviors. Furthermore, if adolescents feel a strong sense of connection to their schools, live in communities with a high degree of social capital, and have access to condoms, then they will be more likely to engage in protective behaviors (Kirby 2001).

Programs targeting these significant community-level influences represent an important strategy for STI/HIV prevention. Such programs would strive to evoke significant changes within the community sphere. One example of a community-level approach is the Prevention Marketing Initiative (PMI) (Kennedy et al. 2000). PMI targeted adolescents less than 20 years of age. The goals of the intervention were to increase adolescents' awareness of STIs, enhance condom use and abstinence, promote parent–adolescent discussions, provide information about STI-related prevention services, and change adolescents' perceptions of norms supportive of STI-preventive behaviors. Using a comprehensive approach, intervention activities crossed multiple levels, affecting individual-level factors, familial factors, and social norms. Evaluation of programmatic impact, conducted in five sites, observed marked increases in STI-preventive behavior (Kennedy et al. 2000).

Another community-level approach is clinic-based screening programs. These programs target adolescents' mesosystem. Recent studies observed that offering repeated STI screening and treatment in clinical settings effectively reduced adolescents' gonorrhea and chlamydia incidence rates (Burstein et al. 1998; Cohen et al. 1999); however, screening programs to be maximally effective need to access a substantial portion of the target population.

In addition to screening programs, other, less intensive strategies, such as setting aside specific clinic hours for adolescents, may enhance accessibility to health care and thereby have an effect on adolescents' sexual behavior and sexual health (Akinbami et al. 2003; Hock-Long et al. 2003; Jaccard 1996). If clinics are not accessible during hours when adolescents are free to visit them, then a barrier is created that reduces the likelihood that adolescents will attend them. All things being equal, the STI rates of the community impact the likelihood of STI among adolescents. Thus, another community-level approach that could also prove to be effective is to target not adolescents per se, but rather their sexual networks (Rothenberg 2001). A sexual network approach is unique in that it increases case findings through "contact tracing" using developmentally appropriate techniques. For example, interviewing one adolescent who tests positive for an STI can serve as the starting point for locating, interviewing, and screening other adolescents within the same network (Rothenberg et al. 1998). This approach also provides an opportunity to promote safer sex behaviors through the education of key members of these sexual networks. Conversely, networks can also exert a positive impact on adolescents' behavior. For example, influencing key venues in adolescents' social networks, such as community and school organizations, so that they feel a greater sense of connection, feel more supported, and have ready access to needed resources such as extracurricular activities, condoms, and sexual education, could also positively impact adolescents' sexual behavior.

Exosystem Approaches

Because adolescents do not interact in the exosystem, exerting influence on their STI/HIV-preventive behavior would be accomplished indirectly. For example, the workplace of adolescents' parents would be one setting that holds promise for reducing adolescent risk behaviors (Schuster et al. 2001). One problem with community-based and school-based family-level interventions is recruiting parents to participate. Parents who work have multiple demands and serious time constraints placed on them making it difficult for them to participate in intervention programs offered in the community in the evening or on weekends. By placing the intervention at the workplace, this problem can be overcome and hopefully "they will come." In fact, Eastman and colleagues (2005) examined whether or not parents would attend worksite-based parenting programs to promote healthy adolescent sexual development. In their focus groups with employed parents of adolescents, they found both parents and employers were supportive of the content that would provide desired education and skills for effectively communicating with and understanding their adolescents.

Although theoretically feasible and practically viable, unfortunately, there is a paucity of worksite-based parenting programs in the literature. One study described the implementation of a one-hour seminar in the workplace ("Project F.A.C.T.S.") that trained parents to communicate effectively with their adolescents about sexuality. The evaluation results showed that following the seminar, more parents reported that they felt they were the primary sexuality educator of their children; more parents indicated that they talked with their children about sex; more parents felt sex discussions should take place openly and more parents discussed sex education of their children with another parent (Caron et al. 1993). Another study described a workplace educational parenting program that although not designed to address adolescent sexual risk, did focus on adolescent substance abuse through two one-hour sessions held at lunchtime over the course of 12 weeks. The results showed that, overall, there were relatively high attendance (74%) and low dropout (16%). Parents who were in the high dosage group (i.e., >80% attendance level) reported significant decreases in child behavior problems, more positive child behavior, less parental punitive behavior, less parental irritability, higher levels of knowledge pertaining to child development, less stress and depression, less work–family conflicts, higher levels of substance abuse knowledge, and less tolerant attitudes toward a friend's substance use and toward substance abuse in general (Felner et al. 1994). In addition to educational programs implemented at the workplace, changes to workplace policies may also have a significant effect on adolescents' STI/HIV behaviors. Policies that enable parents to incorporate more flextime or to telecommute hold the potential to increase the ability of parents to monitor adolescents better, to have more time to engage in family activities, and to communicate with adolescents more often. Indeed, it may be that societal-level practices such as flexibility in the workplace and generally improved living conditions could become precursors of parents' increased vigilance regarding adolescents' health and well-being.

Macrosystem Approaches

The most distal influence of adolescents' STI/HIV-related behaviors is the society in which all of the other influences are embedded. By society, we mean cultural norms and traditions, large-scale policies and laws, economic conditions, and the political climate. One specific pervasive macrosystem characteristic that plays a distinct role in shaping cultural norms and traditions and also, through agenda-setting, and can influence policy and law is the media (Thornburgh and Lin 2002). Whether it is the Internet, movies, television, music videos, or books, research has increasingly demonstrated that media plays a significant role in socialization including the socialization of adolescents and therefore impacts their sexual risk and protective behavior. For example, studies have found that greater exposure to rap music videos and X-rated movies was associated with having multiple sex partners, more frequent sexual intercourse, and testing positive for an

STI (Wingood et al. 2001, 2003). Because of its influence, the media also represents a promising vehicle for the delivery of persuasive health-promoting messages. Mass media campaigns targeting adolescents have been popular in the Netherlands and in Switzerland. Evaluation of a nationwide mass media campaign implemented in Norway indicated that the campaign was effective in changing attitudes and practices relevant to safer sex behaviors (Traeen 1992). In addition, trend analyses of ongoing evaluations of media-based interventions in Switzerland have observed marked reductions in sexual risk behaviors (Hausser and Michaud 1994). In the United States, a four-city study observed lower prevalence of self-report sexual risk behaviors among youth in those cities exposed to "prevention media" relative to adolescents in cities receiving no intervention (Romer et al. 2009; Hennessy et al. 2013; Sznitman et al. 2011).

It is important to note, however, that media campaigns that target a specific subgroup of the population such as adolescents differ significantly from a media campaign that targets the general population. In other words, if the macrosystem represents culture, which comprises the general "majority" culture and the varying subcultures of specific age, gender, race, and ethnic groups, then we must consider whether targeting general cultural norms through a media campaign is the optimal strategy for influencing the cultural norms of specific subgroups although it may result in more widespread societal change. We must consider which macrosystem approach will be more effective. Moreover, achieving social change through macrosystem approaches may not be evident in the short term. Indeed, affecting social change may result in sustaining behavior change in the long-term because of modifying the larger culture in which the subgroups exist; other factors may necessitate targeting subgroups so that shorter term gains can be achieved.

Societal-level changes can also be made by initiating changes to policy. Policies that promote increased accessibility to and acceptability of STI/HIV prevention and control services for adolescents can have a profound effect on sexual health. For example, managed care organizations that provide time and incentives for clinicians to screen, counsel, and educate adolescents at-risk of or diagnosed with STIs could have a tremendous impact on the reproductive rate of the STI epidemic (DiClemente and Brown 1994; Kamb et al. 1998). Healthcare policy should also insure that adolescents receive services for STI/HIV prevention, testing, and treatment despite income disparities. These types of policies should exempt adolescents from obtaining parental consent for the treatment.

Applied Ecological Intervention Example

Perhaps, one of the most poignant examples of an effective ecological approach to HIV prevention occurred in Brazil. Indeed, the Brazilian response to the AIDS pandemic has been described as both comprehensive and progressive (Berkman et al. 2005). At the heart of the approach was a community grassroots movement designed to destigmatize AIDS and demand change and support from law makers—

in other words, change came from the bottom up. Brazilians mobilized and were able to achieve significant social changes through advocacy, the organization of political parties, trade unions, and nongovernmental organizations in collaboration with the government. In fact, the government implemented one of the "most explicit of any governmental information campaign in the world" (Berkman et al. 2005, p. 1168). Longstanding and entrenched cultural values related to sexual behaviors (e.g., premarital sex is morally wrong) began to erode and values supporting open and honest discussion emerged especially regarding the stigma surrounding HIV and AIDS. Indeed, condom sales and distribution rose dramatically in the general population and especially among young people. Subsequently, sexual risk-reduction education programs became more acceptable and were implemented across diverse venues and among diverse populations such as with sex workers and young people. In addition, HIV testing became more socially acceptable, and the treatment for AIDS was viewed as a basic human right. More important were the effects observed in the incidence rates for HIV; they were much lower than projected and mortality rates decreased by 50% (Berkman et al. 2005).

This example is unique. Brazil is one of the few countries that experienced a decline in the incidence of HIV infection and in mortality as a result of social change efforts at the macrosystem level. This approach while effective was different from traditional interventions that have been discussed or published in that the change resulted from unified efforts stemming from a concerned and disenchanted citizenry. Thus, this effort may not be easily replicated in other communities or countries; however, we can learn from the Brazilian experience by focusing on certain aspects that could be replicated elsewhere such as the media campaign messages, the implementation of sexual risk-reduction programs for many subgroups, and the promotion of HIV testing and treatment.

Role of Pediatric Psychologists in STI/HIV Prevention

Pediatric psychologists have an integral role to play in preventing adolescents' STI risk behavior. At each level of the ecological framework, pediatric psychologists can be actively involved in the design, implementation, or evaluation of STI/HIV prevention programs. At the microsystem level, pediatric psychologists, working in clinical venues or community health centers, can provide screening and risk reduction, or psychological counseling, and, if needed, can provide referrals for more detailed psychological evaluation and specialized counseling for adolescents identified with psychological antecedents (i.e., depression, impulsivity, sensation seeking, and substance use) associated with STI/HIV acquisition. At the mesosystem level, pediatric psychologists can work closely with institutions, such as families, to develop programs to enhance parents' ability to supervise their adolescents' behavior or enhance parent–adolescent communication. Both of these factors have been empirically demonstrated to reduce STI/HIV-associated risk behaviors and STI acquisition. Depending on their service agency, pediatric psychologists may recommend periodic parental counseling and long-term follow-up with parents and/or families to monitor the familial relationship and its impact on adolescents' STI/HIV-associated risk behaviors. In addition, some pediatric psychologists may be affiliated with school systems. In their role as a consultant or staff of a school system, they can assist in the design or implementation of school-based STI/HIV prevention programs. These programs would be implemented in schools by teachers, nurses, psychologists, or counselors who have undergone in-service training by pediatric psychologists. At the macrosystem level, pediatrics psychologists can work with broader societal agencies, STI/HIV-preventive interventions as consultants to media, for example, in addressing gender bias and reducing power inequities in relationships that can facilitate the adoption of STI/HIV-associated risk behaviors among young women. The array of opportunities for pediatric psychologists to intervene across the ecological levels is broad. However, adequate systems for financing and provider reimbursement are essential to facilitate the provision of these preventive services.

Future Research

Although the ecological framework described in this article is intuitively appealing, currently, there is a dearth of empirical data that support whether intervening across multiple ecological levels is effective in sustaining behavioral changes. These interventions may draw upon two or more of the ecological levels outlined in this article. For example, testing a small-group educational sexual risk-reduction program (i.e., microsystem) in conjunction with a media campaign (i.e., macrosystem) versus each intervention separately would constitute a test of whether combining multiple levels enhances sustainability of behavioral changes. Thus, future research that incorporates designs to test single-level interventions against multi-level interventions is warranted. Finally, future research should also investigate developmental differences among the various stages that constitute adolescence. Different combinations of the four ecological levels may be more or less effective as a function of adolescents' developmental trajectory.

The central premise of the proposed ecological approach is that none of its levels should function in isolation from the others. Indeed, we suggest that designing effective STI/HIV prevention and control programs can best be achieved by taking full advantage of the "synergy" among the levels that constitute the ecological model. This synergy can amplify and complement isolated intervention approaches, thereby optimizing and sustaining favorable effects (Wingood et al. 2013). Although this approach requires intensified efforts and resources, its returns warrant implementation.

Although expanding investigational and preventive efforts beyond one level may seem daunting, the possibilities are not endless. When thinking about the number of combinations to focus on when conceptualizing research designs, there are approximately 60 potential combinations of factors chosen two at a time from each of five levels of influence. This observation accentuates the point that intervention efforts can and should be creatively tailored to meet the unique needs of adolescents within various environments that influence sexual risk and protective behaviors.

In essence, a need exists to link STI/HIV prevention resources into an efficient network. This network, for example, would consist of key members from families, the community, schools, health providers, local government agencies, and non-governmental agencies or community-based organizations. For example, multiple access points (i.e., recreation centers, after-school programs, physicians' offices, and juvenile justice centers) could be used as opportunity sites for providing STI/HIV prevention information and motivating adolescents to adopt relevant health promotion skills. A key-related question is how to implement this approach in a cost-effective way, while determining which programs work best for various sub-groups of adolescents.

Finally, it is important to note that an ecological approach is proactive. To create "synergy," this approach necessitates complementing the traditional medical model of STI/HIV prevention with theory-guided practice grounded in the developmental context of adolescents' lives. From this perspective, adolescents' STI/HIV risk behavior should not be conceptualized as "individual deficits," but rather more appropriately and favorably viewed as a reflection of their relational, familial, community, and societal environments. Viewed in this manner, it is important to note that the ecological approach could easily be applied to a multitude of other health-related issues that are relevant to adolescents (e.g., pregnancy prevention, the prevention of substance abuse, and avoiding unintentional injury).

Conclusion

This review proposes an ecological framework for understanding the myriad of influences that affect adolescents' risk for acquiring an STI/HIV infection. As a consequence, developing intervention strategies across levels of the ecological framework may, ultimately, provide the preventive synergy that yields more effective and sustainable HIV prevention interventions.

Annotated Bibliography

Berkman, A., Garcia, J., Muñoz-Laboy, M., Paiva, V., & Parker, R. (2005). A critical analysis of the Brazilian response to HIV/AIDS: Lessons learned for controlling and mitigating the epidemic in developing countries. *American Journal of Public Health, 95*(7), 1162–1172. doi:10.2105/AJPH.2004.054593

The authors in this article analyze the Brazilian National AIDS Program, which is one of the most successful examples of an effective ecological approach to HIV prevention. Elements that distinguish Brazil's experiences are discussed to help aid with the development of similar HIV prevention programs in other countries. The authors also discuss the transection of culture and sexuality, politics and public health, and the integration of prevention and treatment.

DiClemente, R. J., Salazar, L. F., & Crosby, R. A. (2007). A review of STD/HIV preventive interventions for adolescents: Sustaining effects using an ecological approach. *Journal of Pediatric Psychology, 32*(8), 888–906. doi:10.1093/jpepsy/jsm056

The authors review the literature on adolescent sexual risk research and outline intervention research suggestive of an ecological perspective. They use various examples from published literature that has investigated preventive interventions using a multilevel approach. The authors find in their study that adolescents are exposed to a diverse array of influences. Therefore, to adequately prevent and maintain the likelihood of adolescents' adopting sexual risk behaviors, intervention efforts should be designed to transect the different factors of causation.

DiClemente, R. J., Brown, J. L., & Davis, T. L. (2013). Determinants of Health-Related Behaviors in Adolescence. In *Handbook of adolescent health psychology* (pp. 107–127). Berlin: Springer. doi:10.1007/978-1-4614-6633-8_8

The authors start by providing an overview of the socio-ecological model of adolescent health behavior by highlighting some key determinants of health outcomes: individual, family, peer, relational, community, and societal. Then they provide examples of interventions designed to address important health determinants and related behaviors at each level of the socio-ecological model. While there is a focus on reproductive health, this article also explores the socio-ecological model in different domains of adolescent health: mortality, unintentional injury, violence, mental health and substance abuse, and chronic disease.

References

Akinbami, L. J., Gandhi, H., & Cheng, T. L. (2003). Availability of adolescent health services and confidentiality in primary care practices. *Pediatrics, 111*(2), 394–401. doi:10.1542/peds.111.2.394

Aral, S. O., & Wasserheit, J. N. (1995). Interactions among HIV, other sexually transmitted diseases, socioeconomic status, and poverty in women. In *Women at risk* (pp. 13–41). Berlin: Springer US. doi:10.1007/978-1-4899-1057-8_2

Bachanas, P. J., Morris, M. K., Lewis-Gess, J. K., Sarett-Cuasay, E. J., Flores, A. L., Sirl, K. S., et al. (2002). Psychological adjustment, substance use, HIV knowledge, and risky sexual behavior in at-risk minority females: Developmental differences during adolescence. *Journal of Pediatric Psychology, 27*(4), 373–384. doi:10.1093/jpepsy/27.4.373

Bandura, A. (1994). Social cognitive theory and exercise of control over HIV infection. In *Preventing AIDS* (pp. 25–59). Berlin: Springer US. doi:10.1007/978-1-4899-1193-3_3

Begley, E., Crosby, R. A., DiClemente, R. J., Wingood, G. M., & Rose, E. (2003). Older partners and STD prevalence among pregnant African American teens. *Sexually Transmitted Diseases, 30*(3), 211–213. doi:10.1097/00007435-200303000-00006

Berkman, A., Garcia, J., Muñoz-Laboy, M., Paiva, V., & Parker, R. (2005). A critical analysis of the Brazilian response to HIV/AIDS: Lessons learned for controlling and mitigating the epidemic in developing countries. *American Journal of Public Health, 95*(7), 1162–1172. doi:10.2105/AJPH.2004.054593

Boyer, C. B., Shafer, M. A., Wibbelsman, C. J., Seeberg, D., Teitle, E., & Lovell, N. (2000). Associations of sociodemographic, psychosocial, and behavioral factors with sexual risk and sexually transmitted diseases in teen clinic patients. *Journal of Adolescent Health, 27*(2), 102–111. doi:10.1016/S1054-139X(99)00113-5

Bronfenbrenner, U. (1979). *The ecology of human development*. Cambridge, MA: Harvard University Press.

Brown, B. B., Clasen, D. R., & Eicher, S. A. (1986). Perceptions of peer pressure, peer conformity dispositions, and self-reported behavior among adolescents. *Developmental Psychology, 22*(4), 521. doi:10.1037/0012-1649.22.4.521

Burstein, G. R., Waterfield, G., Joffe, A., Zenilman, J. M., Quinn, T. C., & Gaydos, C. A. (1998). Screening for gonorrhea and Chlamydia by DNA amplification in adolescents attending middle school health centers. Opportunity for early intervention. *Sexually Transmitted Diseases, 25*(8), 395–402. doi:10.1097/00007435-199809000-00001

Caron, S. L., Knox, C. B., Rhoades, C., Aho, J., Tulman, K. K., & Volovk, M. (1993). Sexuality education in the workplace: Seminars for parents. *Journal of Sex Education & Therapy, 19*(3), 200–211.

Catania, J. A., Coates, T. J., Greenblatt, R. M., Dolcini, M. M., Kegeles, S. M., Puckett, S., … & Miller, J. (1989). *Predictors of condom use and multiple partnered sex among sexually-active adolescent women: Implications for aids-related health interventions.*

Centers for Disease Control and Prevention. (1998). Trends in sexual risk behaviors among high school students–United States, 1991–1997. *MMWR. Morbidity and Mortality Weekly Report, 47*(36), 749.

Centers for Disease Control and Prevention. (1999). *Compendium of HIV prevention interventions with evidence of effectiveness*. Atlanta, GA: Department of Health and Human Services.

Centers for Disease Control and Prevention. (2005). AIDS surveillance report 2005. Vol 17. Rev ed. *Department of Health and Human Services, 500*, 1–46.

Centers for Disease Control and Prevention. (2015). Available at: http://www.cdc.gov/hiv/basics/prevention.html. Accessed 2015.

Cohen, D. A., Nsuami, M., Martin, D. H., & Farley, T. A. (1999). Repeated school-based screening for sexually transmitted diseases: A feasible strategy for reaching adolescents. *Pediatrics, 104*, 1281–1285. doi:10.1542/peds.104.6.1281

Crosby, R. A., DiClemente, R. J., Wingood, G. M., Sionean, C., Cobb, B. K., & Harrington, K. (2000). Correlates of unprotected vaginal sex among African American female adolescents: Importance of relationship dynamics. *Archives of Pediatrics & Adolescent Medicine, 154*(9), 893–899.

Crosby, R., DiClemente, R. J., Wingood, G. M., Sionean, C., Cobb, B. K., Harrington, K., … & Oh, M. K. (2001a). Correct condom application among African-American adolescent females: The relationship to perceived self-efficacy and the association to confirmed STDs. *Journal of Adolescent Health, 29*(3), 194–199. doi:10.1016/S1054-139X(01)00273-7

Crosby, R. A., DiClemente, R. J., Wingood, G. M., Cobb, B. K., Harrington, K., Davies, S. L., … & Oh, M. K. (2001b). HIV/STD-protective benefits of living with mothers in perceived supportive families: A study of high-risk African American female teens. *Preventive Medicine, 33*(3), 175–178. doi:10.1006/pmed.2001.0868

Crosby, R. A., DiClemente, R. J., Wingood, G. M., Cobb, B. K., Harrington, K., Davies, S. L., … & Oh, M. K. (2002a). Condom use and correlates of African American adolescent females' infrequent communication with sex partners about preventing sexually transmitted diseases and pregnancy. *Health Education & Behavior, 29*(2), 219–231

Crosby, R. A., DiClemente, R. J., Wingood, G. M., Harrington, K., Davies, S., & Oh, M. K. (2002b). Activity of African-American female teenagers in black organizations is associated with STD/HIV protective behaviours: A prospective analysis. *Journal of Epidemiology and Community Health, 56*(7), 549–550. doi:10.1136/jech.56.7.549

Crosby, R. A., DiClemente, R. J., Wingood, G. M., Sionean, C., Harrington, K., Davies, S. L., & Oh, M. K. (2002c). Pregnant African American adolescent females are less likely to use condoms than their non-pregnant peers. *Preventive Medicine, 34*, 524–552. doi:10.1006/pmed.2002.1014

Crosby, R. A., DiClemente, R. J., Wingood, G. M., Harrington, K., Davies, S. L., Hook, E. W., et al. (2002d). African American adolescent females' membership in community organizations is associated with STD/HIV-protective behaviors: A prospective analysis. *Journal of Epidemiology Community Health, 23*, 549–550. doi:10.1136/jech.56.7.549

Crosby, R. A., DiClemente, R. J., Wingood, G. M., Lang, D. L., & Harrington, K. (2003). Infrequent parental monitoring predicts sexually transmitted infections among low-income African American female adolescents. *Archives of Pediatrics & Adolescent Medicine, 157*(2), 169–173. doi:10.1001/archpedi.157.2.169

DiClemente, R. J., & Brown, L. K. (1994). Expanding the pediatrician's role in HIV prevention for adolescents. *Clinical Pediatrics, 33*(4), 235–240. doi:10.1177/000992289403300409

DiClemente, R. J., & Crosby, R. A. (2003). *Sexually transmitted diseases among adolescents: Risk factors, antecedents, and prevention strategies.*

DiClemente, R. J., Brown, J. L., Sales, J. M., & Rose, E. S. (2013). Rate of decay in proportion of condom protected sex acts among adolescents following participation in an HIV risk-reduction intervention. *Journal of Acquired Immune Deficiency Syndromes (1999), 63*(0 1), S85. doi:10.1097/QAI.0b013e3182920173

DiClemente, R. J., Crosby, R. A., & Kegler, M. (Eds.). (2002a). *Emerging theories in health promotion practice and research.* San Francisco, CA: Jossey-Bass Wiley.

DiClemente, R. J., Crosby, R. A., & Wingood, G. M. (2002b). Enhancing HIV/STD prevention among adolescents: The importance of parental monitoring. *Minerva Pediatrica, 54*, 171–177.

DiClemente, R. J., Salazar, L. F., Crosby, R. A., & Rosenthal, S. L. (2005). Prevention and control of sexually transmitted infections among adolescents: The importance of a socio-ecological perspective—A commentary. *Public Health, 119*(9), 825–836. doi:10.1016/j.puhe.2004.10.015

DiClemente, R. J., Wingood, G. M., & Crosby, R. A. (2003). A contextual perspective for understanding and preventing STD/HIV among adolescents. In D. Romer (Ed.), *Reducing adolescent risk: Toward an integrated approach* (pp. 366–373). Thousand Oaks, CA: Sage. doi:10.4135/9781452233611.n38

DiClemente, R. J., Wingood, G. M., Crosby, R. A., Cobb, B. K., Harrington, K., & Davies, S. L. (2001a). Parent-adolescent communication about sexuality-related topics and adolescents' risky sexual behaviors, communication with sex partners, and self-efficacy to discuss sexuality-related issues with sex partners. *Journal of Pediatrics, 139*(407), e12.

DiClemente, R. J., Wingood, G. M., Crosby, R. A., Sionean, C., Brown, L. K., Rothbaum, B., … & Davies, S. (2001b). A prospective study of psychological distress and sexual risk behavior among black adolescent females. *Pediatrics, 108*(5), e85–e85. doi:10.1542/peds.108.5.e85

DiClemente, R. J., Wingood, G. M., Crosby, R. A., Sionean, C., Cobb, B. K., Harrington, K., … & Oh, M. K. (2001c). Parental monitoring and its association with a spectrum of adolescent health risk risk behaviors. *Pediatrics, 107*(6), 1363–1368. doi:10.1542/peds.107.6.1363

DiClemente, R. J., Wingood, G. M., Crosby, R. A., Sionean, C., Cobb, B. K., Harrington K., … & Oh, M. K. (2002c). Sexual risk behaviors associated with having older sex partners: A study of black adolescent females. *Sexually Transmitted Diseases, 29*(1), 20–24. doi:10.1097/00007435-200201000-00004

DiIorio, C., Kelley, M., & Hockenberry-Eaton, M. (1999). Communication about sexual issues: Mothers, fathers, and friends. *Journal of Adolescent Health, 24*(3), 181–189. doi:10.1016/S1054-139X(98)00115-3

DiIorio, C., Resnicow, K., Denzmore, P., Rogers-Tillman, G., Wang, D. T., Dudley, W. N., … & Van Marter. (2000). Keepin' it R.E.A.L. A mother-adolescent HIV prevention program. In J. Szapocznik (Ed.), *Working with families in the era of HIV/AIDS* (pp. 113–132). Thousand Oaks CA: Sage Publications Inc.

Doljanac, R. F., & Zimmerman, M. A. (1998). Psychosocial factors and high-risk sexual behavior: Race differences among urban adolescents. *Journal of Behavioral Medicine, 21*(5), 451–467. doi:10.1023/A:1018784326191

Donohew, L., Zimmerman, R., Cupp, P. S., Novak, S., Colon, S., & Abell, R. (2000). Sensation seeking, impulsive decision-making, and risky sex: Implications for risk-taking and design of interventions. *Personality and individual differences, 28*(6), 1079–1091. doi:10.1016/S0191-8869(99)00158-0

Eastman, K. L., Corona, R., Ryan, G. W., Warsofsky, A. L., & Schuster, M. A. (2005). Worksite-based parenting programs to promote healthy adolescent sexual development: A qualitative study of feasibility and potential content. *Perspective on Sexual & Reproductive Health, 37*(2), 62–69. doi:10.1363/3706205.

Ennett, S. T., Federman, E. B., Bailey, S. L., Ringwalt, C. L., & Hubbard, M. L. (1999). HIV-risk behaviors associated with homelessness characteristics in youth. *Journal of Adolescent Health, 25*(5), 344–353. doi:10.1016/S1054-139X(99)00043-9

Felner, R. D., Brand, S., Mulhall, K. E., Counter, B., Millman, J. B., & Fried, J. (1994). The parenting partnership: The evaluation of a human service/ corporate workplace collaboration for the prevention of substance abuse and mental health problems, and the promotion of family and work adjustment. *Journal of Primary Prevention, 15*(2), 123–146. doi:10.1007/BF02197143

Fishbein, M. (2000). The role of theory in HIV prevention. *AIDS Care, 12*, 273–278. doi:10.1080/09540120050042918

Fisher, L., & Feldman, S. S. (1998). Familial antecedents of young adult health risk behavior: A longitudinal study. *Journal of Family Psychology, 12*(1), 66–80. doi:10.1037/0893-3200.12.1.66

Fortenberry, J. D., Tu, W., Harezlak, J., Katz, B. P., & Orr, D. P. (2002). Condom use as a function of time in new and established adolescent sexual relationships. *American Journal of Public Health, 92*(2), 211–213. doi:10.2105/AJPH.92.2.211

Fullilove, R. E. (1998). Race and sexually transmitted diseases. *Sexually Transmitted Disease, 25*, 130–131. doi:10.1097/00007435-199803000-00003

Gollub, E. L. (1995). Women-centered prevention techniques and technologies. In L. S. Jemmott (Ed.), *Women at risk: Issues in the primary prevention of AIDS* (pp. 43–82). New York: Plenum. doi:10.1007/978-1-4899-1057-8_3

Groseclose, S. L., Weinstein, B., Jones, T. S., Valleroy, L. A., Fehrs, L. J., & Kassler, W. J. (1995). Impact of increased legal access to needles and syringes on practices of injecting-drug users and police officers-Connecticut, 1992–1993. *JAIDS Journal of Acquired Immune Deficiency Syndromes, 10*(1), 82–89. doi:10.1097/00042560-199509000-00012

Hausser, D., & Michaud, P. A. (1994). Does a condom promoting strategy (the Swiss STOP-AIDS campaign) modify sexual behavior among adolescents? *Pediatrics, 93*(4), 580–585.

Hawkins, J. D., Catalano, R. F., Kosterman, R., Abbott, R., & Hill, K. G. (1999). Preventing adolescent health-risk behaviors by strengthening protection during childhood. *Archives of Pediatrics & Adolescent Medicine, 153*, 226–234. doi:10.1001/archpedi.153.3.226

Hennessy, M., Romer, D., Valois, R. F., Vanable, P., Carey, M. P., Stanton, B., ... & Salazar, L. F. (2013). Safer sex media messages and adolescent sexual behavior: 3-year follow-up results from Project iMPPACS. *American Journal of Public Health, 103*(1), 134–140. doi:10.2105/AJPH.2012.300856

Hock-Long, L., Herceg-Baron, R., Cassidy, A. M., & Whittaker, P. G. (2003). Access to adolescent reproductive health services: Financial and structural barriers to care. *Perspectives on Sexual and Reproductive Health, 35*(3), 144–147.

Jaccard, J. (1996). Adolescent contraceptive behavior: The impact of the provider and the structure of clinic-based programs. *Obstetrics & Gynecology, 88*(3 Suppl), 57S–64S. doi:10.1016/0029-7844(96)00249-9

Jemmott, J. B., Jemmott, L. S., Spears, H., Hewitt, N., & Cruz-Collins, M. (1992). Self-efficacy, hedonistic expectancies, and condom-use intentions among inner-city black adolescent women: A social cognitive approach to AIDS risk behavior. *Journal of Adolescent Health, 13*(6), 512–519. doi:10.1016/1054-139X(92)90016-5

Jemmott, J. B., III, & Jemmott, L. S. (2000). HIV risk reduction behavioral interventions with heterosexual adolescents. *AIDS Education and Prevention, 14*(Suppl 2), S40–S52.

Jemmott, L. S., Outlaw, F. H., Jemmott, J. B., Brown, E. J., Howard, M., & Hopkins, B. H. (2000). Strengthening the bond: The mother-son health promotion project. In J. Szapocznik (Ed.), *Working with families in the era of HIV/AIDS* (pp. 133–154). Thousand Oaks CA: Sage Publications Inc.

Kahn, J. A., Kaplowitz, R. A., Goodman, E., & Emans, S. J. (2002). The association between impulsiveness and sexual risk behaviors in adolescent and young adult women. *Journal of Adolescent Health, 30*(4), 229–232. doi:10.1016/S1054-139X(01)00391-3

Kamb, M. L., Fishbein, M., Douglas, J. M., Rhodes, F., Rogers, J., Bolan, G., ... & Kent, C. (1998). Efficacy of risk reduction counseling to prevent human immunodeficiency virus and sexually transmitted diseases: A randomized controlled trial. *Journal of the American Medical Association, 280*, 1161–1167. doi:10.1001/jama.280.13.1161

Kennedy, M. G., Mizuno, Y., Hoffman, R., Baume, C., & Strand, J. (2000). The effect of tailoring a model HIV prevention program for local adolescent target audiences. *AIDS Education & Prevention, 12*(3), 225–238.

Kirby, D. (2001). Understanding what works and what doesn't in reducing adolescent sexual risk-taking. *Family Planning Perspectives, 33*(6), 276–281. doi:10.2307/3030195

Ku, L., Sonenstein, F. L., & Pleck, J. H. (1994). The dynamics of young men's condom use during and across relationships. *Family planning Perspectives*, 246–251. doi:10.2307/2135889

Lawrence, J. S. S., Brasfield, T. L., Jefferson, K. W., Allyene, E., & Shirley, A. (1994). Social support as a factor in African-American adolescents' sexual risk behavior. *Journal of adolescent research, 9*(3), 292–310. doi:10.1177/074355489493002

Lesser, J., Verdugo, R. L., Koniak-Griffin, D., Tello, J., Kappos, B., & Cumberland, W. G. (2005). Respecting and protecting our relationships: A community research HIV prevention program for teen fathers and mothers. *AIDS Education & Prevention, 17*(4), 347–360. doi:10.1521/aeap.2005.17.4.347

Li, X., Stanton, B., & Feigelman, S. (2000). Impact of perceived parental monitoring on adolescent risk behavior over 4 years. *Journal of adolescent health, 27*(1), 49–56. doi:10.1016/S1054-139X(00)00092-6

Lindberg, L. D., Ku, L., & Sonenstein, F. L. (1998). Adolescent males' combined use of condoms with partners' use of female contraceptive methods. *Maternal and Child Health Journal, 2*(4), 201–209. doi:10.1023/A:1022304322327

Lown, E. A., Winkler, K., Fullilove, R. E., & Fullilove, M. T. (1993). *Tossin'and tweakin': Women's consciousness in the crack culture* (pp. 90–105). Women and AIDS: Psychological perspectives.

Maton, K. (2000). Making a difference: The social ecology of social transformation. *American Journal of Community Psychology, 28*(1), 25–57. doi:10.1023/A:1005190312887

McNeely, C., Shew, M. L., Beuhring, T., Sieving, R., Miller, B. C., & Blum, R. W. (2002). Mothers' influence on the timing of first sex among 14- and 15-year-olds. *Journal of Adolescent Health, 31*(3), 256–265. doi:10.1016/S1054-139X(02)00350-6

Miller, K. S., Clark, L. F., & Moore, J. S. (1997). Sexual initiation with older male partners and subsequent HIV risk behavior among female adolescents. *Family planning perspectives*, 212-214. doi:10.2307/2953397

Millstein, S. G., & Moscicki, A. B. (1995). Sexually-transmitted disease in female adolescents: Effects of psychosocial factors and high risk behaviors. *Journal of Adolescent Health, 17*(2), 83–90. doi:10.1016/1054-139X(95)00065-Z

Parillo, K. M., Freeman, R. C., Collier, K., & Young, P. (2001). Association between early sexual abuse and adult HIV-risky sexual behaviors among community-recruited women☆. *Child abuse & neglect, 25*(3), 335–346. doi:10.1016/S0145-2134(00)00253-2

Pedlow, C. T., & Carey, M. P. (2004). Developmentally appropriate sexual risk reduction interventions for adolescents: Rationale, review of interventions, and recommendations for research and practice. *Annals of Behavioral Medicine, 27*(3), 172–184. doi:10.1207/s15324796abm2703_5

Pendergrast, R. A., DuRant, R. H., & Gaillard, G. L. (1992). Attitudinal and behavioral correlates of condom use in urban adolescent males. *Journal of adolescent health, 13*(2), 133–139. doi:10.1016/1054-139X(92)90080-U

Pequegnat, W., Bauman, L. J., Bray, J. H., DiClemente, R., DiIorio, C., Hoppe, S. K., ... & Rapkin, B. (2001). Measurement of the role of families in prevention and adaptation to HIV/AIDS. *AIDS & Behavior, 5*(1), 1–19. doi:10.1023/A:1009557103659

Perkins, H. W., & Berkowitz, A. D. (1986). Perceiving the community norms of alcohol use among students: Some research implications for campus alcohol education programming. *International Journal of the Addictions, 21*(9–10), 961–976. doi:10.3109/10826088609077249

Peter, J., & Valkenburg, P. M. (2006). Adolescents' exposure to sexually explicit online material and recreational attitudes toward sex. *Journal of Communication, 56*(4), 639–660. doi:10.1111/j.1460-2466.2006.00313.x

Plichta, S. B., Weisman, C. S., Nathanson, C. A., Ensminger, M. E., & Robinson, J. C. (1992). Partner-specific condom use among adolescent women clients of a family planning clinic. *Journal of Adolescent Health, 13*(6), 506–511. doi:10.1016/1054-139X(92)90015-4

Ramirez-Valles, J., Zimmerman, M. A., & Newcomb, M. D. (1998). Sexual risk behavior among youth: Modeling the influence of prosocial activities and socioeconomic factors. *Journal of Health and Social Behavior*, 237-253. doi:10.2307/2676315

Resnick, M. D., Bearman, P. S., Blum, R. W., Bauman, K. E., Harris, K. M., Jones, J., … & Ireland, M. (1997). Protecting adolescents from harm: Findings from the National Longitudinal Study on Adolescent Health. *Jama, 278*(10), 823–832. doi:10.1001/jama.1997.03550100049038

Robin, L., Dittus, P., Whitaker, D., Crosby, R., Ethier, K., Mezoff, J., … & Pappas-Deluca, K. (2004). Behavioral interventions to reduce incidence of HIV, STD, and pregnancy among adolescents: A decade in review. *Journal of Adolescent Health, 34*(1), 3–26. doi:10.1016/S1054-139X(03)00244-1

Rodgers, K. B. (1999). Parenting processes related to sexual risk-taking behaviors of adolescent males and females. *Journal of Marriage & The Family, 61*(1), 99–109. doi:10.2307/353886

Romer, D., Stanton, B., Galbraith, J., Feigelman, S., Black, M. M., & Li, X. (1999). Parental influence on adolescent sexual behavior in high-poverty settings. *Archives of Pediatrics & Adolescent Medicine, 153*(10), 1055–1062. doi:10.1001/archpedi.153.10.1055

Romer, D., Sznitman, S., DiClemente, R., Salazar, L. F., Vanable, P. A., Carey, M. P., … & Fortune, T. (2009). Mass media as an HIV-prevention strategy: Using culturally sensitive messages to reduce HIV-associated sexual behavior of at-risk African American youth. *American Journal of Public Health, 99*(12), 2150–2159. doi:10.2105/AJPH.2008.155036

Rosenberg, P. S., & Biggar, R. J. (1998). Trends in HIV incidence among young adults in the United States. *Jama, 279*(23), 1894–1899. doi:10.1001/jama.279.23.1894

Rosenthal, D., Moore, S., & Flynn, I. (1991). Adolescent self-efficacy, self-esteem and sexual risk-taking. *Journal of Community & Applied Social Psychology, 1*(2), 77–88. doi:10.1002/casp.2450010203

Rosenthal, S. L., Cohen, S. S., DeVellis, R. F., Biro, F. M., Lewis, L. M., Succop, P. A., et al. (1999). Locus of control for general health and STD acquisition among adolescent girls. *Sexually Transmitted Diseases, 26*(8), 472–475. doi:10.1097/00007435-199909000-00009

Rothenberg, R. (2001). How a net works: Implications of network structure for the persistence and control of sexually transmitted diseases and HIV. *Sexually Transmitted Diseases, 28*(2), 63–68. doi:10.1097/00007435-200102000-00001

Rothenberg, R. B., Sterk, C., Toomey, K. E., Potterat, J. J., Johnson, D., Schrader, M., et al. (1998). Using social network and ethnographic tools to evaluate syphilis transmission. *Sexually Transmitted Diseases, 25*(3), 154–160. doi:10.1097/00007435-199803000-00009

Rotheram-Borus, M. J. (2000). Expanding the range of interventions to reduce HIV among adolescents. *Aids, 14*(Supp. 1), S33–S40. doi:10.1097/00002030-200006001-00005

Schinke, S. P., Orlandi, M. A., & Cole, K. C. (1992). Boys and girls clubs in public-housing developments-prevention services for youth at risk. *Journal of Community Psychology*, 118–128.

Schuster, M. A., Eastman, K. L., Fielding, J. E., Rotheram-Borus, M. J., Breslow, L., Franzoi, L. L., et al. (2001). Promoting adolescent health: Worksite-based interventions with parents of adolescents. *Journal of Public Health Management and Practice, 7*(2), 41–52. doi:10.1097/00124784-200107020-00007

Shafer, M. A., & Boyer, C. B. (1991). Psychosocial and behavioral factors associated with risk of sexually transmitted diseases, including human immunodeficiency virus infection, among urban high school students. *The Journal of pediatrics, 119*(5), 826–833. doi:10.1016/S0022-3476(05)80312-9

Shrier, L. A., Harris, S. K., & Beardslee, W. R. (2002). Temporal associations between depressive symptoms and self-reported sexually transmitted disease among adolescents. *Archives of Pediatrics & Adolescent Medicine, 156*(6), 599–606. doi:10.1001/archpedi.156.6.599

Shrier, L. A., Harris, S. K., Sternberg, M., & Beardslee, W. R. (2001). Associations of depression, self-esteem, and substance use with sexual risk among adolescents. *Preventive Medicine, 33*(3), 179–189. doi:10.1006/pmed.2001.0869

Sieving, R., Resnick, M. D., Bearinger, L., Remafedi, G., Taylor, B. A., & Harmon, B. (1997). Cognitive and behavioral predictors of sexually transmitted disease risk behavior among sexually active adolescents. *Archives of Pediatrics & Adolescent Medicine, 151*(3), 243–251. doi:10.1001/archpedi.1997.02170400029006

Sionéan, C., DiClemente, R. J., Wingood, G. M., Crosby, R., Cobb, B. K., Harrington, K., … & Oh, M. K. (2002). Psychosocial and behavioral correlates of refusing unwanted sex among African-American adolescent females. *Journal of Adolescent Health, 30*(1), 55–63. doi:10.1016/S1054-139X(01)00318-4

Small, S. A., & Luster, T. (1994). Adolescent sexual activity: An ecological, risk-factor approach. *Journal of Marriage and the Family*, 181–192. doi:10.2307/352712

Spencer, J. M., Zimet, G. D., Aalsma, M. C., & Orr, D. P. (2002). Self-esteem as a predictor of initiation of coitus in early adolescents. *Pediatrics, 109*(4), 581–584. doi:10.1542/peds.109.4.581

Stanton, B. F., Li, X., Galbraith, J., Cornick, G., Feigelman, S., Kaljee, L., et al. (2000). Parental underestimates of adolescent risk behavior: A randomized, controlled trial of a parental monitoring intervention. *Journal of Adolescent Health, 26*, 18–26. doi:10.1016/S1054-139X(99)00022-1

Stanton, B., Li, X., Cottrell, L., & Kaljee, L. (2001). Early initiation of sex, drug-related risk behaviors, and sensation-seeking among urban, low-income African-American adolescents. *Journal of the National Medical Association, 93*(4), 129.

Sznitman, S., Stanton, B. F., Vanable, P. A., Carey, M. P., Valois, R. F., Brown, L. K., … & Romer, D. (2011). Long term effects of community-based STI screening and mass media HIV prevention messages on sexual risk behaviors of African American adolescents. *AIDS and Behavior, 15*(8), 1755–1763. doi:10.1007/s10461-011-9946-6

Thornburgh, D., & Lin, H. S. (Eds.). (2002). *Youth, pornography, and the internet*. Washington, DC: National Academy Press.

Traeen, B. (1992). Learning from Norwegian experience: Attempts to mobilize the youth culture to fight the AIDS epidemic. *AIDS Education & Prevention, Fall*, 43–56

Tremblay, R. E., Mâsse, L. C., Vitaro, F., & Dobkin, P. L. (1995). The impact of friends' deviant behavior on early onset of delinquency: Longitudinal data from 6 to 13 years of age. *Development and Psychopathology, 7*(04), 649–667. doi:10.1017/S0954579400006763

Voisin, D. R., DiClemente, R. J., Salazar, L. F., Crosby, R. A., & Yarber, W. L. (2006). Ecological factors associated with STD risk behaviors among detained female adolescents. *Social Work, 51*(1), 71–79. doi:10.1093/sw/51.1.71

Weisman, C. S., Plichta, S., Nathanson, C. A., Ensminger, M., & Robinson, J. C. (1991). Consistency of condom use for disease prevention among adolescent users of oral contraceptives. *Family planning perspectives*, 71-74. doi:10.2307/2135452

Whitaker, D. J., & Miller, K. S. (2000). Parent-adolescent discussions about sex and condoms impact on peer influences of sexual risk behavior. *Journal of Adolescent Research, 15*(2), 251–273. doi:10.1177/0743558400152004

Williams, K. M., Wingood, G. M., DiClemente, R. J., Crosby, R. A., McCree, D. H., Liau, A., … & Oh, M. K. (2002). Prevalence and correlates of Chlamydia trachomatis among sexually active African-American adolescent females. *Preventive Medicine, 35*(6), 593–600. doi:10.1006/pmed.2002.1112

Wilson, M. D., Kastrinakis, M., JD'Angelo, L., & Getson, P. (1994). Attitudes, knowledge, and behavior regarding condom use in urban black adolescent males. *Adolescence, 29*(113), 13.

Wingood, G. M., DiClemente, R. J., Bernhardt, J. M., Harrington, K., Davies, S. L., Robillard, A., … & Hook, E. W. 432(2003). A prospective study of exposure to rap music videos and African American female adolescents' health. *American Journal of Public Health, 93*(3), 437–439. doi:10.2105/AJPH.93.3.437

Wingood, G. M., DiClemente, R. J., Crosby, R. A., Harrington, K., Davies, S. L., & Hook, E. W. (2002). Gang involvement and the health of African-American female adolescents. *Pediatrics, 110*(5), E57. doi:10.1542/peds.110.5.e57

Wingood, G. M., DiClemente, R. J., Harrington, K., Davies, S., Hook, E. W., & Oh, M. K. (2001). Exposure to X-rated movies and adolescents' sexual and contraceptive-related attitudes and behaviors. *Pediatrics, 107*(5), 1116–1119. doi:10.1542/peds.107.5.1116

Wingood, G. M., Rubtsova, A., DiClemente, R. J., Metzger, D., Blank, M. (2013). A new paradigm for optimizing HIV intervention synergy: The role of interdependence in integrating HIV prevention interventions. *Journal of Acquired Immune Deficiency Syndromes, J*

Zimet, G. D., Bunch, D. L., Anglin, T. M., Lazebnik, R., Williams, P., & Krowchuk, D. P. (1992). Relationship of AIDS-related attitudes to sexual behavior changes in adolescents. *Journal of Adolescent Health, 13*(6), 493–498. doi:10.1016/1054-139X(92)90013-2

Chapter 12
HIV-Related Stigma and Children

Anne Stangl and Kirsty Sievwright

Introduction

Over 2.6 million children aged 0–15 are living with HIV globally, the majority of whom reside in low- to middle-income countries, particularly in sub-Saharan Africa (WHO 2015). Most were infected at birth, when antiretroviral therapy (ART) to prevent vertical transmission from mother-to-child was not widely available. Yet, a growing number of adolescents and young people are infected through sexual activity or assault. In 2014 alone, there were 620,000 new HIV infections among youth aged 15–24 (UNICEF 2016). Adolescent girls and young women (AGYW) aged 15–24 are disproportionately affected, experiencing HIV infection rates twice as high as young men and accounting for 22% of all new HIV infections (UNAIDS 2012).

Stigma associated with HIV and AIDS is a constant companion for people living with HIV and their families. From a mother's fear that her child will be excluded from school if the child's HIV status becomes known, to a teenager's worry that his girlfriend will leave him if he discloses his HIV status, and to a young nurse losing her job when her employer learns she is living with HIV. Whether stigma and discrimination are experienced or only anticipated, they often negatively impact a person's quality of life and life chances (Nattabi et al. 2012). Stigma impedes HIV testing and delays entry into care (Rintamaki et al. 2006; Rao et al. 2012; Sabin et al. 2008). Stigma also interferes with adherence to antiretroviral medications

A. Stangl (✉) · K. Sievwright
International Center for Research on Women, Washington, DC, USA
e-mail: alstangl@gmail.com

K. Sievwright
e-mail: kirstysiev11@gmail.com

T. Chenneville (ed.), *A Clinical Guide to Pediatric HIV*,
DOI 10.1007/978-3-319-49704-4_12

(Katz et al. 2013), which is critical for both maintaining good health and preventing transmission to uninfected sexual partners.

Importantly, HIV-related stigma is well understood. We know what drives stigma and how it manifests. We have numerous evidence-based approaches and interventions available to interrupt the stigmatization process or minimize the harmful effects of stigma and discrimination (Stangl et al. 2013). In this chapter, we describe the stigmatization process, demonstrate how stigma impacts children and adolescents living with HIV and their families, and summarize the latest evidence on stigma-reduction interventions. We also highlight key areas for future research and intervention development.

Conceptualizing HIV-Related Stigma

In his 1963 seminal work *Stigma: Notes on the Management of Spoiled Identity*, sociologist Erving Goffman conceptualized stigma as a discrediting attribute that creates a "spoiled identity", which cuts the stigmatized person "off from society and from himself" (Goffman 1963). This fundamental conceptualization has been expanded over the years to articulate each step in the stigmatization process and describe the societal and structural forces that spur it. According to Link and Phelan, discrediting attributes or stigmas are applied when the following components co-occur: (1) a difference is "distinguish[ed] and label[ed]"; (2) the difference is linked to negative stereotypes; leading to (3) a separation of "us" from "them"; followed by (4) "status loss and discrimination" for those identified with the difference (Link and Phelan 2001). Parker and Aggleton added to this conceptualization, highlighting the societal (e.g., gender and wealth inequalities) and structural forces (e.g., punitive laws) that allow the stigmatization process to occur and perpetuate it (Parker and Aggleton 2003). For example, national policies that criminalize HIV transmission maintain stigma against those living with HIV and discourage testing, disclosure, and treatment adherence.

More recently, a global process yielded a practical framework to inform the development and evaluation of interventions to reduce HIV-related stigma and discrimination (Stangl et al. 2013; Stangl et al. 2012). This framework distinguishes between the actionable drivers (e.g., fear of HIV transmission, stereotypes, and social judgment.) and facilitators of stigma (e.g., laws and policies) and the manifestations of stigma, including anticipated stigma, perceived stigma, internalized or self-stigma, experienced stigma, discrimination, and resilience (see Table 12.1). These manifestations can lead to outcomes such as reluctance to test for HIV, delayed entry into HIV care, and poor adherence to antiretroviral therapy (WHO et al. 2011), which in turn can lead to longer term stigma impacts such as poor quality of life and increased morbidity and mortality.

Table 12.1 Manifestations of stigma (Stangl et al. 2012)

1. Anticipated stigma	The fear of negative ramifications should one's HIV status become known, should one associate with a person living with HIV or should one test positive for HIV
2. Perceived stigma	One's perception of the level of stigma that is directed toward people living with HIV
3. Internalized or self-stigma	The acceptance of negative beliefs and feelings associated with HIV and application to oneself, among people living with HIV
4. Experienced stigma	The experience of discrimination based on HIV status or association with a person living with HIV or other stigmatized group that falls *outside* the purview of the law
5. Discrimination	The experience of discrimination that falls *within* the purview of the law
6. Resilience	An individual's ability to overcome and resist or challenge HIV-related stigma when experienced or observed. This is the only positive manifestation of the stigmatization process

Stigma and Child Development

HIV-related stigma affects children living with HIV from gestation to young adulthood (see Fig. 12.1). In this section, we will examine how stigma manifests during each stage of child development.

Pregnancy, Birth, and Infancy

Most women learn they are living with HIV during pregnancy. Antenatal care services (ANC) are often the key point of entry for women into the healthcare system, especially in low- and middle-income countries (Turan et al. 2012, 2015). ANC is also where pregnant women living with HIV can access a series of integrated interventions that can greatly reduce the risk of HIV transmission from mother-to-child, or "vertical transmission." These interventions, known collectively as the preventing mother-to child transmission (PMTCT) "cascade", include antiretroviral treatment, safe birth practices, appropriate infant feeding, and multiple post-natal services. In 2012, the World Health Organization (WHO) updated their guidance on PMTCT to recommend that countries adopt a comprehensive preventative approach called Option B+ for all expectant mothers living with HIV. Option B+ includes the following: lifelong ART provided to all pregnant and breastfeeding women living with HIV regardless of CD4 cell count; daily nevirapine (NVP) or zidovudine (AZT) for infants from birth to 4–6 weeks (regardless of feeding method); early infant HIV testing at six weeks post-partum; and further testing 18 months after breastfeeding ends for a final diagnosis (WHO 2012). Adhering to this protocol can prevent 75% of infant HIV transmissions, as well as most maternal deaths (Kuhn and Coovadia 2012). However, HIV-related stigma

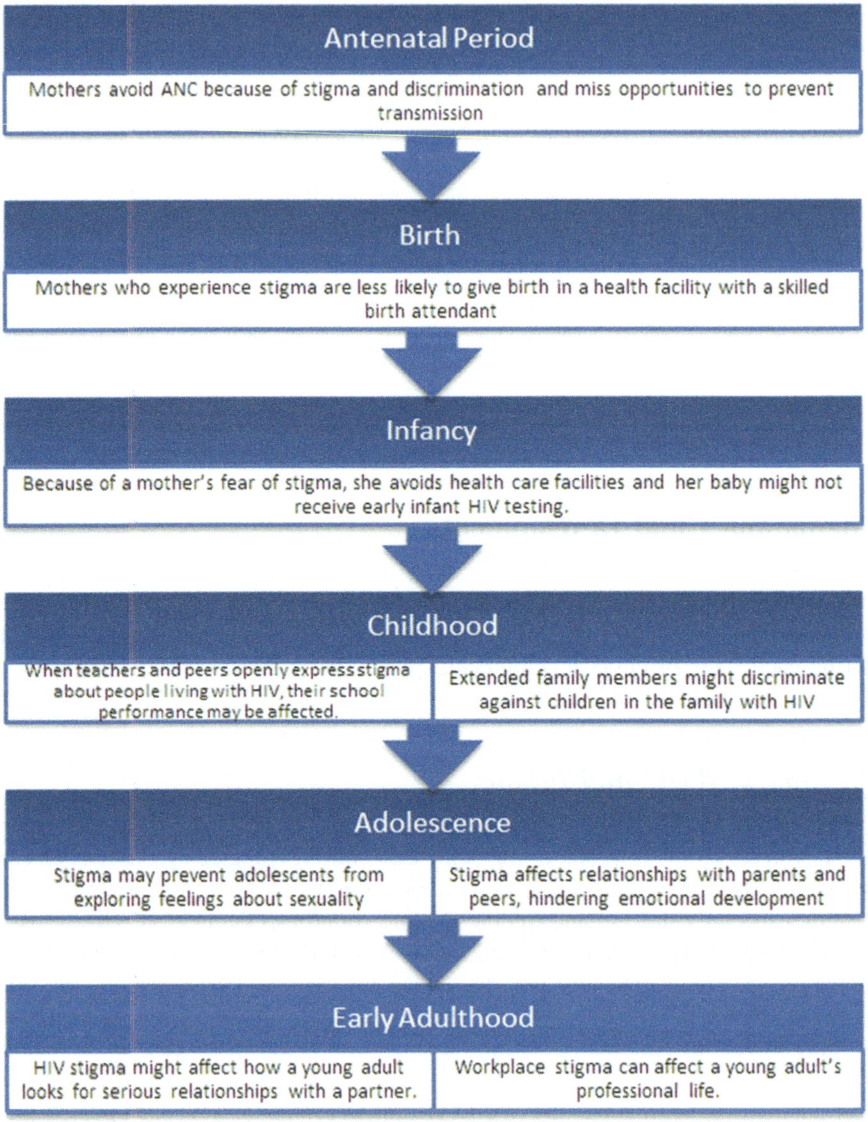

Fig. 12.1 Stigma throughout child development

can act as a barrier at each step in the PMTCT cascade. It has been estimated that more than half of vertical transmissions in some settings can be attributed to the cumulative effect of stigma at each point in the cascade (Watts et al. 2010).

In 2007, the WHO recommended that all countries adopt provider-initiated HIV testing, in which healthcare providers specifically recommend an HIV test to all patients seeking health services, and testing is performed the same day unless the patient declines (WHO 2007). Since these guidelines have been put in place, a growing body of literature suggests that pregnant women, particularly in sub-Saharan Africa, have started avoiding or delaying ANC services to avoid HIV testing and the subsequent stigma associated with HIV (Watts et al. 2010; Bond et al. 2002; Medley et al. 2004). Anticipated stigma, or a woman's fear of experiencing stigma if others learn of her HIV status, can also lead women to refuse HIV testing (Bwirire et al. 2008; Thorsen et al. 2008; Varga and Brookes 2008) or enrollment in PMTCT services (Kilewo et al. 2001; Larsson et al. 2009). One study in Kenya found that pregnant women were concerned that health workers would treat them poorly if they tested positive for HIV and were worried that their test results would not be kept confidential. Thus, women sometimes refused HIV testing and adopted an "ignorance is bliss" attitude to avoid these negative experiences (Turan et al. 2011). The same study also found that non-disclosure of a woman's HIV status was a major impediment to uptake of PMTCT services. Women who had disclosed to anyone were five times as likely as women who had not disclosed to take ART during pregnancy (Spangler et al. 2014). For women who do enroll in PMTCT services, anticipated stigma can impede adherence to ART and retention in care, as women may skip doses or clinic appointments to avoid being identified as living with HIV (Bwirire et al. 2008; Ekouevi et al. 2004; Painter et al. 2005). Anticipated stigma may also lead women to deliver outside of a health facility (Turan et al. 2011), which is the only place to access NVP for infants in many settings. Ultimately, avoidance or delays in care seeking during pregnancy increase the risk of HIV transmission to infants. It is clear that interventions to reduce anticipated stigma, support HIV sero-status disclosure, and ensure non-stigmatizing care at health facilities are needed to ensure uptake and adherence to available PMTCT services for all expectant mothers living with HIV.

Childhood

During childhood, HIV stigma affects parents and caregivers, as well as children living with HIV. Parents and caregivers often struggle with decisions about whom to disclose their child's HIV status to, due to fears of experiencing stigma themselves (secondary stigma) and a desire to protect the child in their care from experiencing stigma and discrimination (Stangl et al. 2015). Disclosure decisions are often based on a "need to know" basis. For example, if a child is going to stay with a relative who will need to ensure the child takes her medication, parents will share her HIV status, but other relatives and siblings are not necessarily told. Similarly, parents sometimes choose to tell a teacher they trust at the child's school but may not disclose to the school administrators, for fear of differential treatment (Stangl et al. 2015).

Parents and caregivers also struggle with when to tell the child that she/he is living with HIV (Sanjeeva et al. 2016; Odiachi and Abegunde 2016). In some cases, a mother or father living with HIV may delay disclosure because of their own guilt about their child's status or worries about being blamed by their child (Stangl et al. 2015). In other cases, parents or caregivers simply do not have enough information on how to explain HIV infection to a child and prefer a healthcare provider to disclose (Wiener et al. 2007). These struggles with disclosure highlight the need for support services for parents and caregivers to help them decide when, how, and who to disclose to.

Children living with HIV may experience stigma within their own families. In the household, having children living with HIV use separate plates, cups, and utensils is unfortunately still common in many settings. Not allowing children living with HIV to stay in the same household or to play with other uninfected children, including siblings and cousins, is another way in which stigma manifests within families. These types of avoidance and isolation behaviors are driven by fear of infection through casual contact with a person living with HIV, which stems from a lack of knowledge about how HIV is and is not transmitted (Ogden and Nyblade 2005). Counseling and support services for family members of children living with HIV would help to minimize these manifestations of stigma in the household.

While overt discrimination at school, such as barring a student from attending, is illegal and uncommon in most settings now, children living with HIV can still face ridicule, gossip, and harassment from peers and teachers if their HIV status becomes known. In formative research we conducted in Zambia, one participant had to switch schools when her status became known to avoid such negative treatment. This is why parents and caregivers often go to great lengths to ensure that their child's HIV status does not become widely known (Stangl et al. 2015).

Adolescence and Young Adulthood

As children living with HIV grow into adolescents, their experiences with HIV and stigma often change. During this phase of child development, many children learn for the first time why they have been taking daily medications their whole life. Learning they are HIV positive is often a shock and is difficult for adolescents to process (Sanjeeva et al. 2016). In addition, adolescents living with HIV are often warned by parents and caregivers not to disclose to anyone, even close friends and relatives, to avoid being treated differently or experiencing stigma and discrimination. While silence may protect adolescents living with HIV from experiencing stigma and discrimination, it also prevents them from sharing their experiences with others and seeking the emotional support they need to cope with their diagnosis (Stangl et al. 2015). This can impair their emotional development and foster internalized stigma.

As adolescents living with HIV begin to question and explore their sexuality, they often receive morally laden advice in "right" and "wrong" terms from both parents and healthcare professionals due to taboos around sex before marriage and transmission fears (Stangl et al. 2015; FHI 360, USAID, and Preventive Technologies Agreement 2013). For example, they may be told not to have sex or not to have children, so they do not transmit HIV to others. Because adolescents living with HIV are expected not to have sex, they are not necessarily given complete information about sexual and reproductive health, family planning, and how to minimize the risk of transmission to uninfected partners or unborn children. For example in Zambia, we found that healthcare workers would often not explain that adhering to ART suppresses viral load, making it virtually impossible to transmit HIV to uninfected sexual partners. In this context, information was held back mainly due to concerns that adolescent girls living with HIV would become promiscuous if they were taught about "treatment as prevention" (Stangl et al. 2015).

A study in South Africa found that young men and women who became infected with HIV during adolescence were very concerned that their parents would view them as irresponsible or careless. Multiple youth in this study stated that disclosing their HIV status to their families would "provide leverage to parents to control their behavior." Importantly, while almost all of the participants in this study reported fear of stigma, very few had experiences that resulted in status loss or discrimination, and many demonstrated resilience and the ability to resist common stigma experiences such as gossip and insults (Abrahams and Jewkes 2012).

Disclosure remains a major challenge for adolescents living with HIV, namely due to fears about retribution from peers if their status becomes known. These fears are heightened in enclosed environments, like schools, and are perpetuated by hearing other students and teachers openly express negative attitudes about people living with HIV (Stangl et al. 2015). Enhanced training programs for secondary school teachers on how to teach about HIV in a respectful and supportive way are urgently needed in many settings. School-wide campaigns to reduce HIV-related stigma and discrimination would also help to interrupt the stigmatization process and might also encourage adolescents living with HIV to seek the emotional support and information they need (Stangl et al. 2015).

Fears of others learning about their HIV status can also interfere with treatment adherence, as adolescents may skip doses if they are not able to take their medication privately (FHI 360, USAID, and Preventive Technologies Agreement 2013). In addition, adolescents living with HIV are especially vulnerable to "treatment fatigue." Coupled with internalized stigma, or the acceptance of negative beliefs and feelings associated with HIV and application to oneself, this fatigue can be severely detrimental to an individual's adherence to medication (UNAIDS 2014). Interventions to help adolescents overcome both internalized and anticipated stigma could help to support treatment adherence and ensure a healthy transition to adulthood.

Case Studies: Experiencing HIV-Related Stigma as an Adolescent

The following case studies exemplify how HIV-related stigma and discrimination can affect adolescents. The first case study is about the life and experiences of Ryan White, one of the first children diagnosed with HIV in the US in the 1980s. The second case study, Mary, was developed based on formative research conducted by the authors in 2015 with adolescent girls living with HIV in urban Zambia. We drew from the experiences of multiple study participants to show how stigma often manifests for adolescent girls in this context (Stangl et al. 2015). The similarities in the experiences of these two young people, experiencing HIV and stigma two decades apart and in two very different contexts, are striking and highlight the persistence of stigma despite the availability of treatment that has turned HIV from a debilitating terminal illness into a manageable chronic condition. The stories of Ryan and Mary also reflect the incredible resilience that often emerges among people living with HIV, even in the face of stigma and discrimination.

Ryan White, Indiana, US

Ryan White was born in Kokomo, Indiana, in 1971 with hemophilia, a hereditary disorder in which blood does not clot normally. This condition required him to have regular blood transfusions, the common procedure for hemophiliacs at the time. Ryan contracted HIV during one of his transfusions and was subsequently diagnosed with AIDS in 1984, a time when HIV and AIDS were thought to be spread chiefly among intravenous drug users and homosexuals, and public fear and uncertainty around HIV were rampant. After he was diagnosed, he stayed home from school due to the severity of his illness. However the following spring, he started feeling better and wanted to return to school to be with his classmates. His desire to return to school was met with protests from parents, teachers, and administrators—resulting in an eight-month legal battle against Ryan and his mother (Health Resources and Services Administration HAB 2015).

In 1986, the Indiana Department of Education ruled that Ryan must be allowed to attend school. On his first day back at Western Middle School, 151 of the 360 students at the middle school stayed home in protest, and many students withdrew shortly after (United Press International 1990). Ryan faced explicit discrimination and was forced to take "precautions," such as using a separate restroom and disposable tableware in the school cafeteria. Further, his classmates wrote obscenities on his locker and shouted insults as he passed in the halls (Johnson 1990). Many thought Ryan had to be gay or was being "punished by God" for some other wrongdoing (Health Resources and Services Administration HAB 2015). Fortunately, when Ryan started high school in Cicero, he was greeted with more supportive peers and administrators who were not afraid to shake his hand or be around him. The school board sponsored several discussions about HIV and AIDS, and the student body president advocated for presentations led by medical experts. People were urged to let common sense and compassion guide their actions, instead of fear.

Ryan died from a respiratory infection in 1990, a month before his high school graduation but left a tremendous legacy behind (Health Resources and Services Administration HAB 2015). In fighting for his rights, Ryan showed the world that HIV and AIDS does not just affect intravenous drug users or the lesbian, gay, bi-sexual, and transgender (LGBT) community, it affects us all. Furthermore, Ryan showed the world that people living with HIV deserve the same rights as everyone else. Ryan's resilience and advocacy in the face of stigma greatly influenced national perceptions about HIV and AIDS and paved the way for federal funding of programs to support PLHIV and raise awareness about HIV. In his memory, The Ryan White Comprehensive AIDS Resources Emergency (CARE) Act was passed. This is the largest federally funded program in the US for people living with HIV (Health Resources and Services Administration HAB 2015).

Mary,[1] Lusaka, Zambia (16 Years Old)

Mary learned that she was living with HIV when she was 12 years old. She found out following several visits to the hospital, for what her family thought was a problem with her tonsils. An HIV diagnosis came as a surprise to Mary and her mother, as neither of Mary's parents were living with HIV. After being questioned by her mother, Mary revealed that when she was a young child a family friend, who had since passed away, sexually abused her. Mary's mother responded to this news by first accusing her of lying and then expressing her frustration that Mary did not tell her this was happening at the time or when the family friend was alive. Mary's mother was not actually upset with her for what happened. Rather she was mad that she was not able to protect her daughter from this abuse, angry that she could not exact justice against the man who put her daughter in this situation, and afraid for her daughter's future knowing how others in the community viewed and treated people living with HIV.

Indeed over the next four years, Mary was faced with a new set of challenges as a result of living with HIV. She had a heightened awareness of the stigmatizing attitudes her family, friends, and community hold regarding HIV. In the classroom, her teacher offered false and stigmatizing information about HIV with statements such as "When you exchange clothes with your friend you can get infected." At church, those living with HIV were referred to as sinners. And now that Mary's

[1]This case study draws from the experiences of multiple participants and does not represent the experiences of one particular individual.

aunt knows she is living with HIV, suddenly Mary cannot share food from the same plate when she visits her aunt's house. After observing and experiencing such attitudes, Mary does not want to risk disclosing to anyone, even her best friend Grace. As a result, Mary has no one she can talk to about her experiences living with HIV.

This fear of disclosure presents another challenge for Mary: adhering to her treatment. For Mary to pick up her medicine, she often has to miss a whole day of school due to the long wait times at the clinic. Mary is concerned about raising suspicion when she misses school and afraid of being seen in line at the clinic by someone she knows. Despite these fears, Mary always makes sure to go to the clinic because she understands how important it is to adhere to her treatment and likes how much healthier she looks when she takes her medicine. But she wishes her experience could be improved. Having someone she could talk openly to about her experiences living with HIV would be greatly beneficial. Despite her experiences with HIV stigma, Mary remains resilient. She will not let HIV hold her back from achieving her dreams. She wants to go to university and study journalism, get married, and have two children.

Stigma-Reduction Interventions: What Do We Know?

In order to reduce HIV-related stigma and discrimination, it is important to revisit the stigmatization process. Figure 12.2, an adaptation of the practical framework developed by Stangl et al. (2012), and Nayar et al. (2014), indicates two main areas for intervention. Ideally, we want to prevent stigma from being applied to an individual or group of people. To accomplish this, we need to target interventions toward the drivers and facilitators of stigma (e.g., trainings to reduce stigmatizing attitudes and behaviors toward PLHIV among health facility staff and communication campaigns to increase knowledge about how HIV is and is not transmitted to reduce transmission fears and avoidance behaviors.). If we are unable to prevent a stigma from being applied, then we need to minimize the harmful effects of that stigma by targeting interventions toward the manifestations of stigma (e.g., helping children living with HIV to overcome internalized or "self-stigma" and providing counseling and disclosure support services to adolescents living with HIV and their families). In many cases, interventions are designed to target both the drivers and manifestations of stigma. This framework also reflects the general consensus among stigma researchers that there is a need to intervene at multiple socio-ecological levels (i.e., individual, interpersonal, organizational, community, and public policy) (Heijnders et al. 2006). Below, we summarize the key approaches for reducing HIV-related stigma and discuss best practices for designing and implementing interventions. We then provide examples of stigma-reduction interventions that have been implemented for children and young people living with or affected by HIV across each socio-ecological level.

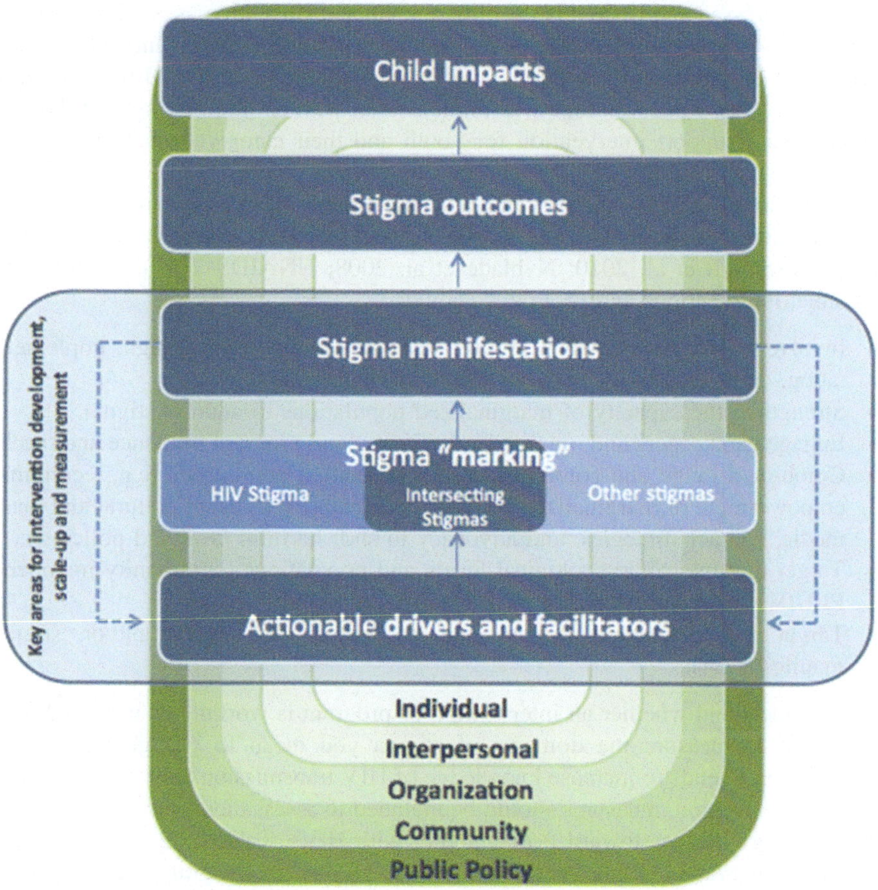

Fig. 12.2 A practical framework to inform interventions to reduce HIV-related stigma. Adapted from Stangl et al. (2013), Nayar et al. (2014)

Previous systematic reviews of the HIV stigma-reduction literature have identified six intervention categories, including (1) information-based approaches (e.g., written information in a brochure); (2) skills building (e.g., participatory learning sessions to reduce negative attitudes); (3) counseling/support (e.g., support groups for PLHIV); (4) contact with affected groups (e.g., interactions between PLHIV and the general public); (5) structural (e.g., strategic litigation, legal, and policy changes); and (6) biomedical (e.g., provision of universal HIV testing and treatment) (Stangl et al. 2013; Brown et al. 2003). Over the last decade, interventions to reduce HIV-related stigma have expanded greatly, with broader geographic representation, multiple target populations (e.g., students, teachers, general community, healthcare providers, PLHIV), more socio-ecological levels addressed, and more domains of stigma addressed (e.g., drivers, facilitators, intersecting stigmas, and manifestations). Of 48 evaluated interventions conducted between 2003 and 2013, 90% demonstrated significant reductions in HIV-related stigma. It should be noted that only one of these interventions was implemented with children living with HIV, a psychosocial support intervention for youth and their caregivers in Haiti (Stangl et al. 2013).

There are several broad programmatic lessons that have emerged over the last two decades that should inform the development of HIV stigma-reduction interventions (Stangl et al. 2010; Nyblade et al. 2008; UNAIDS 2007). As much as possible, interventions and programs should:

- Involve people living with HIV and key populations in the design, implementation, and evaluation of stigma-reduction interventions;
- Strengthen the capacity of marginalized populations to address stigma;
- Engage gatekeepers and opinion leaders to expand program influence and reach;
- Combine a range and combination of intervention approaches (e.g., economic empowerment of marginalized communities, campaigns using cultural and mass media, contact strategies, and advocacy to shift harmful laws and policies.);
- Target multiple socio-ecological levels and populations (community members, PLHIV, healthcare workers, local leaders, etc.); and
- Target the actionable drivers and facilitators of stigma and/or stigma manifestations.

To understand whether an intervention or program is working as expected, it is important to measure the domains of stigma you mean to change (e.g., if an intervention intends to increase knowledge of HIV transmission and reduce fears of casual transmission, measures should be included to assess these outcomes, not just stigmatizing attitudes toward people living with HIV). Table 12.2 provides some examples of evaluated interventions to reduce HIV-related stigma directed toward or experienced by children and adolescents living with HIV.

Table 12.2 Examples of stigma-reduction interventions for youth living with or affected by HIV

Individual	The group-based behavioral intervention, Project ACCEPT (Adolescents Coping, Connecting, Empowering and Protecting Together), works with adolescents and young adults in the US recently diagnosed with HIV. This intervention seeks to promote healthy psychosocial adjustment and improve engagement in medical care through offering HIV-/AIDS-related information, facilitating the acquisition of coping skills and providing contact with other youth living with HIV in order to improve social support. Four aspects of stigma reduction were targeted: (1) decreasing negative feelings toward self and others living with HIV; (2) increasing planned and strategic HIV disclosure to others; (3) building supportive networks to combat fears and feelings of rejection; and (4) building skills to combat HIV-related discrimination and other forms of stigma. Project ACCEPT found overall reductions in personalized stigma, disclosure concerns, and negative self-image (Harper et al. 2014)

(continued)

Table 12.2 (continued)

Interpersonal	In response to the challenge of child disclosure in sub-Saharan Africa and evidence that both healthcare workers and caregivers feel ill equipped to engage in the disclosure process, Namibia's Ministry of Health and Social Services developed and implemented a child disclosure intervention. This multi-pronged intervention aimed to reduce barriers to disclosure and support healthcare workers and caregivers in the disclosure process using: (1) a staged disclosure cartoon book, (2) child and caregiver readiness assessment tools, (3) a monitoring form to track progress over visits, and (4) a healthcare worker training curriculum. The intervention improved confidence and communication skills regarding pediatric disclosure among both healthcare workers and caregivers. Further, both groups of participants reported improved knowledge and ability to support the pediatric patient, improved child understanding of how HIV medications work, increased child hopefulness for their future, and improved child adherence to care and treatment (O'Malley et al. 2015)
Organization	A program in KwaZulu-Natal, South Africa, sought to teach educators how to teach and to handle HIV and AIDS-related issues in the classroom. Educators received training on HIV transmission, risk factors, and actions that educators should know and undertake via either: (1) a CD-ROM-based intervention or (2) attending a two day workshop. Stigma levels of both training groups significantly reduced after the interventions and were significantly associated with improvements in HIV knowledge. It was noted that since teachers are examples for their students and often imitated, the teachers must not only try to exhibit non-stigmatizing behaviors, but they also need to learn how to prevent and mitigate stigma as expressed by others in the school (Chao et al. 2010)
Community and individual combined	African American youth are disproportionately affected by HIV in the US, and knowledge gaps and stigmatizing attitudes have been identified as barriers to HIV prevention among this population. In order to reduce HIV incidence among African American youth, a program in four cities in the US combined a brief, school-based HIV risk-reduction curriculum with a multi-media TV and radio campaign targeted to youth that aired in the evenings over a 12-month period. The aim of these combined interventions was to increase knowledge about HIV, reduce fears of infection through casual contact, and reduce stigma toward people living with HIV among youth. The combined HIV risk-reduction curriculum and culturally tailored media demonstrated some effectiveness in reducing stigma and increasing HIV knowledge (Kerr et al. 2015)
Public policy	The Ryan White Comprehensive AIDS Resources Emergency (CARE) Act offers a comprehensive system of care that includes primary medical care and essential support services for people living with HIV who are uninsured or underinsured. The program works with cities in the US, states and local community-based organizations to provide HIV care and treatment services to more than 512,000 people each year, reaching approximately 52% of all those diagnosed with HIV in the US. While not specific to youth living with HIV, the passage of this Act resulted from the advocacy of a young man living with HIV who shared his story, increased knowledge and awareness of HIV, and ultimately changed public attitudes about HIV and people living with (HIV Health Resources and Services Administration HAB 2015)

Research Gaps

While the field of HIV-related stigma and discrimination has expanded greatly over the past 20 years, the need to understand how stigma is affecting children and adolescents living with HIV and develop and test interventions to reduce stigma among this population has only recently emerged. As such, there are a number of research gaps and areas for further exploration. At the individual level, further research is needed to test interventions to address the emotional and informational support needs of adolescents living with HIV. Interventions could include support groups or other "peer-to-peer" activities, mHealth (or mobile health, a practice of utilizing mobile communication devices to address health priorities) or peer-navigator approaches to provide treatment and emotional support, and economic empowerment and job training to foster resilience.

At the interpersonal level, more support is needed for parents and caregivers of children living with HIV. Such support could address information gaps about HIV, sexual and reproductive health and treatment, disclosure concerns, and how to enable children and adolescents to take part in (or make) decisions related to their care (e.g., allowing young people to take over responsibility for their medication, instead of having a parent or caregiver in control of access to ART).

At the organizational level, it is important to improve the clinic experience. Simple and easy clinical experiences are imperative to adolescent's uptake of services. As such, efforts to minimize wait times and disorganization and improve quality of care at clinics could better facilitate the process and improve testing and uptake of treatment. In schools settings, training programs are needed to train teachers to recognize and challenge stigma in their schools, to talk about HIV in a non-stigmatizing way, and to integrate HIV stigma-reduction into existing curricula on sexual and reproductive health. Creating a nonjudgmental and supportive school environment would encourage more youth and adolescents living with HIV to seek the support they need and adhere to their treatment. Further, it could be beneficial to implement school-wide campaigns promoting compassion and support for people living with HIV, as opposed to inadvertently promoting judgmental attitudes toward people living with HIV.

Lastly, at the policy level, studies are needed to understand how changes in national policy are influencing the experiences of children and adolescents living with HIV. For example, as countries scale-up biomedical approaches such as universal testing and treatment and pre-exposure prophylaxis, how are youth engaged with or affected by these programs? In countries with comprehensive sexuality education curricula with components on gender equality, violence, and stigma, how are these expanded curricula influencing the knowledge, attitudes, and sexual practices of adolescents living with HIV? (Stangl et al. 2015).

Conclusion

In conclusion, researchers, program implementers, and policy makers have a strong foundation upon which to build programmatic approaches to interrupt or minimize the harmful effects of stigma and discrimination toward children living with HIV and their families. The underlying process of stigmatization is the same, regardless of age, and we have a long history of stigma-reduction research to guide intervention development and testing. In order to ensure a healthy transition to adulthood for children and adolescents living with HIV and to reduce new infections among adolescents, it is critical that we tackle stigma and discrimination. To do so, funding for research efforts must keep pace with global demand for evidence-based solutions.

Acknowlegments The authors wish to thank Sabiha Hussain, Hannah Asmail and Sara Doverspike for their support in preparing this chapter, including gathering and organizing references, preparing figures and tables, and gathering information for the case studies. Please direct any comments or questions to Anne Stangl, PhD, Senior Behavioral Scientist, International Center for Research on Women. Email: alstangl@gmail.com.

Annotated Bibliography

Nayar, U. S., Stangl, A. L., De Zalduondo, B., & Brady, L. M. (2014). Reducing stigma and discrimination to improve child health and survival in low-and middle-income countries: Promising approaches and implications for future research. *Journal of Health Communication, 19*(1), 142–163.

This article provides a review of interventions designed to reduce stigma and discrimination related to children's health and well-being in low- and middle-income countries. The authors offer a framework to direct such future research and interventions.

Nyblade, L., Jain, A., Benkirane, M., Li, L., Lohiniva, A. L., McLean, R., … Kwena, Z. (2013). A brief, standardized tool for measuring HIV-related stigma among health facility staff: Results of field testing in China, Dominica, Egypt, Kenya, Puerto Rico and St. Christopher & Nevis. *Journal of the International AIDS society, 16*(3).

This article introduces a brief, standardized tool for measuring HIV-related stigma among staff in health facilities in order to support stigma-reduction efforts in this setting.

Stangl, A. L., Lloyd, J. K., Brady, L. M., Holland, C. E., & Baral, S. (2013). A systematic review of interventions to reduce HIV-related stigma and discrimination from 2002 to 2013: How far have we come? *Journal of the International AIDS Society, 16*(3).

This article provides a systematic review of interventions designed to reduce HIV-related stigma and discrimination, and notes the considerable progress in the stigma-reduction field as well as the remaining challenges and gaps. This article is part of a special issue on HIV-related stigma worldwide.

References

Abrahams, N., & Jewkes, R. (2012). Managing and resisting stigma: A qualitative study among people living with HIV in South Africa. *Journal of the International AIDS Society, 15*(2), 001. doi:10.7448/IAS.15.2.17330

Bond, V., Chase, E., & Aggleton, P. (2002). Stigma, HIV/AIDS and prevention of mother-to-child transmission in Zambia. *Evaluation and program planning, 25*(4), 347–356. doi:10.1016/S0149-7189(02)00046-0

Brown, L., Macintyre, K., & Trujillo, L. (2003). Interventions to reduce HIV/AIDS stigma: what have we learned? *AIDS Education and Prevention, 15*(1), 49–69. doi:10.1521/aeap.15.1.49.23844

Bwirire, L. D., Fitzgerald, M., Zachariah, R., Chikafa, V., Massaquoi, M., Moens, M., et al. (2008). Reasons for loss to follow-up among mothers registered in a prevention-of-mother-to-child transmission program in rural Malawi. *Transactions of the Royal Society of Tropical Medicine and Hygiene, 102*(12), 1195–1200. doi:10.1016/j.trstmh.2008.04.002

Chao, L. W., Gow, J., Akintola, G., & Pauly, M. (2010). HIV/AIDS stigma attitudes among educators in KwaZulu-Natal, South Africa. *Journal of School Health, 80*(11), 561–569. doi:10.1111/j.1746-1561.2010.00542.x

Ekouevi, D. K., Leroy, V., Viho, I., Bequet, L., Horo, A., Rouet, F., … ANRS 1201/1202 Ditrame Plus Study Group. (2004). Acceptability and uptake of a package to prevent mother-to-child transmission using rapid HIV testing in Abidjan, Cote d'Ivoire. *AIDS, 18*(4), 697–700. doi:10.1097/00002030-200403050-00018

FHI 360, USAID, & Preventive Technologies Agreement. (2013). Adolescents living with HIV in Zambia: An examination of HIV care and treatment and family planning. Retrieved from https://www.fhi360.org/sites/default/files/media/documents/zambia-adolescents-living-hiv-integration-family-planning.pdf

Goffman, E. (1963). Notes on the management of spoiled identity. *Englewood Cliffs, New Jersey: Prentice-Hall.*

Harper, G. W., Lemos, D., & Hosek, S. G. (2014). Stigma reduction in adolescents and young adults newly diagnosed with HIV: Findings from the Project Accept Intervention. *AIDS patient care and STDs, 28*(10), 543–554. doi:10.1089/apc.2013.0331

Health Resources and Services Administration HAB. (2015). Who was Ryan White? Retrieved from http://hab.hrsa.gov/abouthab/ryanwhite.html

Heijnders, M., & van der Meij, S. (2006). The fight against stigma: an overview of stigma-reduction strategies and interventions. Psychol Health Med. *11*(3), 353–363. doi: 10.1080/13548500600595327.

Johnson, D. (1990). Ryan White dies of AIDS at 18; His struggle helped pierce myths.

Katz, I. T., Ryu, A. E., Onuegbu, A. G., Psaros, C., Weiser, S. D., Bangsberg, D. R., et al. (2013). Impact of HIV-related stigma on treatment adherence: Systematic review and meta-synthesis. *Journal of the International AIDS Society, 16*(3), 001. doi:10.7448/ias.16.3.18640

Kerr, J. C., Valois, R. F., DiClemente, R. J., Carey, M. P., Stanton, B., Romer, D., et al. (2015). The effects of a mass media HIV-risk reduction strategy on HIV-related stigma and knowledge among African American adolescents. *AIDS Patient Care and STDs, 29*(3), 150–156. doi:10.1089/apc.2014.0207

Kilewo, C., Massawe, A., Lyamuya, E., Semali, I., Kalokola, F., Urassa, E., et al. (2001). HIV counseling and testing of pregnant women in sub-Saharan Africa: Experiences from a study on prevention of mother-to-child HIV-1 transmission in Dar es Salaam, Tanzania. *JAIDS Journal of Acquired Immune Deficiency Syndromes, 28*(5), 458–462. doi:10.1097/00042560-200112150-00009

Kuhn, L., & Coovadia, H. M. (2012). Protecting infants of HIV-positive mothers in Malawi. *The Lancet, 379*(9835), 2405–2407. doi:10.1016/S0140-6736(12)60483-8

Larsson, E. C., Waiswa, P., Thorson, A., Tomson, G., Peterson, S., Pariyo, G., et al. (2009). Low uptake of HIV testing during antenatal care: A population-based study from eastern Uganda. *Aids, 23*(14), 1924–1926. doi:10.1097/QAD.0b013e32832eff81

Link, B. G., & Phelan, J. C. (2001). Conceptualizing stigma. *Annual Review of Sociology, 363–385*, 001. doi:10.1146/annurev.soc.27.1.363

Medley, A., Garcia-Moreno, C., McGill, S., & Maman, S. (2004). Rates, barriers and outcomes of HIV serostatus disclosure among women in developing countries: Implications for prevention of mother-to-child transmission programmes. *Bulletin of the World Health Organization, 82*(4), 299–307.

Nattabi, B., Li, J., Thompson, S. C., Orach, C. G., & Earnest, J. (2012). Between a rock and a hard place: Stigma and the desire to have children among people living with HIV in northern Uganda. *Journal of the International AIDS Society, 15*(2), 001. doi:10.7448/IAS.15.2.17421

Nayar, U. S., Stangl, A. L., De Zalduondo, B., & Brady, L. M. (2014). Reducing stigma and discrimination to improve child health and survival in low-and middle-income countries: Promising approaches and implications for future research. *Journal of Health Communication, 19*(1), 142–163.

Nyblade, L., Hong, K. T., Anh, N. V., Ogden, J., Jain, A., & Stangl, A. (2008). Communities confront HIV stigma in Viet Nam: Participatory interventions reduce HIV-Related stigma in two provinces.

Odiachi, A., & Abegunde, D. (2016). Prevalence and predictors of pediatric disclosure among HIV-infected Nigerian children on treatment. *AIDS Care, 1–6*, 001. doi:10.1080/09540121.2016.1147018

Ogden, J., & Nyblade, L. (2005). Common at its core: HIV-related stigma across contexts. Washington, D.C. International Center for Research on Women. Retrieved from: http://www.icrw.org/wp-content/uploads/2016/10/Common-at-its-Core-HIV-Related-Stigma-Across-Contexts.pdf

O'Malley, G., Beima-Sofie, K., Feris, L., Shepard-Perry, M., Hamunime, N., John-Stewart, G., … MOHSS Study Group. (2015). If I take my medicine, I will be strong: Evaluation of a pediatric HIV disclosure intervention in Namibia. *JAIDS Journal of Acquired Immune Deficiency Syndromes, 68*(1), e1–e7. doi:10.1097/QAI.0000000000000387

Painter, T. M., Diaby, K. L., Matia, D. M., Lin, L. S., Sibailly, T. S., Kouassims, M. K., … Wiktor, S. Z. (2005). Sociodemographic factors associated with participation by HIV-1-positive pregnant women in an intervention to prevent mother-to-child transmission of HIV in Cote d'Ivoire. *International Journal of STD & AIDS,16*(3), 237–242. doi:10.1258/0956462053420158

Parker, R., & Aggleton, P. (2003). HIV and AIDS-related stigma and discrimination: a conceptual framework and implications for action. *Social Science and Medicine, 57*(1), 13–24. doi:10.1016/S0277-9536(02)00304-0

Rao, D., Feldman, B. J., Fredericksen, R. J., Crane, P. K., Simoni, J. M., Kitahata, M. M., et al. (2012). A structural equation model of HIV-related stigma, depressive symptoms, and medication adherence. *AIDS and Behavior, 16*(3), 711–716. doi:10.1007/s10461-011-9915-0

Rintamaki, L. S., Davis, T. C., Skripkauskas, S., Bennett, C. L., & Wolf, M. S. (2006). Social stigma concerns and HIV medication adherence. *AIDS Patient Care & STDs, 20*(5), 359–368. doi:10.1089/apc.2006.20.359

Sabin, L. L., Desilva, M. B., Hamer, D. H., Keyi, X., Yue, Y., Wen, F., et al. (2008). Barriers to adherence to antiretroviral medications among patients living with HIV in southern China: A qualitative study. *AIDS Care, 20*(10), 1242–1250. doi:10.1080/09540120801918651

Sanjeeva, G. N., Pavithra, H. B., Chaitanya, S., Sunil Kumar, D. R., & Rewari, B. B. (2016). Parental concerns on disclosure of HIV status to children living with HIV: Children's perspective. *AIDS Care, 1–7*, 001. doi:10.1080/09540121.2016.1189503

Spangler, S. A., Onono, M., Bukusi, E. A., Cohen, C. R., & Turan, J. M. (2014). HIV-positive status disclosure and use of essential PMTCT and maternal health services in rural Kenya. *JAIDS Journal of Acquired Immune Deficiency Syndromes, 67*, S235–S242. doi:10.1097/QAI.0000000000000376

Stangl, A., Bond, V., Mackworth-Young, C., Sievwright, K., Singh, D., Clay, S., … Konayuma, K. (2015). *Transitioning to a healthy adulthood*. Washington, DC: International Center for Research on Women. Retrieved from http://www.icrw.org/wp-content/uploads/2016/10/FINAL_brief_ALHIV-Zambia.pdf

Stangl, A., Brady, B., & Fritz, K. (2012). *Technical brief: Measuring HIV stigma and discrimination*. Washington, DC: International Center for Research on Women. Retrieved from: http://strive.lshtm.ac.uk/system/files/attachments/STRIVE_stigma%20brief-A4.pdf

Stangl, A., Carr, D., Brady, L., Eckhaus, T., Claeson, M., & Nyblade, L. (2010). *Tackling HIV-Related Stigma and Discrimination in South Asia*. Washington, DC: World Bank. doi:10.1596/978-0-8213-8449-7

Stangl, A. L., Lloyd, J. K., Brady, L. M., Holland, C. E., & Baral, S. (2013). A systematic review of interventions to reduce HIV-related stigma and discrimination from 2002 to 2013: How far have we come? *Journal of the International AIDS Society*, *16*(3), 001.

Thorsen, V. C., Sundby, J., & Martinson, F. (2008). Potential initiators of HIV-related stigmatization: Ethical and programmatic challenges for pmtct programs. *Developing World Bioethics*, *8*(1), 43–50. doi:10.1111/j.1471-8847.2008.00227.x

Turan, J. M., Bukusi, E. A., Onono, M., Holzemer, W. L., Miller, S., & Cohen, C. R. (2011). HIV/AIDS stigma and refusal of HIV testing among pregnant women in rural Kenya: Results from the MAMAS Study. *AIDS and Behavior*, *15*(6), 1111–1120.

Turan, J. M., Onono, M., Steinfeld, R. L., Shade, S. B., Owuor, K., & Bukusi, E. A. (2015). Effects of antenatal care and HIV treatment integration on elements of the PMTCT cascade: results from the SHAIP cluster-randomized controlled trial in Kenya. *Journal Acquired Immune Deficiency Syndromes*, *69*, e172Á81.

Turan, J. M., Steinfeld, R. L., Onono, M., Bukusi, E. A., Woods, M., Shade, S. B., et al. (2012). The study of HIV and antenatal care integration in pregnancy in Kenya: Design, methods, and baseline results of a cluster-randomized controlled trial. *PLoS ONE*, *7*(9), e44181. doi:10.1371/journal.pone.0044181

UNAIDS. (2007). Reducing stigma and discrimination: A critical part of national AIDS Programmes. Retrieved from http://data.unaids.org/pub/Report/2008/jc1521_stigmatisation_en.pdf

UNAIDS. (2012). Adolescents, young people and HIV: Fact Sheet. Retrieved from http://files.unaids.org/en/media/unaids/contentassets/documents/factsheet/2012/20120417_FS_adolescentsyoungpeoplehiv_en.pdf

UNAIDS. (2014). Ensuring that adolescents living with HIV are not left behind. Retrieved from http://www.unaids.org/en/resources/presscentre/featurestories/2014/april/20140430adolescents

UNICEF. (2016). Adolescents are the outliers in the AIDS response. Retrieved from http://data.unicef.org/hiv-aids/adolescents-young-people.html

United Press International. (1990). Ryan White: AIDS victim who fought to go to school. Retrieved from http://www.upi.com/Archives/1990/04/08/Ryan-White-AIDS-victim-who-fought-to-go-to-school/3336639547200/

Varga, C., & Brookes, H. (2008). Factors influencing teen mothers' enrollment and participation in prevention of mother-to-child HIV transmission services in Limpopo Province. *South Africa Qualitative Health Research*, *18*(6), 786–802. doi:10.1177/1049732308318449

Watts, C., Zimmerman, C., Eckhaus, T., & Nyblade, L. (2010). Modelling the impact of stigma on HIV and AIDS programmes: preliminary projections for mother-to-child transmission. *Washington, DC: International Center for Research on Women (ICRW) and London School of Hygiene and Tropical Medicine*. Retrieved from http://citeseerx.ist.psu.edu/viewdoc/download?doi=10.1.1.732.2267&rep=rep1&type=pdf

WHO. (2007). Guidance on provider-initiated HIV testing and counselling in health facilities. Retrieved from http://www.who.int/hiv/pub/vct/pitc2007/en/

WHO. (2012). Programmatic update: Use of Antiretroviral drugs for treating pregnant women and preventing HIV infection in infants. Retrieved from http://apps.who.int/iris/bitstream/10665/70892/2/WHO_HIV_2012.6_eng.pdf

WHO. (2015). HIV/AIDS fact sheet no. 360. Retrieved from http://www.who.int/mediacentre/factsheets/fs360/en/

WHO, UNICEF, UNAIDS. (2011). Progress report 2011: Global HIV/AIDS response. Retrieved from http://www.who.int/hiv/pub/progress_report2011/en/

Wiener, L., Mellins, C. A., Marhefka, S., & Battles, H. B. (2007). Disclosure of an HIV diagnosis to children: History, current research, and future directions. *Journal of Developmental and Behavioral Pediatrics: JDBP, 28*(2), 155. doi:10.1097/01.DBP.0000267570.87564.cd

Index

Note: Page numbers followed by *f* and *t* indicate figures and tables, respectively

T. Chenneville (ed.), *A Clinical Guide to Pediatric HIV*,
DOI 10.1007/978-3-319-49704-4

The manufacturer's authorised representative in the EU is Springer Nature Customer Service Centre GmbH, Europaplatz 3, 69115 Heidelberg, Germany. If you have any concerns regarding our products, please contact ProductSafety@springernature.com

Printed and bound by CPI Group (UK) Ltd, Croydon, CR0 4YY
30/09/2026
02225239-0013